Practical Nuclear Medicine

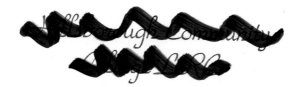

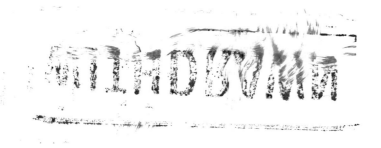

Peter F. Sharp, Howard G. Gemmell
and Alison D. Murray (Eds)

Practical Nuclear Medicine

Third Edition

With 222 Figures including 17 Color Plates

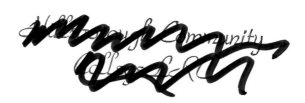

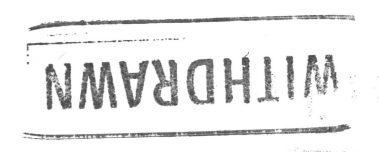

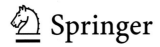 Springer

Peter F. Sharp, PhD, FInstP, FIPEM, FRSE
Department of Biomedical Physics and Bioengineering
Aberdeen University and NHS Grampian, UK

Howard G. Gemmell, PhD, FIPEM
Department of Nuclear Medicine
Aberdeen Royal Infirmary
NHS Grampian, UK

Alison D. Murray, FRCP, FRCR
Department of Radiology
University of Aberdeen, UK

The authors wish to acknowledge their gratitude to OUP for the use of the following figures from the second edition of this book:
1.6, 1.7, 2.1, 2.3, 2.4, 2.5, 2.7, 3.1, 3.3, 3.5, 5.1, 5.2, 5.3, 5.4, 5.5, 5.6, 5.7, 5.8, 5.9, 5.10, 5.11, 5.12, 6.1, 6.2, 7.1, 7.4, 7.5, 7.6, 7.7, 10.1, 10.2, 10.3, 10.4, 10.8, 13.1, 13.10, 13.14, 13.15, 13.16, 14.1, 14.2, 14.3, 14.4, 14.5, 14.9, 14.10, 14.11, 14.12, 14.13, 14.14, 15.1, 15.4

British Library Cataloguing in Publication Data
A catalogue record for this book is available from the British Library

Library of Congress Cataloguing-in-Publication Data
Sharp, Peter F.
    Practical nuclear medicine/Peter F. Sharp, Howard G. Gemmell, Alison D. Murray.–3rd ed.
      p. cm.
    Includes bibliographical references and index.
    ISBN 1-85233-875-X (alk. paper)
    1. Nuclear medicine.   I. Gemmell, H. G.   II. Murray, Alison D.   III. Title.
    R895.S45 2005
    616.07′575–dc22   2004061448

ISBN-10: 1-85233-875-X   3rd edition   Printed on acid-free paper
ISBN-13: 978-1-85233-875-6

First published in 1996 by Oxford University Press; ISBN 0199630321
Second edition published in 1998 Oxford University Press; ISBN 0192628429
Third edition 2005

Printed in Singapore   (TB/KYO)

9 8 7 6 5 4 3 2 1   SPIN 10931226

Springer Science+Business Media
springeronline.com

Foreword

There have been several significant advances in nuclear medicine since the publication of the second edition of *Practical Nuclear Medicine*. The last seven years have seen great strides in instrumentation, including new coincidence detectors, the development of a wider variety of crystals, and the advent of combined anatomical/functional imaging devices, including PET/CT and SPECT/CT. PET imaging with ^{18}F-FDG has become a mainstay of many clinical settings, and other radiotracers are finding their way into the rapidly expanding field of oncologic PET. However, radiopharmaceutical breakthroughs during this period have not been confined to one single imaging modality. Refinements in diagnostic applications of monoclonal antibodies, radiolabeled peptides, neuroreceptors, and a whole spectrum of new molecular targeting agents are steadily strengthening the clinical nuclear medicine armamentarium.

Such a daunting array of changes can present quite a challenge to even the most experienced nuclear medicine practitioner. Consider then the magnitude of complexities that physicians, physicists, and technologists who are just beginning their training in our field are expected to assimilate! That is precisely why this book offers an easily accessible approach to both the basic science groundwork and the clinical applications of nuclear medicine. The third edition presents its material in a very pragmatic manner by disseminating the various contributors' practical experience via detailed instructions. The breadth of this hands-on knowledge and advice will likely benefit readers at all levels of expertise.

The book's concentration on the actual practice of nuclear medicine is particularly discernible in the first few chapters, which address scientific foundations of SPECT, PET, radiopharmaceuticals, etc. Such topics as instrumentation, data processing, and non-imaging radionuclide tests are covered in a way that accentuates specific human interaction; thus, quality assurance is an oft-recurring theme. To reflect the growing importance of PET in the clinical arena, the introductory chapter on this subject has been expanded and a new chapter on current PET radiopharmaceuticals and PET imaging in oncology, neurology, and cardiology has been added. In addition, new contributors have prepared the chapters on the skeletal system, the cardiovascular system, and the urinary tract.

This third edition of *Practical Nuclear Medicine* continues the text's tradition of guiding readers through not only the most commonly performed clinical nuclear medicine tests but the scientific bases on which they were built. In addition, the editors of this version have skillfully weeded out certain procedures and de-accentuated others whose use has lessened in the clinical setting over the last few years. These efforts have produced a clinical manual that clearly addresses many of the diagnostic dilemmas that currently appear in nuclear medicine, which is constantly expanding the limits of its instrumentation, radiopharmaceuticals, and diagnostic capabilities. In the future, many aspects of current molecular imaging research (such as targeting of tumor antigens, receptors, and metabolism; imaging of hypoxia and apoptosis; and antisense targeting for both diagnosis and therapy) will find their way into the clinical setting. Therefore, it is of paramount importance that individuals working in nuclear medicine update their skills today in preparation for the next wave of advanced knowledge and clinical techniques. Fortunately, the third edition of *Practical Nuclear Medicine* will assist members of our community in accomplishing that task, and the editors and contributors are to be commended for making this possible.

Martin P. Sandler, MD
Carol D. and Henry P. Professor and Chairman
Department of Radiology and Radiological Sciences
Vanderbilt University School of Medicine
Nashville, Tennessee, USA

Contents

Contributors

Robert W. Barber, MSc, BSc
Department of Medical Physics, Addenbrooke's
Hospital, Cambridge, UK

Margaret E. Brooks, MB ChB, FRCP, DMRD,
FRCR
Department of Nuclear Medicine, Aberdeen
Royal Infirmary, Aberdeen, UK

Heok K. Cheow, MB ChB, MRCP, FRCR
Department of Nuclear Medicine,
Addenbrooke's Hospital, Cambridge, UK

Gary J. R. Cook, MB BS, MD
Department of Nuclear Medicine and PET,
Royal Marsden Hospital, Sutton, UK

Philip S. Cosgriff, BSc, MSc
Medical Physics Department, Pilgrim Hospital,
Boston, UK

Philip P. Dendy, PhD
Department of Medical Physics, Addenbrooke's
Hospital, Cambridge, UK

James Doherty, BSc, MRPharmS
Pharmacy Department, Aberdeen Royal
Infirmary, Aberdeen, UK

Alex T. Elliott, BA, PhD DSc, CPhys, FInstP,
FIPEM, ARCP
Department of Clinical Physics and
Bioengineering, Western Infirmary, Glasgow,
UK

Howard G. Gemmell, BSc, MSc, PhD, FIPEM
Department of Nuclear Medicine, Aberdeen
Royal Infirmary, NHS Grampian, Aberdeen,
UK

Keith A. Goatman, BEng, MSc, PhD
Department of Bio-Medical Physics and
Bio-Engineering, University of Aberdeen, UK

Karen E. Goldstone, BSc, MSc
Department of Medical Physics, Addenbrooke's
Hospital, Cambridge, UK

David Graham, MSc, BSc, MRPharmS
Pharmacy Department, Aberdeen Royal
Infirmary, Aberdeen, UK

Henry W. Gray MD, FRCP, FRCR
Department of Nuclear Medicine,
Royal Infirmary, Glasgow, UK

Milton D. Gross, MD
Departments of Radiology and Internal
Medicine, University of Michigan Medical
School, Nuclear Medicine Service,
Department of Veterans Affairs Health System,
Ann Arbor, MI, USA

Leslie K. Harding, MB ChB, BSc, FRCP, FRCR
Department of Physics and Nuclear Medicine,
City Hospital NHS Trust, Birmingham, UK

Thomas E. Hilditch, BSc, PhD, FInstP
Department of Clinical Physics and
Bioengineering, Western Infirmary,
Glasgow, UK

Malcohm J. Metcalfe, MD, FRCP
Department of Cardiology, Aberdeen Royal
Infirmary, Aberdeen, UK

William H. Martin, MD
Department of Radiology and Radiological
Sciences, Vanderbilt University Medical Center,
Nashville, TN, USA

Alison D. Murray, MB ChB, FRCP, FRCR
Department of Radiology, College of Life
Sciences and Medicine, University of Aberdeen,
UK

Alp Notghi, MD, MSc, FRCP
Department of Physics and Nuclear Medicine,
City Hospital NHS Trust, Birmingham,
UK

Adrian Parkin, DPhil
Department of Medical Physics, Addenbrooke's
Hospital, Cambridge, UK

Alan C. Perkins, BSc, MSc, Ph.D, FIPEM, ARCP
Department of Medical Physics, Medical
School, Queen's Medical Centre, Nottingham,
UK

A. Michael Peters, MA, MD, MSc, FRCPath,
FRCP, FRCR, FMedSci
Department of Applied Physiology, Brighton
Sussex Medical School, University of Sussex,
Brighton, UK

Martin P. Sandler, MD
Department of Radiology and Radiological
Sciences, Vanderbilt University Medical Center,
Nashville, TN, USA

Peter F. Sharp, BSc, PhD, CPhys, FInstP, ARCP,
FIPEM, FRSE
Department of Bio-Medical Physics and
Bio-Engineering, University of Aberdeen and
NHS Grampian, UK

Roger T. Staff, PhD
Department of Bio-Medical Physics and
Bio-Engineering, University of Aberdeen and
NHS Grampain, UK

Andy Welch, BSc, PhD
Biomedical Physics and Bioengineering, BSc,
PhD, University of Aberdeen, UK

1

Nuclear Medicine Imaging

Peter F. Sharp and Keith A. Goatman

1.1 Introduction

In nuclear medicine clinical information is derived from observing the distribution of a pharmaceutical administered to the patient. By incorporating a radionuclide into the pharmaceutical, measurements can be made of the distribution of this radiopharmaceutical by noting the amount of radioactivity present. These measurements may be carried out either in vivo or in vitro. In vivo imaging is the most common type of procedure in nuclear medicine, nearly all imaging being carried out with a gamma camera (see Section 1.3). Nuclear medicine is intrinsically an imaging technique showing the body's biochemistry, the particular aspect depending upon the choice of the radiopharmaceutical. This is in contrast to other commonly used imaging procedures whose main strengths are showing anatomy.

Where a knowledge of the precise amount of activity present in an organ is required then positron emission tomography can provide this (see Chapter 3), although while its usage is increasing it still remains a specialized technique. If an image of the distribution is not essential, collimated scintillation probe detectors aligned with the organ of interest may be used [1]. If the amount of radioactivity present is very low then high-sensitivity whole body counters, consisting of heavily shielded probe detectors, are necessary [2].

In vitro measurements are made on samples of material taken from the patient, such as breath, blood, urine, and feces, to determine the amount of radiopharmaceutical present. Such measurements are made using the gamma- or beta-sample counting techniques discussed in Chapter 4.

The diagnostic information is provided by the action of the pharmaceutical; the role of the radioactivity is purely a passive one, enabling the radiopharmaceutical to be localized. For this reason it is possible to use low levels of radioactivity and so the potential hazard to the patient can be kept small (see Chapter 6).

1.2 The Ideal Radiopharmaceutical

The specific features looked for in the ideal radiopharmaceutical are summarized in Table 1.1. It must be emphasized, however, that no single radiopharmaceutical actually has all these properties. As the radionuclide label and the pharmaceutical perform different functions, the particular features regarded as desirable for them can largely be considered separately.

1.2.1 Radionuclides

Half-life

The half-life of the radionuclide determines how quickly the radioactivity will decay. Obviously, if the half-life is very short then the activity will have decayed to a very low level before imaging has started. On the other hand, if it is too long then

Table 1.1. Ideal characteristics of a radiopharmaceutical

Half-life should be similar to the length of the test
The radionuclide should emit gamma rays and there should
   be no charged particle emissions
The energy of the gamma rays should be between 50 and
   300 keV
The radionuclide should be chemically suitable for incorpo-
   rating into a pharmaceutical without altering its biological
   behavior
The radionuclide should be readily available at the hospital
   site
The pharmaceutical should localize only in the area of interest
The pharmaceutical should be eliminated from the body with
   a half-life similar to the duration of the examination
The radiopharmaceutical should be simple to prepare

the patient will remain radioactive for a considerable time and in order to reduce the possibility of radiation damage the amount of activity administered will have to be kept low. Roughly, the half-life should be of a similar length to that of the examination, usually a few hours.

Type and Energy of Emission

For imaging it is first necessary that the radiation given off should be sufficiently penetrating to allow it to be detected externally even though it may need to pass through several centimeters of tissue. This limits the choice to gamma rays or X-rays. The energy of the radiation will also affect its ability to penetrate tissue: the higher the energy the better it will be. However, the higher the energy the more difficult it will be to stop the gamma ray in the detector of the imaging device. In practice gamma rays with energies between 50 keV and 300 keV are preferred, about 150 keV being ideal.

The radiation dose received by the patient must also be considered. It is necessary to avoid those radionuclides that have significant particulate (i.e. alpha and beta) emissions which, owing to their short range, will simply increase radiation dose without contributing to the image. As the purpose of radioactive decay is to redress an imbalance in the ratio of protons to neutrons in the nucleus, it is clear that simple gamma decay will be accompanied by the emission of a charged particle, usually a beta particle. There are, however, two decay processes that avoid this problem: isomeric transition and electron capture. Particles will still be emitted, namely Auger and conversion electrons, but at a considerably lower rate than the one per gamma experienced with other modes of decay.

Pharmaceutical Labeling

While the prime consideration in choosing a radionuclide is that its manner of decay should be suitable for in vivo imaging, it must not be forgotten that this material must be incorporated into a pharmaceutical. Unfortunately all the elements of biological interest, such as carbon, nitrogen, and oxygen, do not have radioisotopes meeting the criteria of Table 1.1. These particular elements do, however, have radioisotopes that emit positrons. These positively charged electrons annihilate with an electron to produce a pair of 511 keV gamma rays. While the energy of these gamma rays is such that the sensitivity of detection in the crystal of a standard gamma camera will be low, nevertheless cameras are available that will do both single photon and positron imaging, either by employing a high-energy collimator or, more commonly, by using coincidence electronics. The most effective way of imaging positron emitting radiopharmaceuticals is, however, with specialized equipment, described in Chapter 3.

Despite the potential problems, pharmacists and radiochemists have been very successful in incorporating some of the most unlikely material, such as the widely used radioisotope of technetium, into a large range of pharmaceuticals. This problem will be considered in Chapter 7.

Production of Radionuclides

Radionuclides can be produced from three sources: the nuclear reactor, the cyclotron, or a generator. It is not intended to go into detail about the process of production of radioactive material and the interested reader is recommended to read Ott et al [3].

The reactor radionuclides are produced either by introducing a target of stable material into the neutron flux found inside the reactor, or by separating out fission products from the fuel rods or a uranium target. As neutron irradiation increases the number of neutrons relative to the number of protons in the nucleus, it will produce radionuclides that decay predominantly by beta decay.

The cyclotron produces a beam of charged particles, such as alpha particles or deuterons, which is used to bombard a target material. The resulting radionuclide will have an excess of charge and so will decay either by emission of a positively charged particle (a positron) or by the capture of a negative charge (electron capture). The latter, as has been mentioned earlier, is a particularly useful decay process, as it has a gamma-to-beta ratio greater than unity.

Obviously in most instances radionuclides produced by these two routes will be shipped to the hospital from a central manufacturing site. This creates a problem, since short-lived radionuclides will decay significantly during transportation. For example, carbon-11 is a positron-emitting isotope with a half-life of only 20 minutes, which severely restricts the distance between the cyclotron and the scanner. Fortunately the third mode of production, the generator, provides an answer, at least for certain radionuclides. The generator will be discussed in Section 7.3.2, but basically it depends upon the existence of a long-lived radionuclide which decays into the required short-lived radionuclide. All that is then needed is for this long-lived parent to be supplied in the form of a generator from which the short-lived daughter can be chemically extracted when required. This generator is the source of the radionuclide most commonly used in nuclear medicine, technetium-99m, the parent material in this case being molybdenum-99.

A list of commonly used radionuclides is given in Table 1.2 together with their mode of production and characteristics of decay.

Selection of Pharmaceutical

The most important feature required of the pharmaceutical is that it should be taken up rapidly and completely in the biological system of interest. In practice most radiopharmaceuticals also localize in other parts of the body, and if these are radiosensitive the amount of activity that can be administered will be limited (see Chapter 6). Activity in these other areas may also obscure that in the organ of interest. Tomographic imaging (see Chapter 2) has the advantage that it allows separation of the activity in organs that would be superimposed in the conventional two-dimensional planar image.

The length of time for which the radioactivity remains in the patient obviously influences the radiation dose received. Not only does this depend upon the half-life of radioactive decay (τ_{physical}) but also upon the time taken for the radiopharmaceutical to be excreted from the body, the biological half-life ($\tau_{\text{biological}}$). The total residence time of the radiopharmaceutical, τ_{total}, is given by

$$\frac{1}{\tau_{\text{total}}} = \frac{1}{\tau_{\text{physical}}} + \frac{1}{\tau_{\text{biological}}}.$$

It should be noted that although the physical half-life is known accurately, the biological one may vary considerably, particularly in the presence of abnormal pathology. In seeking to minimize

Table 1.2. Characteristics of commonly used radionuclides

Radionuclide	Mode of production	Type of decay[a]	Principal photon emissions (keV)	Half-life
Imaging tests				
^{67}Ga	Cyclotron	EC	92, 182, 300, 390	78 h
^{123}I	Cyclotron	EC	160	13 h
^{131}I	Reactor	Beta	280, 360, 640	8 days
^{111}In	Cyclotron	EC	173, 247	2.8 days
^{113m}In	Generator	IT	391	100 min
^{81m}Kr	Generator	IT	191	13 s
^{99m}Tc	Generator	EC	140	6 h
^{201}Tl	Cyclotron	EC	68–80[b]	73.5 h
^{133}Xe	Reactor	Beta	81	5.3 days
Non-imaging tests				
^{14}C	Reactor	Beta	–	5760 years
^{51}Cr	Reactor	EC	323	27.8 days
^{54}Fe	Reactor	Beta	1100, 1300	45 days
^{42}K	Reactor	Beta	–	14.3 days

[a] EC, electron capture; IT, isometric transition.
[b] Characteristic X-rays.

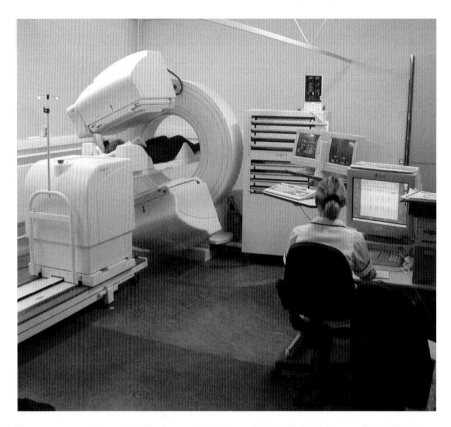

Figure 1.1. The gamma camera. The patient is lying between the detectors of this double-headed system. To the right of the camera is a rack containing extra collimators. The technician is seated at the computer controlling data acquisition and image display.

radiation dose from a radiopharmaceutical it is wise not to place too much reliance on biological excretion, but to use a radionuclide with a reasonably short physical decay time.

1.3 The Gamma Camera System

1.3.1 Introduction

The gamma camera is the principal instrument for imaging in nuclear medicine and is shown in Figure 1.1. As can be seen, it consists of a large detector in front of which the patient is positioned. Gamma cameras with more than one detector are now common, allowing a higher throughput of patients by acquiring two or more views simultaneously. Every aspect of the modern gamma camera is under computer control, allowing the operator to select the study acquisition time, or the number of counts to be acquired, to set the pulse height

analyzers to reject scattered radiation, control the detector and patient bed positions for SPECT and whole body procedures, and display the image. A typical gamma camera image is shown in Figure 1.2.

All gamma camera manufactures sell associated computers and software to process and display the acquired images. The type of computer and the operating system upon which the software functions has, in the past, varied between manufacturers. This has led to a number of problems, which has hindered the transfer of data between systems. However, in recent years, driven by the demand for onscreen reporting of images by clinicians and the need to transfer data to picture archiving and communications systems (PACS), these problems have, in part, been overcome. The solution has been to develop an industry standard data format (DICOM) which, when used with the correct software, will allow the free movement of data between imaging systems. Although

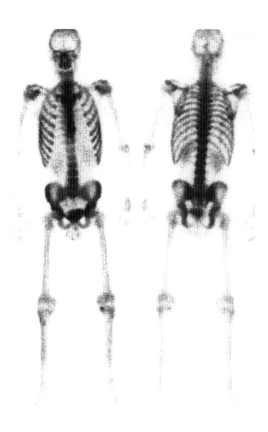

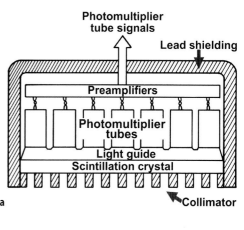

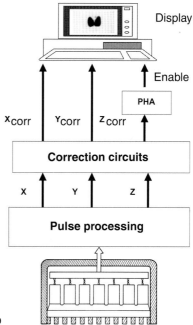

Figure 1.2. Gamma camera images of a bone study. Each spot represents one detected gamma ray.

1.3.2 Mode of Operation of the Gamma Camera

The basic principles of how a camera works are shown in Figure 1.3. The image of the distribution of the gamma-ray-emitting radiopharmaceutical is produced in the scintillation crystal by a collimator. The gamma rays, which are not visible to the eye, are converted into flashes of light by the scintillation crystal. This light is, in turn, transformed into electronic signals by an array of photomultiplier tubes (PMT) viewing the rear face of the crystal. After processing, the outputs from the PMTs are converted into three signals, two of which (X and Y) give the spatial location of the scintillation while the third (Z) represents the en-

Figure 1.3. a Cross-section through the detector head of a gamma camera. Gamma rays emitted from the patient pass through the collimator to form an image in the scintillation crystal. The light from this image is converted into electronic signals by the PMTs. **b** The signals from the camera head are processed to give the X and Y position signals and the Z energy signal. The Z signal goes to a pulse height analyzer and, if it falls within the predetermined range of acceptable energy values, generates a signal which instructs the display system to record a gamma ray as having been correctly detected at the X and Y location.

ergy deposited in the crystal by the gamma ray. To improve their quality these signals then pass through correction circuits. The Z signal goes to a pulse height analyzer (PHA), which tests whether

all manufacturers will promote their products as being fully DICOM compliant, unfortunately a number of specific problems remain.

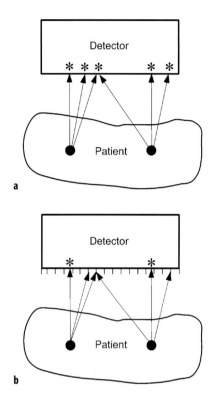

a

b

Figure 1.4. **a** In the absence of collimation there is no relationship between the position at which a gamma ray hits the detector and that from which it left the patient. **b** The parallel-hole collimator forms an image by excluding all gamma rays except those travelling parallel to the hole's axis.

the energy of the gamma ray is within the range of values expected for the particular radionuclide being imaged. If the Z signal has an acceptable value, then a signal is sent instructing the display to record that there has been a gamma ray detected, the position being determined by the X and Y signals. The individual elements of the system will now be considered in more detail.

1.3.3 Collimator

As with all forms of electromagnetic radiation, gamma rays are emitted isotropically. Simply using a detector would not result in an image, as there would be no relationship between the position at which the gamma rays hit the detector and that from which they were emitted from the patient (Figure 1.4a).

In an optical system a lens is used to focus the light but it is not possible to use it with high-frequency radiation such as gamma rays. Instead a much cruder device must be employed, the collimator. The most common type, the parallel-hole collimator, is shown in Figure 1.5a. It consists of a lead plate through which runs an array of small holes whose axes are perpendicular to the face of the collimator and parallel to each other. Only those gamma rays that travel along a hole axis will pass into the scintillation crystal, while those that approach the collimator at an oblique angle

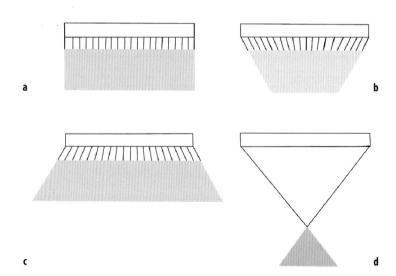

a

b

c

d

Figure 1.5. Different types of collimator. The shaded area shows the field of view of the collimator. **a** The parallel-hole collimator; **b** the converging collimator; **c** the diverging collimator; **d** the pinhole collimator.

will hit the septa and be absorbed (Figure 1.4b). Thus an image is formed by excluding all gamma rays except the small number traveling in the preferred direction perpendicular to the detector.

The two main parameters describing collimator performance are spatial resolution and sensitivity. Resolution is a measure of the sharpness of the image and is approximately equal to the minimum separation needed between two structures if they are to be resolved. A more precise definition is given in Section 5.2.1. Typically the best spatial resolution that can be achieved with a camera fitted with a parallel-hole collimator is about 7 mm. Sensitivity is a measure of the proportion of those gamma rays incident on the collimator that pass through to the detector; the higher the sensitivity, the greater the count rate recorded. Typically the sensitivity for a parallel-hole collimator is only 0.1% (hence 99.9% of photons are absorbed by the collimator and do not reach the detector). The effectiveness of a collimator in producing an image in the scintillation crystal will depend upon the dimensions of the collimator (Table 1.3). Note that not all of these parameters are independent. For example, increasing hole diameter will reduce the number of holes in the collimator.

The first point to note is that image resolution decreases with distance from the collimator. Therefore the resolution will be best for the organ that is closest to the collimator. Imaging must always be carried out with the relevant part of the patient as close to the collimator as possible. Secondly, the sensitivity of the parallel-hole collimator is independent of the distance of the organ from the collimator face. This is only true when there is no attenuating material between organ and collimator. In practice this is rarely the case, and the normal exponential attenuation processes will cause sensitivity to be dependent on distance.

There is a trade-off between collimator spatial resolution and sensitivity; it is not possible to optimize both the spatial resolution and sensitivity

Table 1.3. Factors affecting the performance of a parallel-hole collimator

Parameter that is increased	Resolution	Sensitivity
Number of holes	No change	Increases
Hole diameter	Worsens	Increases
Hole length	Improves	Decreases
Septal thickness	No change	Decreases
Distance of object from collimator	Worsens	No change

Table 1.4. Collimator specifications

Type	Resolution^a (mm)	Sensitivity (cps MBq^{-1})	Energy^b (keV)
Low-energy, high-resolution	6.4	91	140
Low-energy, general purpose	8.3	149	140
Low-energy, high-sensitivity	14.6	460	140
Medium-energy, general purpose	10.8	140	280
High-energy, general purpose	12.6	61	360

^{a} Geometric resolution at 10 cm from collimator face.
^{b} 5% penetration of septa.

of a collimator, and a choice must be made depending upon the type of investigation to be performed. If the test requires high-resolution images and the amount of radioactivity in the patient is sufficiently high so that imaging times will not be unduly long, then the high-resolution design of collimator can be employed. If, instead, the need is for a series of short-exposure images, as in a dynamic imaging study, then resolution may be sacrificed for increased sensitivity.

It is also necessary to have separate collimators for the different energy of radionuclides used: a low-energy (<140 keV), a medium-energy (<260 keV), and a high-energy (<400 keV) collimator. These differ in the thickness of the lead septa between the holes. In practice a department would have available a range of collimators for different circumstances. A list of typical collimators and their relative performance parameters is shown in Table 1.4.

While the parallel-hole collimator is used for most studies, other designs of collimator are available for more specialized applications. The converging collimator has holes that point to a focal spot several centimeters in front of the face of the collimator (Figure 1.5b). The value of this hole geometry is that it will magnify the image of a small organ. Magnification will increase with the distance from the collimator face, and so resolution will not deteriorate as rapidly as with the parallel-hole collimator. Also, sensitivity increases with distance, so helping to compensate for the effect of attenuation. Unfortunately, the image will be distorted, the back of an organ being magnified to a different extent from that of the front, and there will also be variations in resolution across the field of view as the hole geometry varies from highly diverging near the edges to nearly parallel at the center of the collimator. While the converging collimator is rarely used these days, a variant of it, the fan-beam collimator, is used for cardiac and SPECT imaging (see Section 2.2.8). In this collimator the holes in each row converge but in the orthogonal direction they are parallel. Thus they focus to a line rather than a point. The diverging collimator is the opposite to the converging collimator, having holes converging to a point behind rather than in front of the collimator. The result is a collimator that can minify a large object so that it will fit into the smaller detector (Figure 1.5c). This collimator has the same disadvantages of image distortion and sensitivity varying across the field of view found with the converging collimator. The need for such a collimator is rare with modern cameras, but a variation of this design in which the holes diverge in one dimension only is to be found in the so-called fish-tail collimators used with some whole-body scanning cameras. This type of collimator increases the field of view, so allowing the full width of the patient to be imaged. The move to rectangular field of view detectors has made this unnecessary in the modern cameras.

A different concept of collimation is to be found in the pinhole collimator, which forms an image in a way analogous to the optical pinhole camera. It consists of a lead cone with a small hole of a few millimeters in diameter at its apex (Figure 1.5d). It constrains the detected gamma rays to those passing through one particular point; thus each elementary area on the detector sees only a small area of the object and an image is produced in the crystal. The ratio of the size of the image to that of the object will depend upon the ratio of the distance of the hole from the detector to that of the organ from the hole. Its main use is to give an enlarged image of a small organ. The organ must be located near a body surface so that the pinhole can be positioned close to it, the thyroid gland being the organ most commonly imaged in this way. As with all collimators, apart from the parallel-hole type, there is image distortion. For a thick object the magnification of the distant posterior surface will be greater than that of the anterior one. There is a variation in resolution and sensitivity across an organ, and sensitivity falls off quickly with increasing distance of the organ from the collimator.

1.3.4 Detector

While the collimator modifies the gamma ray flux so as to create an image, it is the function of the detector assembly to convert the gamma rays into a form that will, eventually, allow a visible image to be produced. This process takes place in two stages. The first step is the conversion of the gamma rays into visible light by means of a scintillation crystal, while in the second these scintillations are turned into electrical signals by the PMTs. The properties of the ideal scintillation detector are given in Table 1.5.

The scintillation crystal used in gamma cameras is made from sodium iodide with trace quantities of thallium added, NaI(Tl). Its effectiveness at stopping the gammas depends not only on its density but also on the thickness of crystal used (see Figure 1.6).

Table 1.5. Desirable properties of the scintillation crystal

High efficiency for stopping gamma rays
Stopping should be without scatter
High conversion of gamma ray energy into light
Wavelength of light should match response of the PMTs
Crystal should be transparent to emitted light
Crystal should be mechanically robust
Length of scintillation should be short

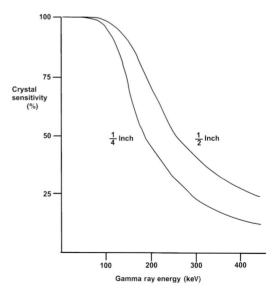

Figure 1.6. The effectiveness of the crystal at stopping a gamma ray as a function of the gamma ray's energy.

Unfortunately, only a small fraction of the energy lost by a gamma ray is converted into light, typically 10%, producing about 3000 light photons at a wavelength of 410 nm for each 100 keV of gamma ray energy absorbed. This wavelength, however, matches quite closely that required by the PMT. The length of each scintillation must be sufficiently short to avoid the overlap of light from consecutive scintillations. In the NaI(Tl) crystal it takes about 0.8 μs to collect most of the light, and this will obviously affect the maximum gamma ray rate that the camera can handle without producing a distorted image (see Section 1.3.8).

NaI(Tl) also suffers from the drawbacks of being expensive to produce as a large crystal, fragile and so needing protection from both thermal and mechanical stresses, and hygroscopic, requiring to be canned to prevent contact with moisture. The latter requirement poses a problem since it is also necessary to ensure that the light emitted in the scintillation is transmitted to the second part of the detector system, the PMT array. While the front face and sides of the crystal are canned, usually with aluminum sufficiently thin so as not to attenuate the incoming gamma rays unduly, the rear crystal surface needs a transparent interface between the crystal and PMTs. This is usually provided by a Pyrex optical plate or light guide a few centimeters in thickness. Despite the obvious problems with using NaI(Tl), it has proved to be the only satisfactory scintillation material for gamma cameras.

While it is possible, at least in theory, to produce an image from the scintillation in the crystal, the main advantage of first converting this image to electrical signals is that pulse height analysis can be used to reduce the effect of scattered photons on image quality.

The PMTs are usually arranged in a close-packed array to ensure that the smallest possible gaps are left between tubes. In recent years, the shape of the crystal has changed from circular to rectangular, as the latter is more suitable for imaging the body. Typically, the crystal size is 60 × 45 cm, giving a field of view of about 55 × 40 cm. About 60 PMTs are needed to cover this rectangular crystal. While PMTs with a photocathode diameter of 3 inches are used mainly, it is also necessary to use some 2 inch diameter tubes.

The PMT not only converts light into an electronic signal but also, as its name suggests, magnifies the electronic signal (typically by a factor of 10^7) to give a sufficiently large current for the subsequent electronics. Even with this signal amplification pre-amplifiers built into the PMT are necessary to ensure a sufficient signal-to-noise ratio.

1.3.5 Signal Processing

Three types of signal processing are to be found in use at present. Analogue circuitry was used in cameras exclusively until about the mid-1990s. Even though so-called digital cameras have been marketed since the mid-1980s, in practice they used analogue circuits to produce the X, Y, and Z signals and digitized them prior to them entering the signal correction and display modules. Only since the mid-1990s has truly digital signal processing been used in commercial cameras, with the signal from the individual PMTs being digitized.

Analogue Systems

The signals from the PMTs are processed to give the three signals required, X and Y providing spatial information and Z the energy. The energy signal is produced simply by summing the outputs from all of the tubes, so measuring the total light produced by the scintillation. The spatial information is more difficult to produce. What is required is that the processed signal should be proportional to the X or Y location of the scintillation. This is achieved by weighting the signals from each tube by passing the output from the PMTs through resistors or capacitors:

$$X = \frac{\sum_i w_i o_i}{\sum_i o_i}$$

where w_i is the weighting factor for the ith PMT and o_i is the output signal. The value of the weighting factor is proportional to the spatial coordinate of the PMT, separate factors being used for the X and Y signals [4]. The divisor, which is equal to the energy of the gamma, is necessary to prevent the X value being dependent upon the energy as well as spatial location of the scintillation.

Digital Systems

Modern camera systems now rely heavily on digital technology, both for correction of the spatial, energy, and temporal information (see Section 1.3.8) and for the analysis of image data. Since this requires the analogue signal to be digitized, there is a strong case for having a completely digital camera. Two general approaches are currently taken; either to digitize the X, Y, and Z signals immediately after these have been computed by analogue circuitry or, in the latest generation of cameras, to completely replace the analogue circuits, the signals from the PMTs being digitized before the X, Y, and Z signals are computed. In the latter case each PMT has an analogue to digital converter located after the preamplifier, and the signal position is calculated from the centroid of the signals from a group of PMTs, usually chosen to be those having the strongest and hence least noisy signals. The Z signal is calculated by summing the outputs from the group of tubes.

Accuracy of Signal Processing

In order to reproduce the image that has been formed in the scintillation crystal the X and Y signals must be proportional to the coordinates of the scintillation. In other words the system must demonstrate good spatial linearity. The detector assembly must be constructed so that small changes in the position of the scintillation alter significantly the relative strengths of the outputs from the PMTs.

While the most obvious solution to optimize the linearity would be to use a large number of PMTs, in practice this would degrade the image in another way. The amount of light incident on the array of tubes is very low, approximately 1000 photons from a 140 keV gamma ray, producing about 25 electrons from the photocathode of each PMT, which are then magnified to give the final output current. In practice the number of photoelectrons will vary randomly about this average value, a feature found in the emission of all quanta including gamma rays. So even if consecutive gamma rays were to be stopped at exactly the same position in the crystal, the PMT outputs would not be identical, but would produce X and Y signals that varied randomly about the true value. The true image of the point would be blurred into a disk. This effect is referred to as the intrinsic resolution of the camera. The total spatial resolution of a camera thus consists of a combination of this intrinsic resolution and the collimator resolution, and is given by

$$R_{total} = \left[R_{collimator}^2 + R_{intrinsic}^2 \right]^{1/2}.$$

Table 1.6. Factors affecting linearity and intrinsic resolution

	Linearity	Resolution
Increasing crystal thickness	Degrades	Degrades
Increasing number of PMTs	Improves	Degrades
Increasing size of photocathode	Degrades	Improves
Improving conversion efficiency of crystal	No change	Improves
Improving PMT conversion efficiency	No change	Improves
Increasing light guide thickness	Improves	Degrades
Using a higher-energy gamma ray	No change	Improves

The paucity of photons will also cause a similar random variability in the energy signal. Typically the energy resolution of a gamma camera is about 10% (see Section 5.2.9).

To produce a high-quality image, both intrinsic resolution and spatial distortion must be considered. Unfortunately, altering the design of the detector to increase the light received by each PMT and so improve resolution will often degrade linearity (Table 1.6). The solution is not necessarily to compromise, as the image can be corrected for poor linearity (see Section 1.3.8). In contrast intrinsic resolution cannot be corrected as it is a random process, in which the correct value for the X and Y signals cannot be determined by some form of calibration. The detector assembly is thus designed to optimize intrinsic resolution.

There are other problems which must be borne in mind when choosing a camera. An improvement in intrinsic resolution may not produce a significant change in the total spatial resolution when the effect of collimator resolution is also taken into account. Only when the resolution of the collimator is good, with objects close to the collimator face or when using a fine-resolution collimator, will the improvement be perhaps noticeable.

Caution must be exercised if the resolution has been improved at the expense of other factors. In particular, the prospective purchaser may be faced with a choice of crystal thickness, a $3/8$ inch is commonly used, but thicknesses between $1/4$ up to 1 inch are used, the higher values being for cameras designed to also do PET imaging. While a thinner crystal will improve intrinsic resolution it also causes a decrease in sensitivity (Figure 1.6). It is debatable whether the overall result is an improvement in performance.

1.3.6 Uniformity

Not only is it desirable that the camera performance be optimized but also performance should not vary significantly between different points in the crystal. Any variability is demonstrated most readily by the image of a uniform distribution of radioactivity, the so-called flood image. Areas of above- or below-average count density are indicative of regions where the camera performance has altered. The effect of variations in linearity and intrinsic resolution is to misposition gamma rays, putting them closer together or further apart than expected. Spatial variations in the value of the Z signal will result in local changes in the apparent sensitivity of the camera as a greater or smaller number of gammas are accepted by the pulse height analyzer. Digital correction circuitry for linearity and the energy signal are found in all modern cameras and will be discussed further in Section 1.3.8.

1.3.7 Pulse Height Analysis

The collimator is responsible for creating an image out of the flux of gamma rays incident on it, yet not all of these gamma rays will carry useful image information. In particular, those rays that have been Compton scattered in the patient, and so appear to come from another location, simply reduce image contrast. Such rays can be identified by the fact that in being scattered they also lose energy, the amount being dependent on the angle through which they were deviated. As the scintillation detector allows the energy deposited by the gamma ray in the crystal to be measured, this information can be used to exclude scattered gamma rays. However, as has already been mentioned, the gamma camera is limited in the accuracy with which it can measure energy, with the result that even in the absence of scatter the gamma rays appear to have a range of energies. The width of this so-called photopeak spectrum, measured at half the maximum height, is about 10% of the true energy. The pulse height analyzer allows the operator to select only the signals from those gammas in which the height of the Z signal, that is, gamma ray energy, has a certain value or range of values. If many useful gammas are not to be excluded from the image, a range of energies must be allowed through the PHA, and typically a window equal to 20% of the peak energy value is used; i.e. for ^{99m}Tc

with a gamma ray of 140 keV those signals with energies between 126 and 154 keV are judged to be acceptable.

While the scattered gamma rays are distinguishable by their lower energy, the spreading out of the photopeak spectrum may mean that the energy of unscattered gammas overlaps that of scattered ones. This overlap of the Compton and photopeak spectrum means that a choice must be made between using a narrow window and so excluding a large proportion of unscattered rays or accepting the presence of some scattered radiation in the image. Usually the latter is chosen, and with a 20% window about 30% of the gamma rays in the image will have been scattered.

When using radionuclides that emit gamma rays at different energies, multiple window analyzers need to be employed. Typically a maximum of three sets of windows is available. In this instance, it is important to remember that scattered radiation from the higher-energy gammas may overlap into the lower-energy photopeaks and this may influence which gamma ray energies should be selected.

1.3.8 Correction Circuits

To improve image quality, real-time compensation is provided for some of the defects in camera performance mentioned above. It is, however, only possible to correct where the cause of the distortion is not random. So, while non-linearity can be corrected, it is not possible to improve the intrinsic spatial resolution of the camera.

Spatial Linearity

Spatial linearity correction is carried out by presenting the camera with an image consisting of a series of parallel straight lines aligned with either the X or Y axis of the camera. The deviation between the true position of each point on the line, as calculated from a best-fit straight line, and the image of the line, is recorded and stored as a correction factor to be applied to subsequently acquired clinical images. To achieve the spatial resolution required to define the straight lines it is necessary for the test pattern to be imaged without the collimator, i.e. placed against the crystal and illuminated with a flood source of gamma rays, usually from a point source of activity placed a long way from the camera. As this requires a phantom

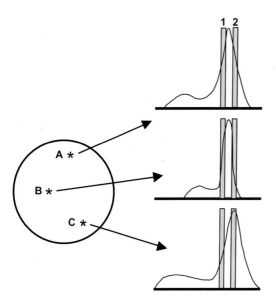

Figure 1.7. Variation of the energy signal with the position of the scintillation in the crystal. At A, the two windows are situated symmetrically around the photopeak. At B, the calculated values for the energy signals are lower than at A and so more events are accumulated in window 1 than 2, while at C the energy signal is higher than at A and there are more events in window 2. Correction factors for the energy signals can be generated by comparing the number of gamma rays in the two windows.

manufactured to high tolerances, the generation of new correction factors is usually done by the manufacturer's service engineer.

Energy

The energy signal may also require correction, as the calculated value is found to vary with the position of the gamma ray across the detector. Shifts in the position of the locally computed energy signal can be measured by comparing the number of gamma rays whose energy falls inside two narrow windows, one set to each side of the average photopeak value (Figure 1.7). Once again the amount of correction required to ensure that the local signal matches the average value, i.e. that there are equal numbers of gamma rays within each window, is stored in a correction matrix to be applied to the subsequent energy signals. This correction is acquired simply by imaging a flood source of radioactivity and can be performed regularly by the user. Typically the average correction should yield a variation in the energy signal of less than 0.2% across the detector.

Scatter Correction

In many clinical studies a significant proportion of the gamma rays in the image will be scattered. The effect is to reduce the contrast since they will, approximately, form a uniform background, and to defeat any attempts to quantify the amount of radioactivity in an organ. Since the amount of scatter will vary within the image depending upon the amount of tissue through which photons need to pass before reaching the detector, any correction will need to be made on a pixel-by-pixel basis. Hence, as was mentioned in Section 1.3.7, the use of the PHA alone is insufficient to remove the scatter.

A number of techniques are offered by manufacturers to remove scatter. They are all based on the removal of a fixed proportion of the photons acquired in a pixel as it is obviously impossible, in the absence of good energy resolution, to identify which particular gammas have been scattered. One class of techniques uses additional energy windows either on either side of the photopeak window, or in a part of the spectrum that is known to include only scattered photons. The proportion of scatter is then calculated from measurement of the number of photons in the various windows [5].

Knowing the energy of the detected photon and the geometry of the scattering medium through which it has passed, it is possible to predict the likelihood that its X and Y coordinates are in error by a particular amount. A second correction technique, employed commercially, uses a correction matrix based on the energy and geometry to predict the probability that, for each photon, the recorded position was the true one [6]. The advantage of such a system is that there is no need to use a pulse height window and so, in theory, all photons can contribute towards the image. The disadvantages are that we do not know the actual energy of the photon, nor the scatter geometry.

Temporal Correction

The typical nuclear medicine study requires the camera to process only a few tens of thousands of counts per second. There are some studies, however, cardiac first pass (see Section 9.5) being the main example, where the count rate can be very high. The probability that successive pulses passing through the camera's electronic circuits will overlap each other becomes unacceptably high. Such pulse pile-up results in incorrect X, Y, and Z signals being produced. Not only will this distort the image, but the recorded energy of these events will be higher than that of the individual pulses leading to them being rejected by the PHA; the detected count rate will no longer increase linearly, or indeed monotonically, with the amount of activity in the camera's field of view. The problem of measuring pulse pile-up effects will be discussed in Section 5.2.8.

The difficulty arises because the pulses coming out of the PMT preamplifiers have a finite length. Electronic pulse shaping can help to reduce the problem and digital arithmetic circuits should be much faster than analogue ones. An online correction circuit has been implemented using a technique known as pulse tail extrapolation [7]. The circuit detects the overlap of two pulses by the failure of the signal to return to its baseline level within a specified time. It then separates the two pulses, the first pulse being without its tail which is now mixed in with the second pulse. By examining the shape of the first pulse the correction circuit extrapolates the truncated tail to recreate its original shape. This extrapolated section is then subtracted from the second pulse, so also restoring it to its original shape.

The effectiveness of correction circuits varies considerably between manufacturers. An image of a flood source often provides a simple test. The prospective purchaser of a camera should check that the correction facilities are usable for all operations with the camera and that the correction works for different radionuclides and for window settings of different energies.

1.3.9 Image Display

Modern camera systems employ digital display systems. If the Z signal corresponding to a particular detected gamma ray falls within the window that has been set on the PHA, then an enable signal is sent and the X and Y signals are recorded.

The most common form of image acquisition is called matrix or frame mode. The camera's field of view is divided into a regular matrix of picture elements or pixels. Each pixel is assigned a unique memory location in the computer. The value stored in this location is the number of gamma ray events that have been detected in the corresponding location on the camera face. The number, and hence the size, of the pixels used is of practical importance and depends on (i) the available computer memory (unlikely to be a prob-

lem with modern systems), (ii) the total number of images to be acquired, (iii) the number of counts contained in each image, and (iv) the required temporal and spatial resolution.

As modern systems can acquire and display static images with array sizes of up to 2048×2048 pixels, image quality is comparable with that of analogue images. Each pixel is typically stored as a 16 bit unsigned integer (allowing count values to range from 0 to 65 535); more bits per pixel would allow higher counts to be recorded, but at the expense of storage space, image transfer rate, and possibly processing time.

The image data are mapped from the array of numbers, representing the number of gamma rays acquired at a specific spatial location, into a viewable image by a look-up table which links the number of gamma rays to a specific value of displayed image intensity. The first question to be addressed is how best to represent image intensity, both gray shades and colors having been used. The human eye can distinguish thousands of different colors, compared with only several tens of gray shades. The use of color to display intensity information, known as pseudo color, should therefore permit a much wider dynamic range to be reproduced. For instance, the so-called "hot body" scale, first proposed for coding ultrasound images [8], uses a gradual variation in hue and intensity to increase the dynamic range of the display; the scale changes from black, through shades of red, to white. Color scales can also make identification of specific ranges of pixel values easier, and are particularly useful for parametric images, which are discussed in Section 1.4.2.

However, there are several serious problems associated with color scales. Firstly, if the scale includes distinct perceptual color steps it can introduce false edges and contours in the image, greatly exaggerating small, and possibly insignificant, changes. Secondly, rather than enhancing the dynamic range, poorly chosen color scales can degrade it and reduce image contrast. Finally, there is the issue as to whether the display device (whether a screen or a hard-copy device) is actually capable of reproducing all the colors in the color scale. Failing to do so can result in large portions of the color scale being reproduced as the same color.

The second question is how to map count density to the chosen gray shades or colors. The simplest case is a linear relationship between the number of counts and the displayed intensity (Figure 1.8a). Other transformations include

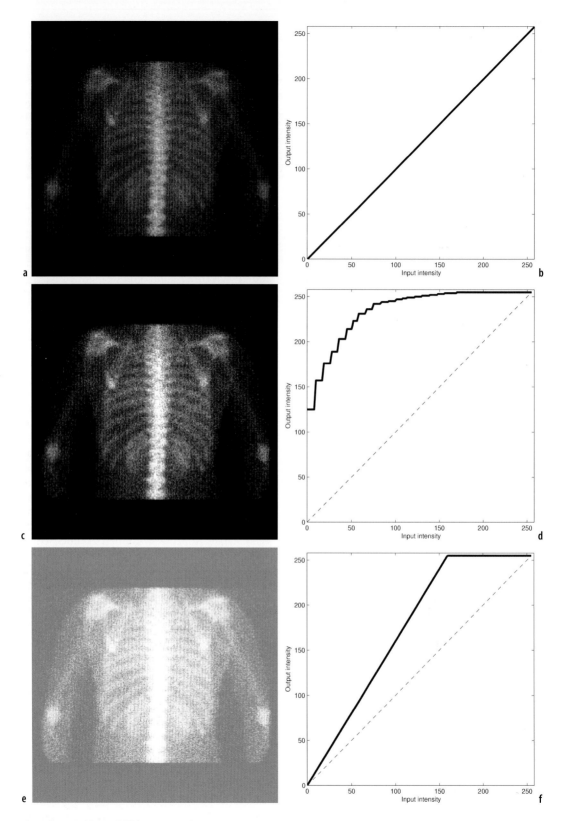

Figure 1.8. Examples of different types of intensity mapping. **a** A linear mapped image; **b** the linear mapping scheme between input (image counts) and output (displayed gray shade) intensity. **c** A histogram equalized image; **d** the histogram equalization mapping scheme. **e** A contrast enhanced image; **f** the contrast mapping scheme.

compression of parts of the scale to increase contrast over a specific count range (Figure 1.8b), and non-linear mappings, such as logarithmic, power law, square root or exponential [9]. Histogram equalization is a non-linear intensity transform which has been applied to nuclear medicine images [10] (Figure 1.8c). Count density is mapped such that each display intensity, gray shade or color, occurs approximately (due to digitization) the same number of times in the image. Although equalization theoretically maximizes image contrast, in practice it is rarely useful. A variation on this, adaptive histogram equalization [11], involves the application of histogram equalization in small sub-areas of the image, rather than globally to the whole image. However, it also tends to amplify image noise, an undesirable property for nuclear medicine images.

One of the simplest ways of manipulating the displayed data is by thresholding (sometimes known as windowing). For example, in bone imaging the radiopharmaceutical is excreted into the bladder, giving an area of very high count density. In the absence of thresholding most of the display levels will be used to display the bladder activity rather than the bones. By applying an upper threshold all areas having counts above a threshold value will be given the same maximum gray shade. This leaves the remaining gray shades or colors to be assigned to those counts found in the bones. Similarly a lower threshold may be applied such that all low count density areas are given the same low gray shade.

1.4 Data Acquisition

1.4.1 Static Studies

Data are acquired for either some pre-selected acquisition time or preset number of counts. The former is effective if the count rate is known not to vary significantly between patients and ensures that patient throughput is predictable. However, if there is an isolated area in the image containing a high level of activity that is not of clinical interest, as for example bladder activity in bone scans, then preset counts may result in very few counts in the areas of potential clinical interest.

1.4.2 Dynamic Studies

In some clinical studies it is not simply the spatial distribution of the radiopharmaceutical that is of interest, but also how this distribution changes with time. In dynamic imaging the camera is set to acquire data either for a preset sequence of frames (where the acquisition time for each frame can be variable) or using list mode.

In list mode acquisition image data are stored as a list of the X and Y coordinates of each detected event along with regular timing data. Some systems also store the Z energy value, allowing post-acquisition energy window selection. In general list mode acquisition requires more memory than matrix mode, since only the individual events are stored whereas matrix mode requires the same amount of memory, irrespective of the number of counts in the image. However, some additional software and time information is required to format such data into suitable matrix mode images for display and subsequent processing.

List mode is of particular value if very good temporal resolution is required, or the required temporal resolution is not known in advance. It has the advantage that several matrix mode studies with different frame times can be produced retrospectively from the original data.

Changes in the distribution of the radiopharmaceutical with time can be measured by drawing a region of interest (ROI) around the features of interest seen in the study, using a cursor under mouse control (sometimes this operation can be automated as described in Section 1.6). The data acquisition system then plots time–activity curves (TACs) showing how the number of counts within the ROIs varies between image frames, i.e. with time. Figure 1.9 shows an example TAC. This

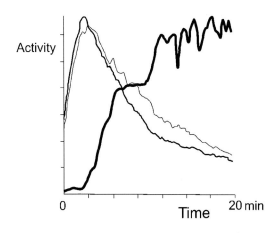

Figure 1.9. Time–activity curves. The number of counts within each of three regions of interest is plotted on the y-axis as activity. The x-axis shows time elapsed after the start of dynamic image acquisition.

technique is of particular value in renography (see Chapter 11).

Gated Imaging

The assumption in nuclear medicine imaging is that the structures being imaged do not themselves move during the imaging time. This is not generally true although, given the relatively poor spatial resolution, the extent of this motion is usually not sufficient to cause significant deterioration in image quality. In the case of cardiac blood pool imaging (see Chapter 9), however, it is desirable to capture images at a sufficiently high rate in order to be able to view the changes in the blood image caused by the beating of the heart.

Given that an average cardiac cycle is about 800 ms in length, to acquire 16 images during the cycle would need an exposure time per image of 50 ms. With a typical count rate of a few tens of thousands of counts per second each image frame would contain only a few hundred counts, far too few to show any structure. The solution is to use a physiological signal, in this case from the electrocardiograph (ECG), to keep image acquisition in phase with the beating heart so that data can be collected over many hundred cardiac cycles. The principle is shown in Figure 1.10.

Data collected in this way can then be displayed in a cine loop, in which the frames are replayed in rapid succession in a continuous loop. The data can be analyzed as a time–activity curve, or parametric images produced.

Parametric Images

While time–activity curves can be analyzed quantitatively, normally they are assessed visually. However, TACs only show the average change in count density within the ROI. In gated cardiac studies there is interest in how wall motion varies at different locations in the left ventricle. One could draw a whole series of small ROIs but this would then produce many TACs needing to be analyzed. Instead each TAC is decomposed into a small number of parameters. For gated cardiac images the parameters are the amplitude of the curve and the phase, the time between maximum and minimum contraction (Figure 1.11a). Thus a TAC can be generated from each pixel in the cardiac study, a pair of parameters produced from each curve and two new parametric images generated in which the number of counts in a particular pixel is replaced by the parameter derived from its TAC (Figure 1.11b).

1.5 Image Filtering

In contrast to the mapping performed with lookup tables to produce a displayed image, image filtering alters the actual count density values. Filtering is used primarily to reduce the effect of

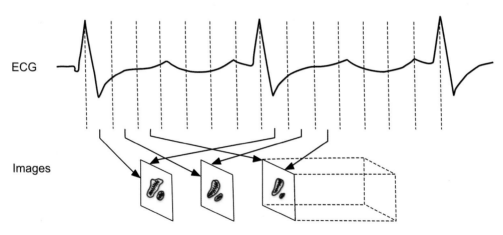

Figure 1.10. Multiple gated cardiac acquisition. In this example a dynamic study of the heart is performed. The start and end of each image is indicated by the broken lines. Image acquisition starts with the arrival of the peak of the ECG and a dynamic study of seven images is collected. With the arrival of the next peak, indicating the start of the next cardiac cycle, data are added to the original set of seven images. This continues over several hundred cardiac cycles. At the completion of the study, each image represents the appearance of the heart at a particular point in the cardiac cycle. Gated cardiac studies are discussed further in Chapter 9.

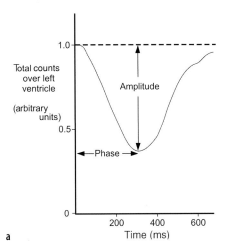

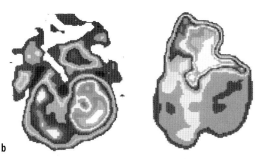

Figure 1.11. a The time–activity curve shows the variation in the amount of radioactivity in the left ventricle of the heart during a cardiac cycle. Such a curve is measured for each image pixel and the length of time to the curve minimum, the phase, and the difference between maximum and minimum activity, the amplitude, are measured. **b** Parametric images. These show the resulting images of the amplitude and phase values for a normal cardiac study.

noise on image interpretation and analysis. It can also, to a certain extent, improve image resolution by compensating for the degradation produced mainly by the gamma camera collimator. Image filtering can be broadly categorized into linear and non-linear techniques.

1.5.1 Linear Filtering

In linear filtering each pixel is replaced with a (usually weighted) linear combination of its surrounding pixels. It may be implemented using convolution, given by

$$g(x, y) = f(x, y) * w(x, y)$$
$$= \sum_{s=-a}^{a} \sum_{t=-b}^{b} f(x - s, y - t)w(s, t)$$

where $f(x, y)$ and $g(x, y)$ are the original and filtered images respectively, $*$ represents the convolution operator, and $w(s, t)$ are the filter coefficients or kernel, which define the filter.

Linear filtering can also be performed in the frequency domain by exploiting the convolution theorem. This states that convolution in the spatial domain is equivalent to multiplication in the frequency domain (and likewise multiplication in the spatial domain is equivalent to convolution in the spatial domain). Hence the convolution above may be performed by taking the Fourier transforms of $f(x, y)$ and $w(x, y)$, applying point-wise multiplication, and taking the inverse Fourier transform of the result to obtain $g(x, y)$, i.e.

$$G(u, v) = F(u, v)W(u, v)$$

where $F(u, v)$, $G(u, v)$ and $W(u, v)$ follow the usual convention that the capitalized form of a variable indicates the Fourier transform (frequency domain form) of the lower case spatial domain function. For larger filter kernels the overhead necessary to calculate the Fourier transform using a fast Fourier transform (FFT) is easily outweighed by the computational complexity of convolution.

The modulation transfer function (MTF) of the gamma camera demonstrates how effectively it reproduces information at different spatial frequencies (see Section 5.2.1). This shows why gamma camera images appear blurred; the MTF decreases rapidly with increasing spatial frequency and consequently fine detail is not recorded. In contrast, the image noise, due primarily to counting statistics, is independent of frequency (and is known as "white noise" by analogy to the energy spectrum of white light). The ratio of the useful image information to the noise, the signal-to-noise ratio (SNR), therefore decreases with increasing spatial frequency. The overall image SNR can be improved quite simply by attenuating the higher spatial frequencies, which are predominantly (or entirely) noise. The simplest solution is to apply a "low-pass filter", which attenuates high-frequency components without affecting the lower-frequency ones. This is particularly important in SPECT imaging where the "ramp filter" required by filtered back-projection also accentuates the noise at high frequencies (see Section 2.2.2). Care should be taken when designing the low-pass filter to ensure that artifacts are not generated by the filter which may be mistaken for abnormalities.

Filters may also be designed that restore some of the image resolution lost due to the MTF of the gamma camera. The simplest approach is to design a filter whose frequency response is equal to the inverse of the camera MTF, a process known as inverse filtering. If $F(u, v)$ and $G(u, v)$ are the Fourier transforms of the true image and the blurred image respectively, then given the MTF, $H(u, v)$, the blurred image is given by

$$G(u, v) = F(u, v) H(u, v).$$

Restoration appears to be straightforward, by simple algebra:

$$F(u, v) = \frac{G(u, v)}{H(u, v)}.$$

In practice this does not work as it is evident that frequencies that are absent in the image cannot be restored by the filter. Inverse filters emphasize the higher spatial frequencies, which are predominantly noise, and thus tend to obscure the true image. Therefore any practical resolution restoration filter needs to employ some form of constraint to control the noise level in the resulting image. Three such methods are Wiener filtering, Metz filtering, and constrained least squares filtering.

1.5.2 Non-linear Filters

The most common non-linear filter is probably the median filter, which replaces each pixel by the median value of its surrounding neighborhood. Since it is not possible to apply Fourier analysis to non-linear filters, it is difficult to predict the effect of the median filter on the spatial frequency content of images. However, in general the median filter behaves like a low-pass filter which preserves some edge detail. It is of limited effectiveness for noisy nuclear medicine images (which do not contain sharp edges) as it can introduce false edge structure and contours to the image and suppress specific spatial frequencies in the image.

A problem with all the preceding filters is that they assume that there is one filter that is best for the whole image. Yet regions with higher numbers of counts will have a higher SNR, and therefore require less smoothing than regions with fewer counts. Adaptive filters attempt to estimate the regional noise level and apply an appropriate degree of smoothing. For instance, one estimate of the

noise level is given by the ratio of the regional standard deviation and mean. In one such filter a median filter has been combined with a local averaging filter and is claimed to be effective for smoothing noisy images containing strong edges.

1.6 Automated Image Analysis

Automated image analysis has the potential, although yet to be fully realized, to increase throughput, ensure consistency, and improve accuracy.

One technique is to make a "normal" or "template" image to which all patient images may be aligned and compared to detect abnormal features. The normal image is usually created from a sample of studies assessed to be clinically normal; the images are registered and the normal inter-subject variations estimated. This approach has been used as the basis for the automated detection of abnormalities in SPECT heart images [12]. Principal component analysis has been used to extract significant modes of variation from such sets of normal images [13].

Another use for the normal template is the automatic location of regions of interest within an image. Once regions have been drawn on the template image (perhaps using higher resolution magnetic resonance images or X-ray CT images as a guide), they may be applied automatically to all subsequent images, either by registering the image to the template and applying the ROIs, or by using the inverse mapping to align the ROIs with the image.

More recently, statistical parametric mapping (SPM) has been used to tackle this problem [14]. Image data are registered and spatially normalized to a standard stereotactic space. A statistical comparison can then be made between groups of images on a pixel or voxel basis. This approach was originally intended for PET and functional MRI brain studies, but has been used by a number of groups with SPECT images. It has the advantage of making no a priori assumptions about the size and location of any differences between groups of images. However, assessment of an individual, as compared to a group of patients, is difficult.

Interest in multimodality imaging [15], to combine the functional information from nuclear medicine and the anatomical information from another modality, has encouraged the development of multimodality registration algorithms and of gamma cameras, and PET imagers, with integrated CT scanners.

1.7 Conclusions

The net effect of the limitations of collimation (see Section 1.3.3), namely its relatively poor spatial resolution and low sensitivity, and the need to limit the amount of radioactivity given to the patient is to produce an image whose appearance compares unfavorably with that achieved by other techniques. However, this is not a problem, as the major advantage that nuclear medicine has over many other medical imaging techniques is in giving images that show physiological function. The effectiveness with which this can be used for clinical purposes is also dependent upon the type of information being provided.

It must be appreciated, however, that the presence of abnormalities in the distribution pattern of a radiopharmaceutical usually does not give a specific clinical diagnosis, but only demonstrates aberrations in the particular physiological process that governs the distribution of this pharmaceutical. So additional information is needed if a more precise diagnosis is to be made and it is important that image interpretation takes account of the wider clinical context. For these reasons it may be that multimodality imaging will be an important development in optimizing nuclear medicine imaging.

References

1. Belcher EH, Vetter H, eds. Radioisotopes in Medical Diagnosis. London: Butterworths; 1971.

2. Brown BH, Smallwood RH, Barber DC, Lawford PV, Hose DR, eds. Medical Physics and Biomedical Engineering. Bristol: Institute of Physics; 1999: 183–184.

3. Ott RJ, Flower MA, Babich JW, Marsden PK. The physics of radioisotope imaging. In: Webb S, ed. The Physics of Medical Imaging. Bristol: Adam Hilger; 1988: 181–193.

4. Barrett HH, Swindell W. Radiological Imaging. The Theory of Image Formation, Detection and Processing, Vol. l. London: Academic Press; 1981.

5. Ichihara T, Ogawa K, Motomura N, Kubo A, Hashimoto S. Compton scatter compensation using the triple-energy window method for single- and dual-isotope SPECT. J Nucl Med 1993; 34:2216–2221.

6. DeVito RP, Hamill JJ, Treffert JD, Stoub EW. Energy-weighted acquisition of scintigraphic images using finite spatial filters. J Nucl Med 1989; 30:2029–2035.

7. Lewellen TK, Bice AN, Pollard KR, Zhu JB, Plunkett ME. Evaluation of a clinical scintillation camera with pulse tail exrapolation electronics. J Nucl Med 1989; 30:1554–1558.

8. Milan J, Taylor KJW. The application of the temperature scale to ultrasound imaging. J Clin Ultrasound 1975; 3:171–173.

9. Metz CE, Chan H-P, Doi K, Shen J-H. Contrast enhancement of noisy images by windowing: limitations due to the finite dynamic range of the display system. Med Phys 1989; 16:170–178.

10. Goris ML, Schiebe PO, Kriss JR. A method to optimise the use of a greyshade scale in nuclear medicine images. Comput Biomed Res 1976; 9:571–577.

11. Pizer SM, Amburn EP, Austin JD, et al. Adaptive histogram equalisation and its variations. Comp Vis Graphics Image Proc 1987; 17:355–368.

12. Peace RA, Staff RT, Gemmell HG, Mckiddie FI, Metcalfe MJ. Automatic detection of coronary artery disease in myocardial perfusion SPECT using image registration and voxel to voxel statistical comparisons. Nucl Med Comm 2002; 23:785–794.

13. Houston AS, Kemp PM, Macleod MA, et al. Use of significance image to determine patterns of cortical blood flow abnormality in pathological and at-risk groups. J Nucl Med 1998; 39:425–430.

14. Friston KJ, Holmes AP, Worsley KJ, et al. Statistical parametric maps in functional imaging: a general linear approach. Hum Brain Mapp 1995; 26:265–277.

15. Hajnal JV, Hill DLG, Hawkes DJ, eds. Medical Image Registration. Boca Raton, FL: CRC; 2001.

2

Single Photon Emission Computed Tomography (SPECT)

Howard G. Gemmell and Roger T. Staff

2.1 Introduction

Although the principles of single photon emission computed tomography (SPECT) have been well understood for many years and several centers were using SPECT clinically in the late 1960s and early 1970s, there has been a dramatic increase in the number of SPECT installations in recent years. It is now unusual to purchase a gamma camera without SPECT capability and most new cameras are dual-headed, which can offer additional advantages in SPECT. A state-of-the-art gamma camera that is well maintained should produce high-quality SPECT images consistently, and even older cameras can produce acceptable images if care is taken. SPECT is essential for imaging the brain with either cerebral blood flow agents, such as ^{99m}Tc-HMPAO, or brain receptors, such as ^{123}I-FP-CIT, and for imaging myocardial perfusion with either ^{201}Tl or the technetium-labeled agents MIBI and tetrofosmin. SPECT is also now widely used in some aspects of skeletal imaging and can be helpful in tumor imaging with, for example, ^{123}I-MIBG, ^{111}In octreotide, or ^{99m}Tc NeoSPECT.

What is the purpose of SPECT and what is its advantage over planar imaging? Planar imaging portrays a three-dimensional (3-D) distribution of radioactivity as a 2-D image with no depth information and structures at different depths are superimposed. The result is a loss of contrast in the plane of interest due to the presence of activity in overlying and underlying structures, as shown in Figure 2.1. Multiple planar views are an attempt to overcome this problem but SPECT has been developed to tackle the problem directly. SPECT also involves collecting conventional plane views of the patient from different directions but many more views are necessary, typically 64 or 128, although each view usually has fewer counts than would be acceptable in a conventional static image. From these images a set of sections through the patient can then be reconstructed mathematically. Conventionally SPECT images are viewed in three orthogonal planes – transaxial, sagittal, and coronal – as shown in Figure 2.2. Usually the transaxial images are directly obtained from SPECT data; a particular row of pixels in each image obtained with a rotating gamma camera corresponds to a particular transaxial section. The other planes are derived from a stack of transaxial sections.

2.2 Theory of SPECT

In this section the emphasis will be on gamma camera SPECT. The fact that these systems can also be used for conventional imaging makes them an attractive option for any nuclear medicine department. Owing to the cost and lack of flexibility of dedicated tomographic devices producing single or multiple sections with higher resolution and better sensitivity, they are likely to remain the

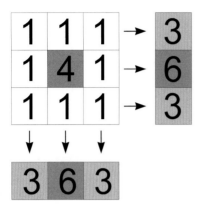

Figure 2.1. A contrast of 4:1 in the object becomes a contrast of 2:1 in planar imaging.

Table 2.1. Operator choices in SPECT

Acquisition	Size of image matrix
	Number of angular increments
	180° or 360° rotation
	Collimator
	Acquisition time
	Uniformity correction
	Center of rotation correction
	Scatter correction
Reconstruction	Method
	Filter
	Attenuation correction or not
	Attenuation correction method

choice of specialist centers only. Now that gamma camera SPECT is well developed commercially and relatively inexpensive, it seems certain that interest in longitudinal or limited-angle SPECT will continue to decline and so this will not be considered further.

The aim here is to consider the theory of SPECT only in sufficient detail to enable the user to understand the principles involved and to make any necessary decisions on an informed basis. A list of likely areas for decisions by the user is given in Table 2.1.

2.2.1 Projection, Back-projection

In order to obtain transaxial sections of the distribution of radioactivity within a patient, projections of that distribution must first be

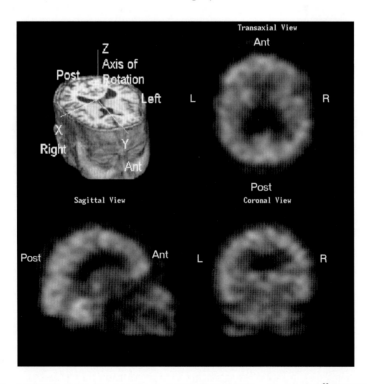

Figure 2.2. Orientation in SPECT. The three orthogonal planes conventionally used are demonstrated using ^{99m}Tc-HMPAO cerebral blood flow images.

The simplest and most common method of reconstructing an image of the original distribution is by "back-projecting" each profile at the appropriate angle on to an image array in the computer as shown in Figure 2.3b. In other words, a constant value equal to the profile element is assumed for each point along that line in the image array. This procedure is carried out for each profile in turn and an image is built up numerically. This image is, however, of poor quality; regions of higher activity show up well but the back-projected image is blurred and has a structured background. This background includes the "spoke" or "star" artifact whose shape and magnitude will depend on the number of projections. These problems are fundamental to the projection/back-projection procedure but can, to some extent, be dealt with by filtering the profiles prior to back-projection.

In practice back-projection is not carried out over 360° as shown in Figure 2.3b. Instead, although data are generally acquired over 360°, it is usual to average opposite projections and then back-project only over 180°. The advantage of this is that it partially compensates both for the drop in spatial resolution with distance from the camera face and for attenuation. Projections can, under certain circumstances, be collected over only 180° rather than the full 360°; when this is done the data are back-projected without prior averaging.

2.2.2 Filters

The problems of blurring and the high background in the reconstructed image are tackled by back-projecting negative numbers adjacent to the positive numbers which represent the object in the original profile. This is achieved by operating on the profile with an appropriate filter as demonstrated in Figure 2.4. After a sufficiently large number of profiles have been back-projected, these negative numbers tend to cancel out the positive background in the image.

Using the mathematical technique known as Fourier analysis it is possible to describe images in terms of their spatial frequencies; these have units of 1/distance, that is cm^{-1}. This is known as working in "frequency or Fourier space" as opposed to "real" space. In the image of a distribution of radioactivity, for example, fine detail is associated with the higher spatial frequencies and coarser structures with the lower spatial frequencies.

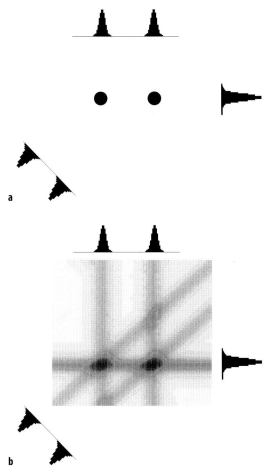

Figure 2.3. a Profiles relating to a single transaxial section from a distribution of radioactivity comprising two point sources. **b** Back-projection of these profiles builds up an image of the point sources by superimposition but at the expense of a high background.

collected at a series of positions around the patient. In Figure 2.3a, 1-D projections or profiles of a distribution of radioactivity comprising two point sources are shown for three positions of the detector. These correspond to a single transaxial section and are obtained from the same single row of pixels on each of the gamma camera images. Each element in each profile therefore represents the sum of the activity along a line perpendicular to the profile, that is perpendicular to the camera face. This profile element is often referred to as the line integral, being the integral along that line of the 2-D function which describes the variation of radioactivity with position.

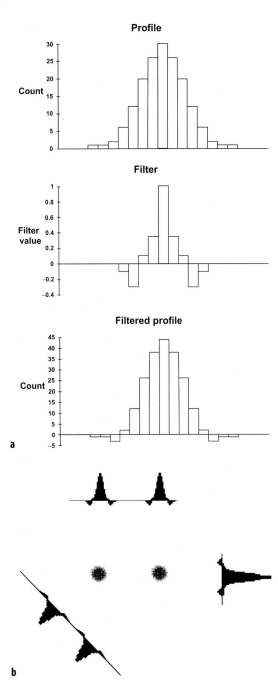

Figure 2.4. a The filter acts on each point in the profile in turn. The values obtained are added to obtain the filtered profile, which includes negative as well as positive points. **b** When the negative values associated with the positive values in each profile are back-projected they tend to cancel out the positive background shown in Figure 2.3b.

Using a modern gamma camera, the upper limit for spatial frequencies recorded in planar images without scatter is about 2 cm^{-1}. How the filters are designed and selected is best appreciated in frequency space, hence its introduction at this point, but it is not necessary to be familiar with the mathematics involved in Fourier analysis. For those wishing to consider this topic in more detail, the text by Brigham [1] offers an excellent introduction to the concepts involved. In Figure 2.5 three important situations are described in both real and frequency space. In an idealized line spread function (LSF) or delta function, all spatial frequencies are present with equal amplitude (upper images), but in a more realistic LSF there is a loss of signal at the higher spatial frequencies (middle images). Also shown (lower images) is a filter similar to many used in SPECT. Any process that results in a loss of signal at the higher spatial frequencies is said to smooth the signal. A filter that has this effect is described as a smoothing filter, and so back-projection itself can be said to act as a smoothing filter, as does the filter shown in Figure 2.5. The projection/back-projection procedure filters the image by a factor $1/f$ where f is the spatial frequency. Hence the higher the spatial frequency, the more the signal is suppressed and so a smoother image is produced.

This effect is overcome by using a ramp filter in which each spatial frequency is amplified in proportion to the value of that frequency up to a maximum frequency, f_{max}, which is determined by data sampling. This filter will, of course, enhance the higher spatial frequencies, the aim being to restore higher spatial frequencies lost by the back-projection process. There are two problems with using the unmodified ramp filter. The first is that with real data, especially at the count densities encountered in clinical imaging, the higher spatial frequencies will be mainly noise rather than fine spatial detail. This noise is enhanced by the ramp filter producing a poor quality or "noisy" image. Secondly, the sharp cut-off at f_{max} produces "ringing" in the filter in real space; instead of the filter going negative and then tending to zero (Figures 2.4, 2.5) it will oscillate about the axis, going successively negative and positive. This reflects the difficulty of computing a sharp cut-off in frequency space with a finite, preferably fairly small, number of terms. Ringing will produce structured distortion of the reconstructed image.

SINGLE PHOTON EMISSION COMPUTED TOMOGRAPHY (SPECT)

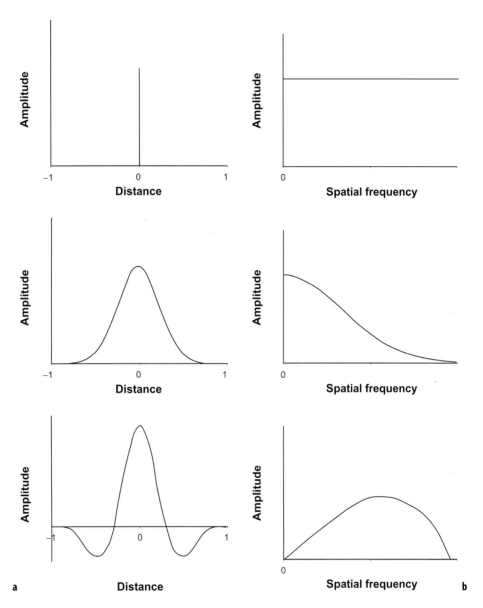

Figure 2.5. An idealized line spread function (top), a realistic line spread function (middle) and a filter typical of those used in SPECT (bottom) are shown in **a** "real" and **b** "frequency" space.

It is usual, therefore, to use a filter that is ramp-shaped at the lower spatial frequencies but rolls off at the higher spatial frequencies. This filter is produced by multiplying the ramp by a second filter, which causes the rolling off at higher spatial frequencies thus suppressing the noise. This technique is known as windowing. There are several possible options for this second filter and all manufacturers include a choice of filter in their SPECT

software. Popular filters include the Butterworth, Hamming, and Shepp-Logan filters. Within each filter a number of options are available to control the amount and type of smoothness that the filter can apply. All SPECT filters require a cut-off value. The high-frequency content of an unfiltered back-projected SPECT image is almost exclusively noise and adds nothing to the quality of the image. The cut-off value is the spatial frequency above which

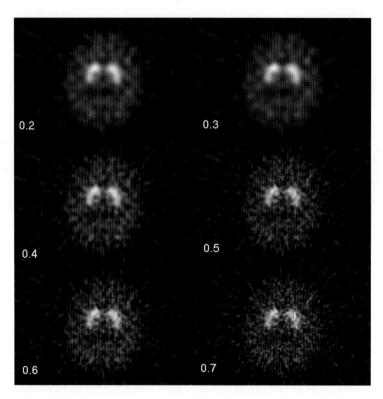

Figure 2.6. Normal ^{123}I-FP-CIT SPECT images reconstructed using a Butterworth filter with cut-off values ranging from 0.2 to 0.7 cycles/cm.

all of the spatial content is removed. Figure 2.6 shows the effect on a normal ^{123}I-FP-CIT SPECT image of using different cut off values in a Butterworth filter. Filters like the Butterworth and Hanning have additional parameters that change the shape of the filter, promoting and suppressing different frequencies within the image. Note that different computing systems express cut-off frequencies in different ways, cycle per cm, cycles per pixel or fractions of the Nyquist frequency, so it is important to be aware that a cut-off of 0.4 on one system may not give the same image on a different system.

The various filters each have their advocates, but it is difficult to predict simply by imaging resolution phantoms which filter will produce the "best" clinical images. In most centers the type of filter and the degree of smoothing incorporated in it will be decided empirically from the clinical images they produce. Usually an optimum filter can be agreed on amongst the users concerned and this will only be altered when the count rates vary either for a particular patient or for

a different study. At one time the Hamming filter was popular despite its fairly high degree of smoothing because the major problem in SPECT was felt to be lack of counts. With the widespread use of multiple-headed gamma cameras this is now less of a problem and a sharper Butterworth filter is the more usual choice. An exception to this is quality assurance (see Section 5.3.4) when the ramp filter itself is used to optimize resolution. This is because higher count rates and longer collection times are possible when imaging test phantoms.

An alternative to introducing smoothing when filtering the profiles is to smooth the original data before carrying out the reconstruction process and then use a less smooth (or sharper) filter on the profiles prior to back-projection. This is known as pre-filtering or pre-smoothing. Several different methods have been proposed but none has really become established clinically. It is now usual is to carry out 2-D filtering of the data after back-projection rather than the 1-D filtering process described in Figure 2.4.

2.2.3 Data Sampling

In any consideration of data sampling both translational and angular sampling must be taken into account. The translational data sampling frequency is determined by the size of the pixels in the image array; for example, if the pixel side length is 5 mm then there are two samples per centimeter and so the sampling frequency is 2 cm^{-1}. Sampling theory states that, if "aliasing" artifacts are to be avoided, only data containing frequencies of less than half this sampling frequency should be transmitted through the system. This upper limit is known as the Nyquist frequency, f_N. The cutoff frequency, f_{max}, of the filters described above is often made equal to f_N, thereby setting any frequencies greater than f_N in the input signal to zero and so ensuring that "aliasing" is avoided. Although a modern gamma camera can record spatial frequencies up to 2 cm^{-1}, in the presence of scattered radiation the upper limit is often less than 1 cm^{-1}. If we set f_N to 1 cm^{-1} the sampling frequency should be at least 2 cm^{-1} and so the image pixels should have a side length of 5 mm. For a 40 cm field-of-view gamma camera this implies that a 128 × 128 matrix should be used for data acquisition rather than a 64 × 64 matrix because in the latter case the pixel size is greater than 6 mm. The use of a 128 × 128 matrix instead of a 64 × 64 matrix for acquisition will, of course, cause the counts per pixel to drop by a factor of 4, thereby increasing noise. There will also be an increase in computing time, although nowadays this should not be a problem.

There is no point in the angular sampling being finer than the translational sampling discussed above, since the characteristics of the overall system, in particular spatial resolution, will be determined by the poorest component. If the number of translational sampling points is N and the number of projections used for reconstruction is M, then

$$M = \frac{\pi}{2} \cdot N. \tag{2.1}$$

This implies that, if data acquisition is on a 64 × 64 matrix, then about 100 projections should be used to reconstruct the data. As was mentioned above, the number of projections used in reconstruction will usually be only half the number acquired since opposite views are averaged. Equation 2.1 therefore implies that, when collecting over 360°, 200 angular increments are required to match a 64 × 64 acquisition. Since there are still situations when only 64 views are acquired it must be asked whether this represents adequate sampling. It has been shown that the magnitude of the residual background artifact becomes acceptable at around 64 views. Since 64 views are only just adequate, 128 views are probably indicated but, as ever, the question is whether any improvement in image quality would be maintained at clinical count rates.

An alternative approach is to use the spatial resolution in the final image to determine what constitutes adequate sampling. The sampling interval should be one-third of the resolution in the final reconstruction image where the resolution is defined as the full width at half maximum (FWHM) of the line spread function (see Section 5.2.1). A translational sampling interval of 6 mm for a 64 × 64 acquisition therefore implies a resolution of 18 mm. This is rather coarse, even when the effects of scattered radiation at distances comparable to the typical radius of rotation are taken into account. This again indicates that finer sampling is required. To apply a similar argument to angular sampling it is necessary to know the distance D of the camera face from the axis of rotation. The arc length for each angular sample is $\pi \cdot D/M$, and this should be around 6 mm to match the translational sampling. Since D cannot be much less than 20 cm, this implies that at least 100 projections should be collected, suggesting once more that 64 views are not sufficient.

The preceding discussion has shown that 128 views on a 128 × 128 matrix are required to optimize image quality. With the current generation of computers there will be no difficulty in handling the increased amount of data but the problem of lack of counts per pixel remains. The time spent collecting data, up to 30 min, is as long as patients can reasonably be expected to remain still, so increasing collecting times to improve counting statistics is not an option. However, most departments are now opting to purchase dual-headed gamma cameras and these can be used to double the counts although sometimes the priority will be to increase throughput. With these devices acquiring 128 views on a 128 × 128 matrix becomes a realistic option. Each clinical situation should be taken on its merits and many centers, particularly those with single-headed gamma cameras, will continue to acquire 64 views on a 64 × 64 matrix. However, 128 views on a 128 × 128 matrix are required for SPECT quality control (see Section 5.3.4) when lack of counts is not a problem. In practice $64 \times 64 \times 64$ is generally used for cardiac SPECT, while $128 \times 128 \times 128$ is used for brain SPECT, reflecting the lower resolution images required in cardiac SPECT.

2.2.4 Attenuation Correction

The preceding discussion has ignored the effect of the attenuation of photons by overlying tissue. If no correction for attenuation is made, superficial structures are emphasized at the expense of deeper structures and there is a general decrease in count density from the edge to the center of the image. There are, however, some situations when it is quite reasonable to use uncorrected images. In the case of myocardial perfusion imaging there is an ongoing debate as to the necessity for attenuation correction, with some centers arguing that it can introduce artifacts so the disadvantages outweigh any benefits. However, in the case of brain SPECT, most would accept that attenuation correction is necessary.

Quantitation of the uptake of radioactivity in an organ raises different problems. SPECT clearly has the potential to provide true quantitation, in units of MBq g^{-1}, and attenuation correction is a necessary prerequisite for this. Considerable effort has gone into developing algorithms for attenuation correction but their value in clinical practice is, as yet, unproven. In practice, most users will restrict themselves to whatever attenuation correction software is supplied, but it is important that the underlying assumptions and limitations are appreciated, especially if some form of quantitation is to be attempted. Also since no attenuation correction method has yet established itself as the method of choice, and many methods require significant additional operator time to draw body outlines, the option of no correction should be seriously considered where SPECT is to be used simply for imaging.

The most easily implemented method of attenuation correction is pre-processing. In this method the attenuation correction is incorporated into the back-projection by multiplying each element in each profile by a factor that will correct it for attenuation. For each element this factor will depend on the thickness L at the appropriate angle of the object being imaged (Figure 2.7). For clinical imaging, this means that the patient's shape must be known. The shape is generally assumed to be elliptical and so the size of the major and minor axes of the appropriate ellipse must be specified prior

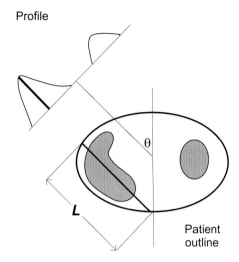

Profile

Figure 2.7. In the pre-processing attenuation correction method the correction factor applied to each element in the profile collected at angle θ will depend on the patient thickness L at the appropriate angle.

to reconstruction. A further assumption is that the radioactivity is uniformly distributed along L and that the attenuation is constant, in other words that a large extended source is being imaged. Finally, the factor will depend on whether opposite projections are averaged with an arithmetic or geometric mean. In the former case, which is more common, the correction factor is

$$\mu L / [1 - \exp(-\mu L)] \qquad (2.2)$$

where μ is the linear attenuation coefficient. The value of μ used must take scatter into account, and is usually determined empirically using a known distribution of radioactivity. For ^{99m}Tc a value of around 0.12 cm^{-1} is often used. Equation 2.2 also assumes that the ellipse is centered on the axis of rotation and so, if this is not the case, the original data must be adjusted accordingly; this adjustment will usually be included in the attenuation correction software. Not surprisingly, given the underlying assumptions, the pre-processing method is rather ineffective when applied to distributions comprising small discrete sources of radioactivity, but gives satisfactory results for large sources, including those found in many clinical situations. This method requires less computing power than any of the alternatives.

Another popular method of attenuation correction is that of Chang [2]. This is a post-processing method in which the transverse section is first reconstructed by filtered back-projection and then corrected pixel by pixel using a correction matrix. This correction matrix is obtained by calculating the attenuation of a point source at each point in the matrix and again requires knowledge of the body outline and the attenuation coefficient. It also assumes narrow beam conditions. Usually a uniform attenuation coefficient is assumed but μ can vary with position within the body. This procedure can be regarded as a first-order correction and is often referred to as "first-order Chang". Being based on the point source response, this method is better than the pre-processing method for small sources, but is less effective for larger sources, which will be over-corrected or under-corrected depending on their position within the image. To compensate for this, a second stage can be included. In this the first-order correction image is re-projected to form a new set of profiles. These are subtracted from the original profiles to form a set of error profiles. Filtered back-projection of this error set produces an error image that must be attenuation corrected as in the first-order Chang. The corrected error image is then added to the first-order image to obtain the final image. This second stage is similar to the step repeated in many of the iterative methods of attenuation correction but in the Chang method the single iteration converges so quickly that further iterations are unnecessary. A useful approach in situations where the assumption that μ is uniform cannot be made, for example in cardiac imaging, is to use information about the distribution of μ. This can be obtained from either CT or transmission images. The latter method, often using gadolinium (^{153}Gd) line sources to produce the transmission image, is available on several multiple-headed gamma cameras and one manufacturer supplies a dual-headed gamma camera with a CT mounted on the same gantry. This latter option is more expensive but has the additional advantage that the CT images can be fused with the SPECT images for reporting.

2.2.5 Iterative Reconstruction

Although filtered back-projection (FBP) remains the reconstruction method most used in routine clinical SPECT, as computing power has increased other options have become available and should be considered. Iterative reconstruction methods, not based on filtered back-projection, such as MLEM (maximum likelihood, expectation maxi-

mization) and particularly its accelerated version OSEM (ordered subsets, expectation maximization), offer potential advantages over FBP because they can model the emission process [3]. The iteration is similar to the process described above for the Chang attenuation correction (Section 2.2.4) and it is possible to include attenuation and other corrections in the iterative process. Iterative reconstruction tends to handle noise better than FBP and will reduce the streak artifacts caused by high count areas. OSEM is now available on most nuclear medicine computers and so is easy to implement, although the user will notice that, unlike FBP, iterative reconstruction does take a little time, typically a minute or two with modern systems. The value of OSEM is probably fairly task dependent, that is better suited to some tasks than to others, and there is no general agreement as to the parameters used, for example the number of iterations or the number of subsets. For these reasons OSEM is still mainly the choice of the specialist rather than the routine SPECT user.

2.2.6 Scatter

At 140 keV most photons will have been scattered rather than absorbed so a true scatter correction would go a long way towards solving the attenuation problem. A number of different approaches have been proposed and tested in recent years [4]. These include dual/multi energy window methods and deconvolution techniques. As yet, there is no agreed method even for planar imaging (see Section 1.3.8). A fundamental problem is that each method is again rather task dependent. However, most vendors now offer a scatter correction technique and these are worth investigating. Scatter correction is probably essential if attenuation correction is planned.

2.2.7 Noise

Noise is, of course, a fundamental problem in nuclear medicine, but it presents a much greater problem with SPECT than in planar imaging. The main reason is that the reconstruction process will itself amplify the noise, but it should also be borne in mind that, even with a 30 min total collection, the counts per pixel in each projection will be lower than in a conventional static image and so the percentage uncertainty per pixel will be greater. It has been shown that the noise amplification factor in tomography can be approximated by

$$\%\text{rms uncertainty per pixel} = N^{-\frac{1}{2}} \cdot n^{\frac{1}{4}} \quad (2.3)$$

where N is the counts per pixel and n is the number of pixels in each projection [5]. The first factor is familiar to anyone who has considered Poisson noise in conventional images, but the second factor shows that the noise increases with the number of pixels. It is clear that the effect of changing data collection from 64 views at 64 × 64 to 128 views at 128 × 128 will be marked. N will drop by a factor of 8 and n will increase by a factor of 4, so the uncertainty will increase by a factor of 4.

When noise is a problem, it can be worth compromising between resolution and sensitivity by choice of collimator as described in the next section. It should also be remembered that the choice of filter will have a significant effect on noise and that in SPECT generally it is always difficult to separate out the many factors affecting the quality of the final image.

2.2.8 Collimation

As in planar imaging it is necessary to strike a balance between resolution and sensitivity with the choice of collimator. Because of the improved contrast in SPECT images it is possible to use a high-resolution collimator without loss in image quality more often than one might expect [6]. An option that increases both sensitivity and resolution is to use a fan-beam collimator (see Section 1.3.3), in which the holes are parallel in the direction of the axis of rotation but converging in the other direction, thereby using the crystal more efficiently [7]. Because of the change in geometry, however, different software is required to reconstruct data collected with these collimators.

2.3 Instrumentation

2.3.1 Rotating Gamma Cameras

Single-headed rotating gamma camera systems have been in use for routine SPECT throughout the world for many years but are increasingly being replaced by dual-headed systems. All gamma camera manufacturers now offer SPECT systems as part of their model range. Although all these systems do basically the same thing, namely move the camera head through 360° around the patient, there are variations in system design. These variations mainly reflect differences in conventional camera design, in particular how the head is moved and supported. Most SPECT systems were originally modifications of the manufacturer's basic models but current models have usually been designed with SPECT in mind.

Dual-headed and even triple-headed rotating camera systems are now commercially available, their attraction being the increase in sensitivity giving the option of improved image quality and/or shorter imaging times. Dual-headed systems have become particularly popular in recent years as they present a cost-effective alternative to a single-headed systems. This is because, although around 50% more expensive in capital costs, they occupy no more space and require no more staff. They, therefore, have the potential to increase patient throughput and/or image quality at little additional revenue cost. Most systems are now "variable angle" in that the heads can be positioned at various angles relative to each other (Figure 2.8), for example positioning the heads at 90° to each other so the benefits of two heads can still be applied to 180° acquisition is popular in myocardial perfusion imaging.

A number of modifications to the standard rotating gamma camera have resulted from the recent emphasis on cerebral SPECT imaging. Ideally the radius of rotation should be as small as possible and values of around 15 cm can be achieved when imaging the brain. One way of reducing this further is to remove the safety pad from the camera face, although a risk assessment should be carried out before doing this; it may be an option for some patient groups but not for others. In practice the limiting factor is often the patient's shoulders, since it is difficult to avoid these while keeping the patient's head in the field of view, and the radius of rotation can be as large as 25 cm. Since the body outline is closer to an ellipse than a circle, a camera rotating on a circular orbit will be further from the patient than necessary most of the time. Many rotating cameras have the option of a non-circular orbit or of following the patient contour; depending on the camera design, an easier option is often to retain the circular motion of the camera but move the couch during the study to minimize the patient–camera distance. Other systems combine head and couch movement during acquisition. Modifications of this type are probably more relevant to body rather than

SINGLE PHOTON EMISSION COMPUTED TOMOGRAPHY (SPECT)

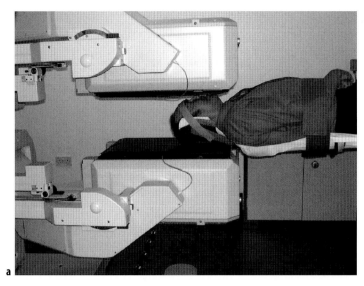

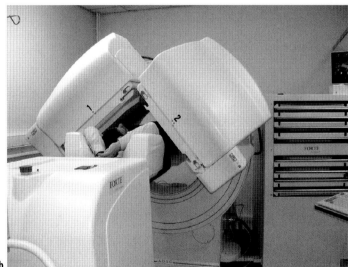

Figure 2.8. Dual-headed gamma cameras with the heads at **a** 180° for brain imaging and **b** 90° for myocardial perfusion imaging.

head imaging, but have been shown to improve resolution.

2.3.2 Single- or Multiple-section Devices

These devices produce either single or multiple transverse sections using one or more rings of focused detectors respectively. In these systems the detectors are usually moved laterally and then rotated to produce the profiles used for back-projection. The advantage of these devices over rotating gamma cameras is improved spatial resolution and increased sensitivity per section. This permits high-quality sections to be obtained in a few minutes, and so dynamic SPECT studies are possible. Most clinical SPECT is, however, carried out on stable distributions of radioactivity, and so this potential advantage has yet to be realized. A weakness of these systems is that the section or sections being imaged have to be selected either from anatomical landmarks or from a rectilinear scan; this can be a problem and often wastes time. Given that the spatial resolution of the latest SPECT cameras is only slightly poorer than the much more expensive single-section devices, these systems seem likely to be restricted to a few specialist centers.

2.4 Quality Issues

The quality control requirements for gamma cameras to be used for SPECT are much more stringent than for planar use. SPECT quality control will be considered in Chapter 5; it is not intended to repeat the detailed advice given there, but rather to consider how image quality can be optimized.

2.4.1 Data Correction

Advances in camera design, in particular linearity and energy corrections and the use of μ-metal shields to screen the photomultiplier tubes from magnetic fields, have improved gamma camera uniformity considerably. As a result the emphasis has changed from data correction to improve SPECT image quality to quality assurance (QA) to maintain SPECT image quality. Despite these improvements, circular artifacts (holes and rings) caused by camera non-uniformity may still be seen on transaxial sections through a uniformity phantom (see Section 5.3.5), although their amplitude should be less than with older cameras. When a correction for a displacement of the center of rotation is available it should always be implemented; the camera should, of course, be set up to minimize any such displacement (see Section 5.3.3). The routine QA on the gamma camera must include the regular acquisition and assessment of a total performance phantom such as the Jaszczak phantom.

2.4.2 The Role of the Operator

The emphasis on the technical aspects of SPECT image quality can obscure the important role of the operator. Good technique in setting up the patient and the camera head is vital. In particular, the radius of rotation, that is the distance between the face of the camera and the patient, must be kept to a minimum. As in planar imaging the closer the camera is to the patient the better the spatial resolution will be. Figure 2.9 shows how the

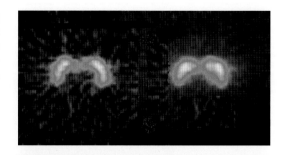

Figure 2.9. The effect of varying the radius of rotation on transaxial images of an FP-CIT brain phantom. On the left the radius of rotation is 135 mm while on the right it is 185 mm.

image quality deteriorates as the radius of rotation increases.

After each SPECT acquisition the operator should check for patient movement. The simplest way to do this is by inspecting a cine loop of the acquired projections. A popular alternative is to display the "sinogram" as the first stage of the reconstruction process. This is a single composite image which is generated by stacking the profiles from the same row, often the middle row, from each of the acquired projection images. This should demonstrate the smooth progress of the camera head around the patient: any discontinuity indicates patient movement. If patient movement has taken place the original projection images can be shifted laterally to reduce its effect. Users should ensure that their nuclear medicine software includes a user-friendly image shifting routine.

2.4.3 The Couch

One aspect of rotating gamma camera systems that receives less attention than it should is the effect of couch and head-rest design on image quality. The convention for transaxial brain imaging in all modalities is to image parallel to the orbito-meatal line; this is impossible without an adjustable head-rest. The data can be realigned post-reconstruction to compensate but substantial realignment will cause additional smoothing of the data. Another problem with couches is their tendency to vibrate because support is at one end only; for cerebral imaging, some centers use an additional couch support. Finally, although a narrow couch is essential for SPECT, patient comfort is also important and it is not obvious that the best compromise has been achieved – an uncomfortable patient is less likely to stay still for 30 minutes. Patient comfort can be increased by using some form of support below the knees.

2.4.4 Limited Angle Acquisition

In cardiac SPECT projections are often only collected over 180°. There is good justification for this when imaging the myocardium with ^{201}Tl. This is because the stress images should be obtained within 30 min of exercise because of redistribution, and so the time is best spent with the camera near the heart, data usually being collected from −60° to +120° relative to the vertical. This argument is particularly strong for ^{201}Tl, whose low-energy gamma rays are readily attenuated as they pass through tissue. This is not a significant effect when the detector is near the heart but most of the gamma rays recorded in images collected over the other 180° will have been scattered and so these data would detract from the quality of the reconstructed data. However, 180° acquisition is also preferred for cardiac SPECT with ^{99m}Tc agents, even though the energy is higher, and there is some experimental evidence to support this approach [8]. In SPECT contrast is improved with 180° acquisition but there is some distortion of the reconstructed data; it is a matter of judgment as to the best compromise. An extension of this approach for centers with dual-headed, variable geometry gamma cameras is to carry out a 90° acquisition with the detector heads at 90° degrees to each other, thereby giving 180° acquisition. Similarly some workers have successfully used 180° acquisition when carrying out SPECT of the lumbar spine.

2.5 Conclusion

Having considered the implications of the operator choices listed in Table 2.1, new users should now be able to make the required decisions on an informed basis. Although the requirements of SPECT, in both a technical and procedural sense, are more demanding than for planar nuclear medicine, they are not as formidable as they might seem, especially for those with modern equipment.

References

1. Brigham OD. The Fast Fourier Transform. Englewood Cliffs: Prentice Hall; 1988.
2. Chang LT. A method for attenuation correction in radionuclide computed tomography. IEEE Trans Nucl Sci NS 1978; 25:638–643.
3. Hutton BF, Hudson HM, Beekman FJ. A clinical perspective of accelerated statistical reconstruction. Eur J Nucl Med 1997; 24:797–808.
4. Rosenthal MS, Cullom J, Hawkins W, et al. Quantitative SPECT imaging: A review and recommendations by the Focus Committee of the Society of Nuclear Medicine Computer and Instrumentation Council. J Nucl Med 1995; 36:1489–1513.
5. Budinger TF, Derenzo SE, Greenberg WL, Gullberg GT, Huesman RH. Quantitative potentials of dynamic emission computed tomography. J Nucl Med 1978; 19:309–315.
6. Muehllehner G. Effect of resolution improvement on required count density in ECT imaging: a computer solution. Phys Med Biol 1985; 30:163–173.
7. Jaszczak RJ, Chang LT, Murphy PH. Single photon emission computed tomography using multi-slice fan beam collimators. IEEE Trans Nucl Sci NS 1979; 26:610–618.
8. Maublant JC, Peycelon P, Kwiatkowski F, et al. Comparison between 180° and 360° data collection in technetium-99m MIBI SPECT of the myocardium. J Nucl Med 1989; 30:295–300.

3

Positron Emission Tomography

Peter F. Sharp and Andy Welch

3.1 Introduction

While the advantages of PET imaging over conventional single photon nuclear medicine imaging are widely acknowledged (Table 3.1), until recently the high cost of the equipment and operating expenses had limited it to relatively few centers. With a clearer appreciation of the clinical value of PET ([1] and Chapter 17) and reimbursement by agencies such as Medicare in the USA, PET is now to be found widely in many countries, although its acceptance by the NHS in the UK has been slower. This chapter will concentrate on the technology behind PET. The clinical applications will be discussed in detail in Chapter 17.

While the cost of a dedicated imager is now within reach of many of the larger nuclear medicine departments, the problem of producing radiopharmaceuticals still remains. The introduction of commercial production centers provides a partial answer to this problem allowing the longer-lived positron emitters, mainly 2-[^{18}F] fluoro-2-deoxyglucose (^{18}FDG), to be made available to a wide range of users.

3.2 Principles of PET Imaging

PET imaging is not a new concept; it was first proposed in the early 1950s and the first imaging devices were developed by Brownell and by Anger in the 1950s. The main reason for the interest in PET is to be found in the nature of the positron decay process. Positrons are positively charged electrons emitted from nuclei that have an excess of protons. As the positron encounters negatively charged electrons it quite quickly loses the energy that it is carrying. Eventually, when nearly all the energy has been lost, it will combine with an electron, forming a positronium. The positronium will quickly annihilate forming two 511 keV gamma rays that travel in diametrically opposite directions. By surrounding the patient with a detector system, the simultaneous arrival of these two gamma rays can be recorded. The origin of the emission can then be assumed to lie along the line joining the two points at which the gamma rays hit the detector. This line is known as the line of response (LOR). The total number of coincident events acquired by a pair of detectors is related to the integral of the activity along the LOR that joins the two detectors. By measuring the integral of the activity along sets of LORs we can acquire projection data that can be reconstructed to produce an image of the distribution of positron emitter within the object (Figure 3.1a). Note that there is no need to use collimation. A typical PET imager and image are shown in Figure 3.2.

While the simplicity of the imaging process is attractive, the need to record the simultaneous arrival of photons while excluding random coincidences poses a challenge for the designers of the PET imager. Before discussing this difficulty and the resulting effect on the performance of the imager, one must consider two other fundamental limitations to the ability to locate the origin of the decay. By detecting the origin of the emission of the gammas, one is identifying the location of

Table 3.1. Advantages and disadvantages of PET imaging

Advantages	Disadvantages
Does not require a lead collimator	Many radionuclides require to be produced on site from a cyclotron
Uses biologically interesting radionuclides, such as ^{11}C, ^{15}O, ^{13}N	Cost of cyclotron, imager and radiochemistry facility high
Can accurately measure the amount of radiopharmaceutical present in a region of the body	
Spatial resolution of about 5 mm	

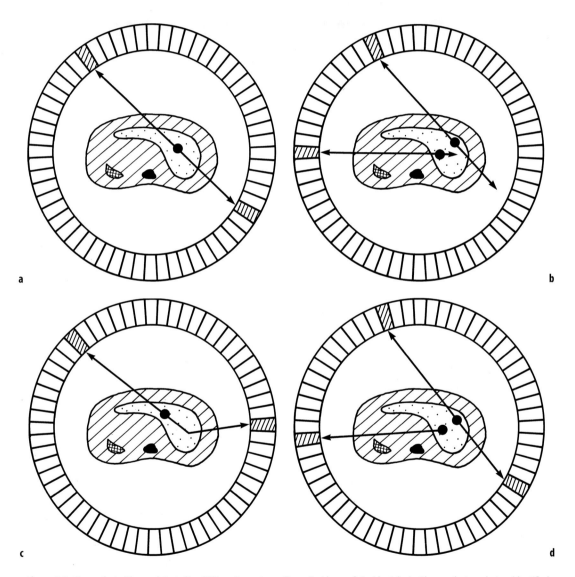

Figure 3.1. Types of coincidences detected in a PET imaging system. **a** True coincidences. **b** Accidental coincidences, the two photons identified as arriving in coincidence have originated from different disintegrations. **c** Scatter, one of the photons has undergone Compton scattering prior to being detected. **d** Multiple coincidences. More than two photons arrive in coincidence. Apart from the true coincidences, all others will result in incorrect spatial information.

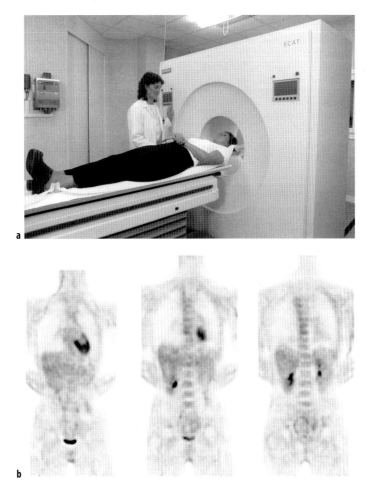

Figure 3.2. **a** Typical PET imager. **b** FDG image.

the positronium; depending upon its energy, the positron will travel a few millimeters through tissue before decaying. Secondly, if the positron still has some energy when it annihilates then conservation of momentum will mean that the angle between the two gammas will not be exactly 180°, indeed the error can be up to ±6°. The combined effect of these two factors is to limit the potential resolution of a PET system to between 1.5 and 3 mm, still considerably better than that achieved with a single photon system.

3.3 The PET Imager

In the conventional gamma camera single photon imaging quality is mainly restricted by the need to employ collimation; in the PET imager the major problem is to achieve the good temporal resolution to facilitate coincidence detection at the high data rates that are encountered.

3.3.1 The Detector

The main limiting factor for PET imager performance is that of the crystal. Table 3.2 summarizes the features required of a good detector material while Table 3.3 shows the properties of the main types of crystals that have been used for PET. Sodium iodide with thallium doping NaI(Tl), the crystal used in the gamma camera, has the best light output but the worst stopping efficiency. Bismuth germanate (BGO) was, until recently, the material used in most PET imagers. It has a

Table 3.2. Requirements for PET detector material

Good stopping power for 511 keV gammas, i.e. high density
Quick reaction time, i.e. short fluorescence decay time
Good energy resolution, i.e. high number of light photons per MeV energy stopped
Low Compton scatter inside detector crystal
Matching of wavelength of fluorescence to response of light detector

Table 3.3. Principal detector materials that have been used in PET

Scintillator	Chemical name	Density (g/cm³)	λmax (nm)	Photons/ MeV	Decay time (ns)
Sodium iodide	NaI(Tl)	3.67	415	38 000	230
Bismuth germanate	$Bi_4Ge_3O_{12}$ (BGO)	7.13	480	8 200	300
Barium fluoride	BaF_2	4.89	195, 220	1 800	0.8
Gadolinium orthosilicate	Gd_2SiO_5(Ce) (GSO)	6.70	430	10 000	30–60
Lutetium orthosilicate	Lu_2SiO_5(Ce) (LSO)	7.4	420	30 000	40

high density but has the lowest light output and the longest decay time. Barium fluoride (BaF_2) is the fastest but has very low density and efficiency. The latest generation of imagers use lutetium orthosilicate (LSO) or gadolinium orthosilicate (GSO) which have a shorter decay time and higher light output than BGO.

Most dedicated PET systems employ an array of block detectors, each block viewed by a number of photomultiplier tubes (PMTs) to improve spatial resolution. A typical block detector (Figure 3.3) consists of a single detector crystal divided into an array of between 8×8 and 13×13 distinct crystal elements, each element having a side length between 6.4 and 4 mm. The crystal element in which the scintillation is located is determined from the amount of light received at each of four PMTs. Each block is grouped into a cassette, or bucket, containing a number of blocks (Figure 3.3b), and the buckets are then arranged in a ring around the patient (Figure 3.3c). The number of detector rings used varies; typically a three-ring system would be between 24 and 39 detectors deep, producing between 47 and 81 slices. Typically the axial field of view is between 15 and 18 cm.

3.3.2 Electronics

The calculation of the location of the positron depends upon accurately determining the coincident arrival of the pair of photons. Although the term "coincident" is used, in fact there will be a small time difference for all emissions that do not originate at the center of the system. For a torso the difference is of the order of 2 nanoseconds.

Because of the response time of the detector material a time window, the so-called prompt channel, is used such that any photons arriving within that window are judged to be coincident. For systems using BGO this window is typically 12 nanoseconds, while for the faster LSO it is 5 nanoseconds.

In addition to a true coincidence, the image may be degraded by artifactual coincidences. These can be classified as three types (Figure 3.1b, c, d):

- *accidentals or randoms*, the two photons identified as arriving in coincidence have, in fact, originated from different disintegrations,
- *scatter*, one of the photons has undergone Compton scattering prior to being detected,
- *multiple coincidences*, more than two photons arrive in coincidence.

Apart from the true coincidences, all others will result in incorrect spatial information. Thus the coincidence system must be designed to keep processing time to a minimum and to reduce the effect of false coincidences.

The recorded count rate will be a combination of true coincidences, randoms and scatter. A delayed time window is used to estimate the random events. These randoms are then subtracted from the events in the prompt channel, leaving trues and scatter. A lower level energy discriminator (LLD), usually between 300 and 435 keV depending on the detector material, is used to reduce the number of scatter coincidences and also random coincidences since the latter result from photons with a range of energies. Unfortunately, increasing the

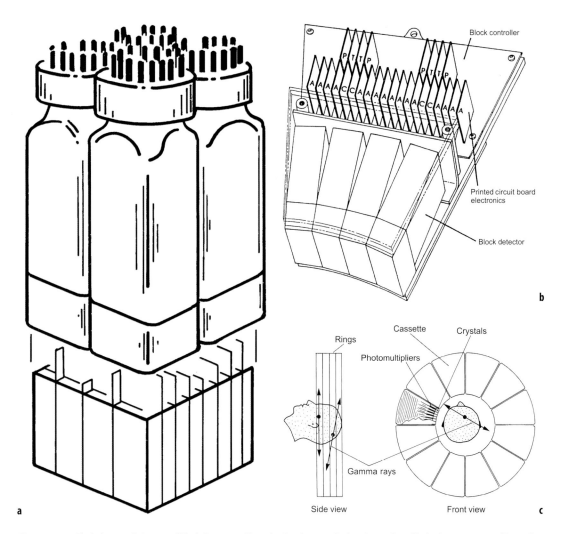

Figure 3.3. a Block detector. **b** A group of blocks is arranged into a bucket detector sharing electronics. **c** The buckets are arranged into a ring of detectors around the patient.

LLD also reduces the number of true coincidences by removing those in which the 511 keV photons undergo Compton scatter in the detector crystal.

The number of unwanted coincidences may also be reduced by electronically limiting the number of pairs of detectors in a ring which can detect photons in coincidence and the number of detector rings. Lead or tungsten disks, known as septa, may be inserted between detector planes so reducing in-plane and out-of-plane scatter (Figure 3.4a). The outer septa are thicker than those between planes to remove extraneous singles and scatter photons from outside the imaged area and the room. This form of imaging is referred to as two-dimensional (2-D) imaging. With detector crystals showing better energy resolution some cameras now do without the septa, which increases sensitivity by a factor of about 6 (Figure 3.4b). As these data are acquired as a volume rather than a series of slices, this form of imaging is called 3-D and is discussed further in Section 3.3.4.

3.3.3 Correction

Attenuation Correction

One of the strengths of PET is its ability to accurately quantify the amount of radioactivity in

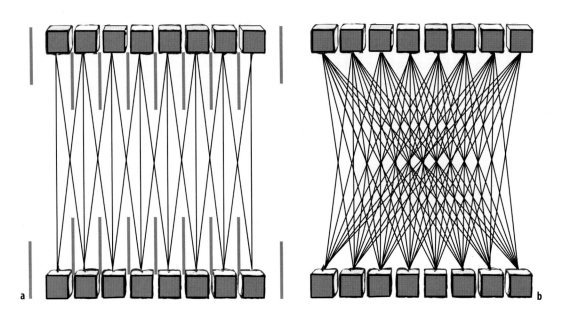

Figure 3.4. a 2-D imaging. **b** 3-D imaging without lead septa between rings of detectors.

an organ or region of interest. Consider a source located at a distance x from one detector and let the total thickness of material through which both photons pass be D. Then, since we are dealing with a pair of photons traveling in opposite directions, the number of pairs of photons detected, N, will be related to the number emitted, N_0, by the relationship

$$N = N_0 \, e^{-\mu x} \times e^{-\mu(D-x)}$$
$$= N_0 \, e^{-\mu D}. \tag{3.1}$$

So N depends upon the effective attenuation coefficient of the material, μ, through which it passes and on the total thickness of tissue through which the two photons traveled, but not on the location of the source in the body.

Attenuation is corrected by the acquisition of a "blank scan" before the patient is placed in the detector and a "transmission scan" when the patient is in position. This can be performed using an external positron source, usually ^{68}Ge which has a half-life of 275 days, or by taking an X-ray CT scan. The positron source is either in the form of a ring or rods; in the latter case the rods rotate around the patient with the position of the rods being correlated with the detectors receiving coincidences. For each LOR the attenuation is measured. The process takes about 5 minutes.

Many modern cameras incorporate a CT scanner and the transmission information is derived from the CT image [2]. This significantly reduces the time needed to correct the attenuation image data from 5 to 15 minutes for each bed position, to about one minute for a 100 cm axial view. Thus, combined with the more sensitive LSO detector, the total time for a typical body scan has been halved. As the CT scan is acquired at a lower photon energy than the PET, typically 70 keV compared with 511 keV, the CT correction factors require scaling before they can be used. The value of the scaling factor depends on the elemental composition of the tissue; in practice the factor varies little between tissues but is significantly different for bone. In current PET/CT scanners only two scaling factors are used, a threshold being used to distinguish between bone and non-bone material.

A further problem arises when iodinated contrast media is used. Contrast enhanced areas of the image may have their attenuation factors incorrectly scaled, so leading to artifacts. In practice it would appear that intravenous contrast has little effect but oral contrast does.

In addition the PET/CT scanner provides an anatomical image which can easily be superimposed on the functional PET image; see Chapter 17.

Normalization/Uniformity Correction

There are a three main non-uniformities inherent in a PET scanner that have to be corrected. These arise from the geometry of the detector arrays or response variations between detectors.

Firstly, it is inevitable that in a system containing thousands of crystals their response will vary. Intrinsic crystal efficiency can be measured using a uniform phantom, rod sources or plane source.

Secondly, a correction has to be made for geometric profile or arc correction. In order to build up the sinogram, data from a radial array of detectors is projected onto a linear data set. At the center of the flat array the effective width of the detectors increases and the effective detector density decreases. The effect is to reduce the count rate towards the center of each projection.

The final normalization correction is crystal interference. This again is due to the geometric problems of mapping radial data acquired from a ring of detectors, onto a square image array. Photons obliquely incident on a crystal not only have a lower probability of being stopped by the crystal but may also interact with an adjacent crystal. The combined effect of these two factors is measured during the normalization process after the crystal efficiency and the geometric arc correction have been performed.

Scatter Correction

Scattered coincidence events occur when one of the photons released from a positron-electron annihilation is deflected due to Compton scattering. The lower level energy discriminator imposed on the detector will help reduce the effect of scatter. However, problems still exist, particularly when imaging in the 3-D mode. A number of techniques have been developed to correct for this problem including:

- Using septa between image planes.
- Multiple energy windows in which a second lower energy window is used. It is then assumed that the number of scattered events measured in the lower energy window is proportional to those measured in the upper one.
- Fitting a curve to data outside the object. It is assumed that the object being imaged can be identified and confined to a region on the sinogram. Signals arising from outside this region are assumed to be scatter

and a curve is fitted to the scatter distribution based on the regions that contain only scattered events.

- Convolution methods. A point source is used to measure the scatter function, which is then convolved with the image to give the scatter distribution. The distribution is scaled and subtracted from the image.
- Calculation/simulation. A calculation or Monte Carlo simulation is used to model the scatter using the emission and attenuation image as the input data.

Randoms Correction

As mentioned in Section 3.3.2, random coincidence events occur when two photons arising from different positron decays hit the detector ring within the timing window. If a second coincidence window with a delayed input is used, then this will measure only random events because of the delay introduced to one input. If many events are recorded then statistically the number of randoms recorded by the delayed coincidence window will be the same as those recorded in the normal coincidence window. Random correction is made by subtracting the counts measured in the delayed window from those measured by the trues window.

3.3.4 Reconstruction

2-D Reconstruction

In this imaging mode data are acquired with the interplane septa in place. For each coincidence pair there is a line of response (LOR) joining the two detectors. Each LOR is identified by the angle it makes with the scanner axis and the offset distance from the axis. This data is stored in a sinogram, a 2-D data array in which each location represents the number of LORs with a particular offset (array column position) and angle (row position). Before reconstruction the sinogram data are corrected for detector non-uniformity and for attenuation; corrections are also made for random coincidences, count rate response (see Section 5.2.1) and scatter (see Section 3.3.3).

Nearly all of the methods currently in use for image reconstruction fall into one of two classes: analytic and iterative. The former method treats the object and projection data as continuous variables, which are linked via their Fourier transforms and include the filtered back-projection technique, which is the most widely used reconstruction algorithm (see Section 2.2). The main advantage of filtered back-projection is that it is fast. However, it suffers from two main drawbacks. Firstly, it amplifies high frequencies, which can result in very noisy images. In practice the noise properties of the algorithm can be improved by modifying the filter with a window function that is "rolled-off" at high frequencies, but this affects spatial resolution. Secondly, the algorithm can only be applied to a particular geometry, i.e. one in which the projection data are line integrals along sets of parallel lines.

Iterative algorithms start from the assumption that both the object and the measured data are discrete and that the data are a linear sum of the object elements with weighting factors being used to represent the probability that an event emitted at one location is detected at another. This representation is inherently flexible in that it can be used to represent any geometry and the weights can be modified to incorporate physical effects such as attenuation, scatter, and geometric response. The aim is to find the object that best fits the measured data assuming some model for the imaging system (i.e. a set of weights). The definition of "best fit" can include some knowledge of the statistical properties of the data leading to a class of algorithms known as maximum likelihood techniques, which include the popular expectation maximization, maximum likelihood (EM-ML) method. Iterative methods such as the EM-ML algorithm have much better noise properties than the filtered back-projection method and are, therefore, becoming more popular. However, they are inherently slower. In order to reconstruct an image the data must be projected and back-projected at least once (and usually more than once). With the filtered back-projection algorithm the data are only back-projected once. Since projection and back-projection take a similar amount of time the iterative algorithms take at least twice as long as the filtered back-projection method to produce an image and usually an order of magnitude longer. However, as computational speed has increased, these issues have become less important and the algorithms have gained acceptance for clinical use.

3-D Reconstruction

In 3-D PET imaging the projection data contain information from multiple transaxial slices so 3-D algorithms are required. As described above, the iterative algorithms are inherently flexible and can easily be extended to deal with 3-D data. However, 3-D projection and back-projection operations are much slower than 2-D ones.

The analytic algorithms can be extended to three dimensions. Since sensitivity and both axial and transaxial resolution are not spatially invariant, simple back-projection from the sinogram data is not accurate. If a complete set of 2-D data is also acquired (as is the case with dedicated PET imagers) then a 3-D dataset can be produced by first reconstructing the 2-D data and then projecting through this image to fill in the missing 3-D data. However, this technique requires at least one 3-D projection and back-projection operation so in practice it may not be significantly faster than the iterative methods, which also have the advantage of better noise properties.

An alternative to a full 3-D reconstruction is to rebin the 3-D data into a 2-D dataset. This approach is popular in PET where an exact method based on the 2-D Fourier transform of the projection data has been developed.

3.4 Performance of PET Imagers

Clearly, there are many similarities between those measurements required for SPECT imagers (see Section 5.3) and for PET systems. The principal differences are to be found in the effect of accidental coincidences and attenuation correction. A set of performance tests has been proposed by the International Electrotechnical Commission (IEC) in Europe [3] and, more recently, by a joint group of the Society of Nuclear Medicine and the National Electrical Manufacturers Association (SNM/NEMA) in the USA [4]. Unfortunately there are differences between the two standards. The SNM/NEMA standards are described in outline below. Typical values for the performance parameters are taken from references [5] and [6].

With the exception of the spatial resolution measurements, most performance parameters can be measured using a phantom. The intention is to use a phantom that approximates to the conditions under which PET imaging is carried out. In recent years there has been a concentration on whole body imaging and the consequent development of imagers with larger fields of views. So in its latest standard NEMA have proposed using a phantom 70 cm in length consisting of a solid polyethylene cylinder of outside diameter 20 cm. Activity is placed in a line source running parallel to the central axis at a radius of 4.5 cm.

In addition, an image quality test has been introduced using an IEC body phantom containing simulated lesions.

3.4.1 Spatial Resolution

Measurements are made with a point source, whose dimensions are less than 1 mm in any direction, containing ^{18}F and the data are reconstructed with a ramp filter. Measurements are taken of the full width at half maximum (FWHM) and full width at tenth maximum (FWTM) of the point spread function (see Section 5.2.1), in the transverse slice in two directions radially and tangentially, and in the axial direction.

In the axial direction two slices are selected, one at the center of the axial field of view and one at $^1/_4$ of the axial field of view. In each axial slice the source is positioned at (i) 1 cm vertically from the center, (ii) 10 cm vertically from the center and (iii) 10 cm horizontally from the center. Radial and tangential resolution are averaged over all slices to give the transverse resolution.

Typically values for the transaxial resolution are 6.3 mm at 1 cm and 6.9 mm at 10 cm, and for the axial resolution 4.5 mm at 1 cm and 6.1 mm at 10 cm in 2-D mode. Similar results are found in the 3-D mode.

3.4.2 Scatter Fraction

This is a measure of the sensitivity of the system to scattered radiation. If measurements are made at low count rates so that random coincidences are negligible, then:

Scatter fraction, SF
    = scattered events/total events.   (3.2)

Data are acquired with a phantom consisting of a 20 cm diameter solid polyethylene phantom, 70 cm long. A line source, approximately 2.3 mm internal diameter, running parallel to the axis of the cylinder at a radius of 4.5 cm, is filled with ^{18}F. The phantom is positioned so that the line source is closest to the surface of the imager couch.

The sinogram profile (see Section 3.3.4) is then used to calculate the number of scatter events. The true counts are assumed to be those within ±2 cm

of the peak; the pedestal on which the profile of true counts stands is then defined as the scatter counts. Measurements of counts are made assuming a field of view of 24 cm. The sinogram profile is analyzed as a function of angle and the results averaged. The scatter fraction for each slice and the average of the slice scatter fractions are recorded. Typically SF is 10% in the 2-D mode and 45% in the 3-D.

While this is a useful measure for comparing scanners, the value will depend greatly on the body organ being imaged, increasing with the size of the body section.

3.4.3 Sensitivity

In the past sensitivity has been measured by recording the count rate from a known amount of activity in a cylindrical phantom. With the larger field of view of some PET imagers, particularly gamma cameras, it is no longer practicable to use a large phantom. In the NEMA standard measurements are made with a 70 cm long line source. In order to provide material in which the positrons can annihilate, the source is surrounded by a metal shield. However, as this material will also attenuate the gamma rays it is necessary to compensate for this. By plotting a curve showing how the count rate, R(x), varied with sleeve thickness, x, the effective attenuation coefficient, μ, and the count rate in the absence of attenuation, R(0), can be calculated by fitting the simple formula

$$R(x) = R(0)\, e^{-2.\mu.x}. \qquad (3.3)$$

The total sensitivity is then calculated from the ratio of R(0) to the activity. The sensitivity for a particular slice is calculated as the ratio of total sensitivity to the fraction of total counts contained in that slice when the thinnest sleeve is used.

Sensitivity is measured both with the line source at the center of the field of view and 10 cm radially from the center. Typical values are 2 cps/kBq for the 2-D mode and 9 cps/kBq in 3-D mode.

3.4.4 Count Rate Losses

The line source in the 70 cm cylinder is filled with a high level of activity, sufficient that the peak trues rate and peak noise equivalent count (NEC) can be measured. The line source is positioned as in Section 3.4.1. Measurements are made of the total count rate within a 24 cm field of view as the radioactivity decays and continued until the randoms and dead-time are negligible.

The randoms and scatter background is calculated as in Section 3.4.1. The true rate, R_{true}, is calculated by simply subtracting the randoms plus scatter background from the total rate, R_{total}. The separate random and scatter rate are then calculated from:

$$R_{random} = R_{total} - \frac{R_{true}}{1 - SF} \qquad (3.4)$$

$$R_{scatter} = R_{true} \frac{SF}{1 - SF} \qquad (3.5)$$

where SF is the scatter fraction.

The NEC is a global measure of the scanner count rate which defines an effective true count rate by accounting for the additional noise from the scatter and random coincidences.

$$NEC = \frac{R_{true}^2}{R_{total}}. \qquad (3.6)$$

The square root of the NEC is proportional to the signal-to-noise ratio in the image.

Count rate performance can be expressed by plotting the total, true and randoms, scatter and NEC rates against the effective activity concentration, i.e. total activity in the line divided by the total volume of the phantom.

Typical peak true counting rate is 270 kcps at 114 kBq/cm^3 in 2-D mode and 292 kcps at 20 kBq/cm^3 and peak NEC rates are 81 kcps at 64 kBq/cc in 2-D and 66 kcps at 15 kBq/cm^3 in 3-D.

3.4.5 Accuracy of Corrections

The accuracy of corrections for dead-time losses and randoms is assessed from the count rate performance measurements (Section 3.4.4). The data are reconstructed with the corrections applied. An 18 cm diameter ROI is defined and the residual error, ΔR, as a function of activity concentration is given by

$$\Delta R = \frac{R_{true}}{R_{extrap}} - 1 \qquad (3.7)$$

where R_{extrap} is determined by linearly extrapolating from the low count rate data where losses are negligible. The largest and smallest errors for all slices are plotted as a function of effective activity concentration. Typical values for maximum loss are 7% (2-D) and 2% (3-D).

3.4.6 Image Quality Measurement

This test is designed to study how all aspects of scanner performance interact to give the overall image quality. A modified IEC body phantom containing hot and cold spheres is used to mimic an FDG tumor study. A 5 cm insert having an attenuation coefficient approximately equal to that of lung tissue is placed in the center of the phantom.

The background is filled with ^{18}F at a concentration of 5.3 MBq/ml, typical of that seen in a patient. The hot spheres are filled with a concentration of 8 times that of the background and the measurements repeated with a concentration of 4 times the background. The 70 cm phantom used previously is placed adjacent to the torso to give the situation of activity outside the field of view of the scanner. The line source is filled with activity at an effective concentration equal to that in the torso.

Data are acquired as if scanning an axial distance of 100 cm in 60 min. The acquisition time per slice must include emission and transmission time.

After reconstruction using the normal corrections and reconstruction algorithms, image quality is quantified by drawing ROIs around the spheres and throughout the background. Twelve background ROIs are drawn in the central slice, as well as slices 1 and 2 cm away, giving 60 in total. Background variability is measured from the coefficient of variation of these background ROIs as a function of size. The hot and cold sphere recovery coefficients, CRC_{hot} and CRC_{cold}, respectively, are given by:

$$CRC_{hot} = \frac{(C_{hot}/C_{cold} - 1)}{(A_{hot}/A_{bkgd} - 1)} \qquad (3.8)$$

$$CRC_{cold} = 1 - (C_{cold}/C_{bkgd}) \qquad (3.9)$$

where A_{hot}/A_{bkgd} is the ratio of activity in the hot sphere and background. Typical values are 20% CRC_{hot} for a 10 cm diameter sphere and 69% for a 22 cm one.

The accuracy of attenuation and scatter corrections are measured by drawing an ROI over the lung insert. The error for each slice, ΔC, is given by:

$$\Delta C = C_{lung}/C_{bkgd} \qquad (3.10)$$

where C_{lung} is the average of the counts over the lung insert. Typical values are 24% (2-D) and 17% (3-D).

3.5 The Gamma Camera for PET Imaging

The strengths and weaknesses of NaI(Tl) for the detection of 511 keV photons have been described in Section 3.3.1. With the widespread use of dual-headed gamma cameras for routine nuclear medicine imaging, their development into PET imaging systems becomes technically attractive. PET imaging can be carried out either by employing collimators designed for use at 511 keV or, more commonly, by coincidence detection utilizing dual-headed detectors without collimators.

The collimated system is conventional SPECT imaging and does not, for example, give the advantage of quantitative accuracy found in coincidence PET imaging. Also, in practice the collimated system has been shown to offer both poor spatial resolution, approximately 15 mm FWHM in the reconstructed image for ^{18}F, and low sensitivity, of the order of a factor of 15 lower than conventional PET imagers operating in the 2-D mode. As a result, coincidence detection gamma camera systems are now the standard.

There are two issues to be considered if the gamma camera is to be used for PET imaging. Firstly, the gamma camera employs NaI(Tl) detectors, which have a lower density and hence stopping power than BGO or LSO. There is a limit on increasing crystal thickness to compensate for this as it would compromise resolution and linearity (see Table 1.6). Typically a camera designed to do PET would have a crystal thickness of between 15 and 25 mm. Although the high light output of NaI(Tl) gives it an excellent energy resolution, about 9%, the use of an energy window to reduce scatter reduces the detection efficiency to about 10%.

The second significant difference is that the gamma camera uses an area detector rather than individual crystal localization, although some manufacturers have used a segmented crystal design. This means that the camera operates in 3-D mode and so is very sensitive to scatter coincidences from radiation emitted outside the field of view of the detectors. This is more of a problem with body imaging than brain imaging. The mechanism of localization of the scintillation in an area detector also means that the maximum count rate is restricted, bearing in mind that the camera will also be processing a high singles rate.

3.6 Production of Radiopharmaceuticals

3.6.1 Production of Radionuclides

The Cyclotron

Cyclotrons have been designed specifically for use in PET imaging. By tailoring the cyclotron design to meet the specific requirements for the production of the most common positron emitting radionuclides, it has been possible to build machines that are simple to operate in the hospital environment. Such, so called, baby cyclotrons are now very compact, the typical room size being 7 m by 7 m, and can be self-shielding, so minimizing the amount of extra radiation shielding needed in the cyclotron room. An example of a medical cyclotron is shown in Figure 3.5.

The mode of action of the cyclotron is to be found in many texts and will not be described in detail here. Charged particles are repeatedly accelerated through intermediate voltages to achieve high energy. Particle acceleration takes place inside hollow metal cavities known as Dees; medical cyclotrons use either two or four such Dees. An RF electric field across the gap between the Dees, operating at typically 72 MHz, ensures that the particle encounters an accelerating force each time it crosses the gap. The Dees are located in a magnetic field, of about 1.2 T, generated by an electromagnet which ensures that the particle moves in a circular orbit. The maximum orbit diameter is about 1 m.

Most medical cyclotrons now use negative ions created by the ionization of a gas, usually hydrogen or deuterium, in the center of the Dees. Earlier generations of cyclotrons accelerated positive particles but this had the disadvantage that should part of the beam hit any component of the cyclotron then it could be made radioactive.

After the particles have been accelerated to their final energy they pass through thin carbon stripper foils, which remove two electrons so giving a positively charged particle beam, a few millimeters in diameter, which will be deflected by the magnetic field out the chamber and onto the target. Typically the maximum particle energy will be 11 MeV for H$^+$ and 5 MeV for D$^+$ with beam currents of about 40 μA.

Self-shielded cyclotrons are surrounded by their own radiation shields, so removing the need for

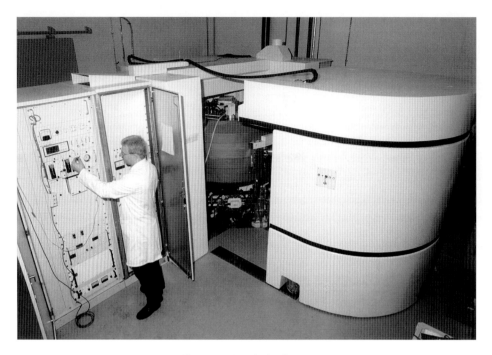

Figure 3.5. A medical cyclotron.

a heavy shielded cyclotron vault. The inner layer of the shield is made out of a mixture of lead and boron. This reduces the energy of the 1–2 MeV neutrons, absorbs most of the prompt gamma radiation from the target reactions, and the thermalized neutrons. A 70 cm thick outer shield of polyethylene and boron carbide loaded concrete moderates neutrons, through collisions with the water and polyethylene, which are eventually absorbed by the boron.

Target Irradiation

The particle beam is deflected onto a target where it interacts with the target material to produce an altered nucleus which is unstable. The main considerations of target design are:

1. That the target volume should be as small as possible to ensure a high specific activity of the radionuclide, but sufficiently large to utilize a large proportion of particles in the beam.
2. The target material should be of sufficient purity that radioactive by-products are not produced by irradiation of the impurities.

3. Significant quantities of heat must be dissipated or there will be a danger of the target rupturing and releasing the radioactive material.
4. There needs to be a mechanism for the automatic extraction of the radionuclide to the radiochemistry laboratory for labeling.
5. Some typical reactions and yields are shown in Table 3.4. The gaseous or liquid targets are pressurized, which allows the products of the irradiation to be transferred by pressure through shielded small bore tubing to the radiochemistry laboratory.

3.6.2 Production of Radiopharmaceuticals

One of the main attractions of PET imaging is the wide variety of radiopharmaceuticals that can be produced. Some of the commonly used ones are listed in Table 3.5. Automated production modules are offered by cyclotron manufacturers for the production of the most commonly used radiopharmaceuticals, such as $H_2{}^{15}O$, $C^{15}O_2$, and

POSITRON EMISSION TOMOGRAPHY

Table 3.4. Typical reactions and yields from a medical cyclotron

Target material	Reaction	Product	Irradiation time	Yield
5 mmol ethanol in H_2O	$^{16}O\,(p,\alpha)\,^{13}N$	Aqueous ammonium ion	10 min	4 GBq
^{18}O enriched water	$^{18}O\,(p,n)\,^{18}F$	Aqueous fluoride ion	60 min	40 GBq
N_2 + trace O_2	$^{14}N\,(p,\alpha)\,^{11}C$	Carbon dioxide gas	50 min	56 GBq
^{15}N enriched N_2 + 1–5% O_2	$^{15}N\,(p,n)\,^{15}O$	Oxygen gas	10 min	74 GBq

Table 3.5. Some commonly used PET radiopharmaceuticals

Radiopharmaceutical	Process	Clinical studies
^{18}FDG	Glucose metabolism	Cerebral glucose utilization
		Myocardial glucose metabolism
		Tumor detection and assessment of cell metabolism
$^{13}NH_3$	Perfusion	Myocardial muscle perfusion
$^{15}O_2$	Oxygen metabolism	Cerebral oxygen metabolism
^{11}C methionine	Amino acid uptake and protein	Study of protein synthesis in tumors
^{11}C thymidine	synthesis	
H_2O_{15}	Blood flow	Brain activation. Organ blood flow
$C^{15}O$	Blood volume	Cerebral blood volume
		Myocardial blood volume

^{18}FDG. There is, however, a need for specialized radiochemistry facilities to permit the development of automated radiolabeling, using high levels of radioactivity, for more complex molecules, in particular those labeled with ^{11}C. The problems of radiochemistry will not be considered in this chapter.

3.7 Data Analysis in Clinical Studies

For reasons discussed in Section 3.3.3, it is possible to accurately measure the amount of radiopharmaceutical in an area of tissue, so allowing comparison to be made of radiotracer uptake between different patients or in a longitudinal study. Perhaps the most common measure of the amount of radiotracer in tumor tissue is the standardized uptake value (SUV). This is defined as:

$$SUV = \frac{\text{tracer activity in the tumour per unit mass}}{\text{amount of injected radioactivity per unit body mass}}. \tag{3.11}$$

This measure represents, of course, the fraction of the administered radiopharmaceutical taken up by the tumor at the time that the measurement was made. If this measure is to be of clinical value it must not only reflect the metabolic or other activity of the tumor, but the tracer must have reached a steady state of concentration by the time of measurement. For tumors other than the brain, a number of studies (see [7]) have indicated that a steady state may not be reached until after several half-lives of the radionuclide, making such a measurement impractical.

The most useful quantitative measures are to be found when it is possible to model the behavior of tracer uptake by tissue. The most common models are the linear compartment ones where rate constants are used to describe the rate of exchange of material between the various biological compartments. To deduce the rate constants it is necessary to know the blood activity input function and the output function, i.e. the tissue time–activity curve. The input function is usually found by taking a series of arterial blood samples and the output one from time–activity curves generated from a region of interest over the image of the organ of interest. By curve fitting using the input and output functions, the rate constants can be calculated. These constants can then be used to determine the physiological parameters of interest, such as glucose metabolism [8] and blood flow [9].

The success of the model approach depends upon the complexity of the model and how sensitive the derivation of the rate constants is to noise. Noise usually limits the application of tracer models to generating parametric images (see Section 1.4.2) in which a value for the biological parameter is derived for each pixel in the image. For any tracer that is irreversibly trapped in the tissue space then the Patlak plot [10] can be used to generate parametric images. This involves taking a sequence of images from 20 to 60 min post-injection. A plot is then made of the concentration of the tracer in tissue, normalized by that in plasma, against the integral of the plasma concentration from the start of the study to the present time, as a fraction of the current plasma concentration. The slope of the resulting straight line graph, the fraction of blood activity taken up by tissue per unit time, will give a value equal to a mixture of the rate constants. With ^{18}FDG as the tracer, the regional metabolic rate of glucose uptake can be calculated from the slope [11]. The technique has also been applied to the measurement of myocardial blood flow using ^{13}NH$_3$ [12].

Other techniques include factor analysis [12] and spectral analysis [13].

References

1. Bradbury I, Bonnell E, Boynton J, et al. Positron Emission Tomography (PET) in cancer management. Glasgow: Health Technology Board for Scotland; 2002: Health Technology Assessment Report 2.
2. Townsend DW, Carney PJ, Yap JT, Hall NC. J Nucl Med 2004; 45:4S–14S.
3. International Electrotechnical Commission. EC Standards 61675-1: Radionuclide Imaging Devices – Characteristics and Test Conditions. Part 1. Positron Emission Tomographs. Geneva: International Electrotechnical Commission; 1998.
4. National Electrical Manufacturers Association. NEMA Standards Publication NU 2-2001: Performance Measurements of Positron Emission Tomographs. Rosslyn: National Electrical Manufacturers Association; 2001.
5. Daube-Witherspoon ME, Karp JS, Casey ME, et al. PET performance measurements using the NEMA NU-2-2001 standard. J Nucl Med 2002; 43:1398–1409.
6. Bettinardi V, Danna M, Savi A, et al. Performance evaluation of the new whole-body PET/CT scanner: Discovery ST (2004). Eur J Nucl Med Mol Imaging 2004; 31:867–881.
7. Keyes JW. SUV: standard uptake or silly useless value. J Nucl Med 1995; 36:1836–1839.
8. Phelps ME, Huang SC, Hoffmann EJ, et al. Tomographic measurement of local cerebral glucose metabolic rate in humans with (F-18) 2-fluoro-2-deoxy-D-glucose: validation of method. Ann Neurol 1979; 6:371–388.
9. Sharp PF. The measurement of blood flow in humans using radioactive tracers. Physiol Meas 1994; 15:339–379.
10. Patlak CS, Blasberg RG. Graphical evaluation of blood-to-brain transfer constants from multiple-time uptake data. J Cereb Blood Flow Metab 1985; 5:584–590.
11. Gambhir SV, Schwaiger M, Huang S-C, et al. Simple non invasive quantification method for measuring myocardial glucose utilization in humans employing positron emission tomography and flourine-18 deoxyglucose. J Nucl Med 1989; 30:359–366.
12. Wu HM, Hoh Ck, Buxton DB, et al. Quantification of myocardial blood flow using dynamic nitrogen-13-ammonia PET studies and factor analysis of dynamic structures. J Nucl Med 1995; 36:2087–2093.
13. Cunningham VJ, Jones T. Spectral analysis of dynamic PET studies. J Cereb Blood Flow Metab 1993; 13:15–23.

4

Non-Imaging Radionuclide Investigations

Alex T. Elliott and Thomas E. Hilditch

4.1 Introduction

Some 12% of nuclear medicine investigations carried out in the UK do not involve imaging and, although being replaced by methods not involving the use of radioactivity, a number of laboratory tests still utilize radioimmunoassay.

The counting of samples is a neglected area and the aim of this chapter is to cover the essentials of this topic in addition to describing the actual investigations.

4.2 Instruments for the Assay of Radioactivity

The standard method for assaying low levels of radioactivity in samples or organs is scintillation spectrometry. Energy deposited in the detector by incident radiation is converted to light photons which are viewed by a photomultiplier tube (PMT). This converts the light into an electrical pulse and provides amplification. Pulse height analysis enables separation of photopeak from scatter events in the detector. For each of the clinical investigations described below, it is assumed that the appropriate energy window is selected and that the energy calibration of the counting system has been checked.

4.2.1 Gamma Counters

A basic counting system consists of the detector assembly (sodium iodide detector and PMT), high voltage supply, amplifier, single- or multichannel pulse height analyzer and a scaler/timer; in modern systems, the latter two components are provided via a computer. For low-energy photon counting, the entrance window of the detector encapsulation may be made of thin beryllium.

For in vivo counting, the crystal is a solid cylinder and the detector assembly is fitted with a collimated shield and mounted on an adjustable stand. In sample counting, the crystal is of the well or diametrical through-hole types and the detector assembly is placed in a shielded enclosure.

Where there are large numbers of samples to be assayed, it is essential to have an automatic counter. A modern system may have up to 10 detectors and a sample capacity of over 1000. Computerized systems afford the opportunity of assaying batches of samples containing different radionuclides and assaying samples containing more than one radionuclide.

With a through-hole type of detector, samples are transported by elevator, allowing position to be adjusted to produce optimum counting efficiency for the specific sample volume, which is entered into the system for a particular batch of samples.

Care requires to be exercised in the choice of automatic gamma counter. Many systems are designed specifically for the assay of samples containing [125]I. The shielding around the detector will be sufficient to minimize low-energy cross-talk from adjacent samples, but would be inadequate in the case (for example) of the 320 keV photons from [51]Cr. Additional shielding should be specified where it is known that the counter will be used for a range of radionuclides.

An interesting feature of larger through-hole detectors is the increased likelihood of observing sum coincidence peaks (due to the simultaneous detection of two events) in the spectrum. Coincidence counting can be put to good use in determining the absolute activity of a sample. Eldridge and Crowther [1] have applied this specifically to [125]I. There are two peaks, the first corresponding to the detection of a single photon of energy 27.4–35 keV and the second smaller sum peak corresponding to the simultaneous detection of two photons. The absolute disintegration rate (R_a) can be obtained from the observed counting rates in the singles channel (R_1) and the coincidence channel (R_2) from

$$R_a = (R_1 + 2R_2)^2/4R_2.$$

In practice, this is a highly effective means of determining the absolute activity of a sample of ^{125}I, taking into account the relative emission probabilities and assuming equal counting efficiency for the energies involved.

4.2.2 Liquid Scintillation Counters

Liquid scintillation counters are used primarily to assay pure beta emitters such as ^{3}H, ^{14}C, and ^{32}P, but are also an effective means of measuring low-energy photon emitters such as [55]Fe. The radioactive sample is dissolved in the detecting medium (the liquid scintillator) or, if the sample is insoluble, it may be suspended as a fine dispersion or in a gel. Liquid scintillators are solutions of materials that are scintillators (fluors) in their solid phase. Organic aromatic solvents, such as alkylbenzene, pseudocumene, and xylene, are used in preference to the more hazardous toluene (which has a lower flash point and higher vapor pressure). There are typically two fluors in solution, primary and secondary; the primary fluor is the scintillator, emitting light photons on absorption of energy from ionizing events, while the secondary fluor absorbs the light from the primary fluor and re-emits it at a wavelength matched to the photocathode of the PMT. Secondary fluors are also referred to as wavelength shifters.

The most commonly used primary and secondary fluors are PPO (2,5-diphenyl oxazole) and bis-MSB (1,4-bis-(2-methylstyryl)-benzene) respectively. These are preferred because of their superior stability and counting efficiency. The fluor concentration is usually of the order of a few grams per liter of solvent: lower concentrations lead to loss of counting efficiency due to insufficient mass of fluor, while higher concentrations lead to loss of counting efficiency due to self-absorption of the fluorescence radiation. The choice of liquid scintillator depends on the particular application; some scintillators are best suited to aqueous samples, others to organic samples. Another consideration is compatibility with the solvent that is sometimes required for solubilization. Tissue solubilizers in common use include hyamine hydroxide (1 N quaternary ammonium hydroxide solution in methanol) and soluene (0.5 N quaternary ammonium hydroxide solution in toluene).

A feature of liquid scintillation counting is the problem of quenching, either chemical or color, which results in a decrease in the intensity of light transmitted to the photomultiplier tube. This leads to a downward shift in the detected energy spectrum with a resultant loss in detection efficiency. Chemical quenching occurs during the transfer of energy from the solvent to the scintillator where there is non-radiative dissipation of energy due to chemical contamination of the solution by the sample. Color quenching occurs when there is attenuation of the light photons due to colorization of the solution. In practice, it is necessary to correct for quenching and this is achieved by making use of a quench correction curve, which is the relationship between counting efficiency and a parameter (the spectral index) which characterizes the spectrum from the sample or an external standard. The spectral index may be the ratio of counts in two counting channels or, as in more modern systems, a parameter based on the whole spectrum such as the mean pulse height or a transform of the spectrum. Irrespective of which parameter or whether sample or external standardization is chosen, the quench correction curve is obtained by counting a series of standards in the chosen liquid scintillator, each with a different level of quenching, and noting the value of the quench indicating parameter for each. Different levels of quenching can be produced by increasing the amount of material to be assayed, supplemented by the addition of sub-milliliter quantities of quench agents such as carbon tetrachloride or acetone.

The method of choice for most applications is to use a quench correction curve based on an external standard which is a low activity (800 kBq) gamma source such as ^{133}Ba, ^{137}Cs or ^{152}Eu. When the external standard is placed adjacent to the sample, a pulse height spectrum is produced by the Compton electrons generated in the sample. Although the spectrum is different to that from a pure beta-emitting radionuclide, it is affected by quenching and can be characterized by a quench-indicating parameter. For unknown samples, the external standard is placed adjacent to each sample for about 15 seconds and the quench-indicating parameter obtained from the resultant spectrum. Quench correction using an external standard is not affected by the statistical variations that would affect correction methods based on the sample's own spectrum, particularly for low activity samples.

A further complication of liquid scintillation counting is the problem of luminescence, which is the generation of unwanted light photons within the sample. Chemiluminescence is caused by chemical reactions in the sample and photoluminescence by excessive exposure to light. Luminescence can be short-lived and its effect may be reduced by delaying counting and by dark adaptation. Cooling the sample may help also.

Recent techniques for detecting and correcting for luminescence make use of the fact that luminescence (the spectrum of which has a different shape to that of the radionuclide in the sample) affects the quench-indicating parameter of the sample differently to that of the external standard. The unwanted contribution is removed by spectral stripping.

In use, the unknown sample is mixed with the liquid scintillator (less than 20 ml) in a transparent glass vial or a translucent polyethylene vial. The former is chemically inert and is not permeable to the solvent. Plastic vials can be permeable to some solvents but have the advantage of a lower background due to absence of natural radionuclides. The light output is viewed by two opposing photomultipliers whose outputs are passed through a coincidence unit; an event is recorded only when a signal is received simultaneously from both PMTs, thereby reducing the random noise background counting rate. The thermal noise from the PMTs can be reduced further by cooling and so the detector assembly and samples are contained in a refrigerated compartment.

A typical liquid scintillation counting system will be fitted with an automatic sample changer capable of holding some 400×20 ml vials (or larger numbers of smaller vials). Operation of the counter is computer-controlled and it will incorporate a multichannel analyzer; the latter offers the advantage of basing quench and luminescence corrections on the whole spectrum. Dual or multichannel counting capability is provided.

4.3 Errors in Measurement of Radioactivity

4.3.1 Random Nature of Radioactive Decay

All measurements of radioactivity are influenced by the random nature of radioactive decay, whether in the source being measured or in background radiation. Nuclear disintegrations follow a Poisson distribution so that if a radioactive source were measured a large number of times for a fixed period and the observed number of counts (n) plotted as a frequency histogram, the distribution would be described by (ignoring radioactive decay of the source):

$$P(n) = 1/n! \, e^{-M} \, M^n$$

where M is the mean value of the distribution. When M is small, the distribution is asymmetrical but for $M > 30$ the asymmetry is negligible and the distribution becomes virtually identical to a Gaussian distribution with mean M and standard deviation of $\sqrt{M}$. Thus 68.3% of the observations will lie in the range $M \pm \sqrt{M}$, 95.4% in the range $M \pm 2\sqrt{M}$ and 99.7% in the range $M \pm 3\sqrt{M}$.

In practice, the source will be measured once only and the observed count becomes the best estimate of the mean. For practical purposes, $\sqrt{n}$ is a good estimate of the standard deviation of the distribution. The true mean has a 68.3% probability of lying in the range $n \pm \sqrt{n}$ etc, thus giving an estimate of the precision of the estimate. For an observed count of 100, the fractional (relative) standard deviation is 10%, reducing to 1% for an observed count of 10 000. It is clear, therefore, that errors due to the random nature of radioactive decay depend upon the source activity and the counting time.

4.3.2 Propagation of Errors

In general, if $U = f(x,y,z \ldots)$, then

$$(\Delta U)^2 = (df/dx.\Delta x)^2$$
$$+ (df/dy.\Delta y)^2 + (df/dz.\Delta z)^2 + \ldots$$

Thus, when two quantities are added or subtracted, the error in the result is given by

$$\Delta U = \sqrt{(\Delta_x^2 + \Delta_y^2)}$$

where Δx and Δy are the errors in the individual values. This rule is particularly important in the measurement of radioactivity, where the contribution from background radiation always has to be subtracted from the sample count. If the count with the sample in place is N_t and that with the sample removed is N_b over the same time period, the standard deviation of the net sample count N_s ($= N_t - N_b$) is

$$s(N_s) = \sqrt{(N_t + N_b)}.$$

If the count obtained from the sample is much greater than that from the background, the latter has little effect on the accuracy of the measurement – thus steps should always be taken to minimize the background counting rate.

In the case of the quotient, Q, (or product) of two quantities x and y, the fractional standard deviations are added in quadrature, i.e.

$$s(Q)/Q = \sqrt{((s(x)/x)^2 + (s(y)/y)^2)}.$$

This rule can be applied to show that the standard deviation of a counting rate, R, is

$$s(R) = \sqrt{N}/t = \sqrt{Rt}/t = \sqrt{(R/t)}$$

where N counts are observed in time t and the error in t can be neglected.

4.3.3 Optimum Division of Counting Time

For the special case of measuring radioactivity in a single sample, it is possible to derive the optimum division of counting time between the sample in place (T_t) and removed (T_b) in order to minimize the standard deviation of the net count rate ($s(R_s)$). If the background counting rate is R_b and the total counting rate is R_t, then

$$T_t/T_b = \sqrt{(R_t/R_b)}.$$

The resulting standard deviation is given by

$$s(R_s) = (\sqrt{R_t} + \sqrt{R_b})/\sqrt{T}$$

where T ($= T_t + T_b$) is the total counting time available. Previous knowledge of R_t and R_b is required; this can be obtained by counting each for a short period before conducting the definitive assay.

In practice, it is more likely that a batch of samples will require to be assayed, using a system with an automatic sample changer. The batch should include an absolute minimum of two blanks to determine the background counting rate and two standard sources to determine the counting efficiency, one of each at the start and at the end of the batch. Several different approaches to the counting procedure are possible:

1. each sample (including each blank) is counted for the same period of time, T;

2. each sample (including each blank) is counted until the same preset number of counts, N, has been accumulated;

3. each sample is counted until either a preset number of counts has accumulated or a preset time has elapsed.

In the first case, the relative standard deviation in the net sample counting rate is

$$s(R_s)/R_s = \sqrt{(R_t + R_b/k)}/(\sqrt{T}.(R_t - R_b))$$

where k is the number of times background is counted in the assay sequence.

In method 2:

$$s(R_s)/R_s = \sqrt{(R_t^2 + R_b^2/k)}/(\sqrt{N}(R_t - R_b)).$$

In this case, all samples having a counting rate much greater than background will have the same relative standard deviation.

Option 3 is a practical compromise in that time will not be wasted counting higher activity samples while ensuring that counting of lower activity samples and background is time-limited.

4.3.4 Errors due to High Counting Rates

Radiation detection systems require a period of time to process an event prior to being able to process the next event. This interval is known as the dead time, or resolving time. Detector systems fall into two classes – paralyzable and nonparalyzable. The latter type will not respond at all to a second event occurring within the dead time following the first event. In a paralyzable system, a second event occurring within the dead time due to the first event will not be recorded but will also initiate a new dead time. This means that not only will the recorded counting rate be less than the true counting rate but that, at high sample activities, the recorded counting rate will begin to decrease and eventually reach zero.

If D_t is the system dead time, the observed counting rate R_o is related to the true counting rate R_t in a paralyzable system by

$$R_o = R_t \exp(-R_t D_t).$$

In a non-paralyzable system, the relationship is

$$R_o = R_t/(1 + R_t D_t)$$

where the maximum observable count rate is $1/D_t$. The equation can be rearranged to yield

$$R_t = R_o/(1 - R_o D_t).$$

This equation holds also for a paralyzable system, provided that $R_o.D_t \ll 1$.

In counting systems incorporating a multichannel analyzer (MCA), dead times can vary from 1 μs to 10 μs or more, dependent on the analogue-to-digital converter (ADC). Some utilize a fixed dead time but in others the dead time is a function of the energy of the detected radiation (since higher energies give rise to higher channel numbers). Irrespective of the type of system, there will be a separate MCA clock which will increment only when the ADC is available to process pulses; this corrects automatically for dead time, permitting data collection for a given "live" time.

It is good practice, nevertheless, to operate at counting rates where the dead time losses are minimal (<5%) since this will minimize problems of pulse pile-up also. The latter arises when pulses from two separate radiation events become superimposed on each other, leading to distortion of the pulse height spectrum. Some systems incorporate pulse pile-up rejection circuitry.

4.3.5 Radioactive Decay During Counting

If the counting period is much shorter than the half-life of the radionuclide, it is sufficiently accurate to assign the result to a time corresponding to the midpoint of the counting period. When measuring a short-lived radionuclide, it is necessary to correct for radioactive decay during the counting

period. If N counts are acquired in a counting interval T, the counting rate at the start of the interval, R_s, is given by:

$$R_s = N\lambda/(1 - e^{-\lambda T})$$

where λ is the decay constant.

It is important also to note that if an ultrashort-lived radionuclide is being assayed in an automatic counter, there is a time delay between samples due to operation of the sample changer.

4.3.6 Multiple Radionuclide Counting

Situations may arise where it is necessary to count samples containing two (or more) radionuclides. As a general rule, if there are n separate counting channels, it is possible to determine the activity of n radionuclides, provided it is possible to count a pure sample (standard) of each radionuclide. The problem reduces to solving n simultaneous equations in n unknowns.

Taking the simplest case of two radionuclides, let Y_1 and Y_2 be the net counting rates in the two channels. If the counting rates due to the first radionuclide are a_1 and $a_1.X_{21}$ in the two channels (the factor X_{21} being obtained by counting the standard of the first radionuclide) and those from the second radionuclide are $a_2.X_{12}$ and a_2 respectively, then

$$Y_1 = a_1 + a_2 X_{12} \quad \text{and} \quad Y_2 = a_1 X_{21} + a_2.$$

These can be solved to yield

$$a_1 = (Y_1 - X_{12} Y_2)/(1 - X_{12} X_{21})$$
$$a_2 = (Y_2 - X_{21} Y_1)/(1 - X_{12} X_{21}).$$

The general expression for the counting rate in the nth channel is

$$Y_k = \Sigma_j(a_j X_{kj}) \, k = 1 \text{ to } n : X_{11} = X_{22}$$
$$= X_{22} \ldots = 1$$

with the solution

$$a_j = |X'(j)|/|X|.$$

The denominator is the determinant of the X matrix, the numerator being the determinant of the matrix formed by substituting the jth column by the Y matrix.

In practice, it is important to ensure that information is to hand about the purity of the radionuclide to be assayed. On occasions, it is necessary to delay counting of high activity samples of short-lived radionuclides in order to avoid dead-time problems (see Section 4.3.4), but this may introduce another error if there is a long-lived contaminant, the relative activity of which will increase with time.

4.3.7 Source Geometry and Self-absorption

Care must be taken to ensure that there are as few differences as possible between different samples and standards to minimize such errors.

Large volume inhomogeneous samples (e.g. feces) pose considerable practical problems and these are best assayed between two large opposing scintillation detectors. The significance of self-absorption within the sample depends on the volume and nature/energy of the radiation. Problems are encountered commonly in the assay of ^{125}I, which emits low-energy photons in the range 27–35 keV.

As a general rule, it is good practice to ensure that all samples and standards have identical volumes and are counted in identical positions.

4.4 Blood Volume

Measurements of blood volume are required in patients with hematological disorders such as polycythemia rubra vera. It is possible to obtain estimates of plasma volume using ^{125}I human serum albumin (HSA) and red cell volume using ^{51}Cr-autologous red cells. Determination of both components by direct measurement of just one requires an assumption to be made about the relationship between venous hematocrit (PCV) and whole body hematocrit.

PCV may be measured using a Wintrobe tube spun at $1500g$ for 30 min and the value corrected for trapped plasma:

whole body hematocrit (PCV_{corr})
$$= 0.91 \times 0.96 \times PCV.$$

4.4.1 Direct Measurement of Plasma Volume

(a) No patient preparation is necessary, but note height (m) and weight (kg). Determine whether any other radionuclides have been administered recently and, if so, obtain a background blood sample.

(b) Obtain 0.15 MBq of ^{125}I-HSA in 7 ml saline.

(c) Administer 0.11 MBq (5 ml) of ^{125}I-HSA intravenously using a 19-gauge needle, taking care to avoid extravasation. If using a butterfly, flush with 5–10 ml saline. Note time of administration.

(d) Ten minutes post-injection withdraw a 7 ml blood sample from the contralateral arm into a heparinized tube. Mix gently.

(e) Prepare standard solution by diluting 1 ml from dose vial into approximately 50 ml of water containing one pellet of sodium hydroxide (to hydrolyze the HSA and so prevent sticking). Make up volume to exactly 100 ml and mix well. Withdraw two 2.5 ml aliquots into counting tubes as standards.

(f) Use a Pasteur pipette to remove 0.5 ml from the blood sample and place into a Wintrobe tube. Obtain PCV_{corr} as noted above.

(g) Centrifuge remainder of blood sample for 10 min at $1500g$. Withdraw 2.5 ml plasma into a counting tube. If there is insufficient plasma, note the actual amount and make up the sample volume to 2.5 ml with water.

(h) Using result from standard, calculate total counts per minute (cpm) injected.

(i) Calculate plasma volume (PV) from:

PV = total cpm injected/
cpm per ml plasma.

The normal range for plasma volume is relatively wide (35–45 ml/kg) [2], with a mean value of 40 ml/kg for both males and females. Regression equations to predict normal plasma volume are:

female PV (ml) $= 284.8 \times \text{weight}^{0.425}$
$$\times \text{height}^{0.725}$$
male PV (ml) $= 329.3 \times \text{weight}^{0.425}$
$$\times \text{height}^{0.725}.$$

4.4.2 Direct Measurement of Red Cell Volume

(a) No patient preparation is necessary, but note height (m) and weight (kg). Determine whether any other radionuclides have been administered recently and, if so, obtain a background blood sample. Refer to local Standard Operating Instructions for patients with HIV, hepatitis B or C.

(b) Obtain 1 MBq of ^{51}Cr-sodium chromate in 1 ml (in 30 ml vial).

(c) Heparinize a 20 ml syringe by drawing up 5000 units of heparin, washing the inside of the syringe and discarding the residue.

(d) Using a 19-gauge needle, withdraw 20–22 ml blood from the patient and mix gently. Remove the needle and attach a sterile cap to the syringe.

(The following labeling steps should be carried out under appropriate aseptic conditions, e.g. in a laminar flow cabinet. Transfers from and to the vial should utilize a 19-gauge needle and a bleed needle to equalize internal pressure.)

(e) Add the blood sample to the 30 ml vial containing the ^{51}Cr-sodium chromate. Mix well and leave for 35–40 min at room temperature to incubate.

(f) Spin the vial at 600g for 5 min and then withdraw as much of the supernatant plasma as possible.

(g) Replace the supernatant with an equal volume of sterile isotonic saline (0.9% wv), mix gently, spin as before and remove the supernatant. Perform this washing procedure twice more.

(h) Resuspend the labeled red cells in 10–12 ml sterile isotonic saline. Mix gently.

(i) Remove 1 ml and add to approximately 50 ml of water. Make up to exactly 100 ml, shake well and withdraw 2 × 2.5 ml aliquots into counting tubes as standards.

(j) Reinject the labeled red blood cells into the patient, taking great care not to extravasate and noting the volume injected. It may be a local requirement for this step to be performed by a member of medical staff.

(k) Ten minutes post-injection, withdraw a 10 ml blood sample into a heparinized tube from a site other than that used for administration.

(l) Use a Pasteur pipette to remove 0.5 ml from the blood sample and place into

a Wintrobe tube. Obtain PCV_{corr} as noted above.

(m) Hemolyze the sample with a sprinkling of saponin powder and withdraw 2.5 ml into a counting tube.

(n) Using result from standard, calculate total cpm injected.

(o) Calculate red cell volume (RCV) from:

$$RCV = \text{total cpm injected}/ \text{cpm per ml red cells.}$$

The 95% confidence range for red cell volume is 25–35 ml/kg for adult males and 20–30 ml/kg for adult females [3]. In polycythemia rubra vera, red cell volume is >36 ml/kg for males and >32 ml/kg for females. Regression equations to predict normal red cell volume are:

$$\text{female RCV (ml)} = 169.7 \times \text{weight}^{0.425} \times \text{height}^{0.725}$$
$$\text{male RCV (ml)} = 222.2 \times \text{weight}^{0.425} \times \text{height}^{0.725}.$$

4.4.3 Indirect Measurements

(a) When carrying out either of the above procedures, remove 0.5 ml of the patient blood sample and place into a Wintrobe tube. Calculate PCV_{corr} as detailed in Section 4.4 above.

(b) If measuring PV, calculate RCV and total blood volume (TBV) from:

$$RCV = (PV \times PCV_{corr})/(100 - PCV_{corr})$$
$$TBV = (100 \times PV)/(100 - PCV_{corr}).$$

(c) If measuring RCV, calculate PV and TBV from:

$$PV = (RCV(100 - PCV_{corr}))/PCV_{corr}$$
$$TBV = (100 \times RCV)/PCV_{corr}.$$

4.5 ^{14}C-Urea Breath Test for *Helicobacter pylori* (*H. pylori*)

H. pylori in the stomach is believed to be responsible for the occurrence of duodenal ulcers. Eradication of the bacterium with antibiotics has proven to be an effective treatment. If ^{14}C-urea is given orally, the urease produced by *H. pylori* catalyzes the test dose into ^{14}C-labeled CO_2 and ammonia.

The labeled CO_2 diffuses into the blood supply and is then exhaled; measurement of ^{14}C radioactivity in a breath sample is thus a means of determining the presence of the bacterium.

The procedure described here involves the administration of 0.1–0.2 MBq of ^{14}C-urea after a test meal. Alternative methods using a lower activity and no test meal are used in some centers.

4.5.1 Preparation of Individual Dose

(a) Dissolve 37 MBq freeze-dried ^{14}C-urea in 6.5 ml sterile water and empty into flask.

(b) Rinse vial twice with 5 ml sterile water each time.

(c) Make up to 250 ml with sterile water and mix thoroughly

(d) Dispense 1 ml aliquots into screw-capped plastic vials.

(e) Put aside three vials to determine activity and to use as counting standards (see Section 4.5.3).

(f) Store dispensed doses in a refrigerator (shelf life up to 6 weeks).

4.5.2 Preparation of Indicator Solution

(a) Dissolve 60 mg thymolphthalein in 500 ml hyamine hydroxide 10-X in methanol.

(b) Make up to 1000 ml with ethyl alcohol and mix well.

(c) Dispense 2 ml aliquots into scintillation vials.

When neutralized with 1 mmol CO_2, color changes from blue to clear, indicating that a sufficient breath sample has been obtained.

4.5.3 Preparation of Standards and Background Samples

(a) Dilute each of three doses to 50 ml with ethyl alcohol and mix well.

(b) From each diluted dose, withdraw 3 × 1 ml aliquots into scintillation vials.

(c) Add 1 ml hyamine hydroxide 10-X to each vial.

(d) Add 10 ml liquid scintillator to each vial and count in a liquid scintillation counter (all should lie within 5% of the mean value, which should fall in the range 0.2–0.3 mBq).

(e) Retain two of these aliquots as counting standards.

(f) Prepare two background samples by neutralizing 2 × 2 ml indicator solution in scintillation vials with non-radioactive breath. Add 10 ml liquid scintillator to each vial.

4.5.4 Test Procedure

(a) Fast patient from 21.00h on day previous to test.

(b) Weigh patient (kg).

(c) Ask patient to brush his/her teeth without swallowing any water and discarding all rinsings into running water in the basin.

(d) Show the patient how to give a breath sample. Obtain baseline sample and add 10 ml of liquid scintillator to the vial.

(e) Give patient test meal of 200 ml citric acid solution (containing 4g citric acid monohydrate plus 25 mg Canderel powder) to drink (or 200 ml Fortisip or 200 ml milk).

(f) Administer test dose of ^{14}C-urea (made up to 25 ml with water), then two rinsings of 25 ml water. Note time.

(g) Ask patient to re-brush teeth as in (c).

(h) Obtain breath sample at 20 min post-administration and add 10 ml of liquid scintillator to vial.

(i) Using result from standard, calculate total cpm administered.

(j) Calculate the parameter A_e, a measure of exhaled activity adjusted for patient weight, from

$$A_e = \text{net sample cpm} \times \text{weight(kg)} \times 10^4/\text{cpm administered.}$$

If $A_e < 20$, test is negative for *H. pylori*.
If A_e is 20–40, result is equivocal.
If $A_e > 40$, test is positive for *H. pylori*.

4.6 Other Breath Tests

While the ^{14}C-urea breath test is much more common, other tests also employ the measurement of exhaled $^{14}CO_2$.

4.6.1 ^{14}C-Glycocholic Acid Breath Test

Bacterial colonization of the small bowel can be investigated using ^{14}C-glycocholic acid, which is deconjugated into ^{14}C-glycine and cholic acid if bacteria are present. After oxidation of the labeled glycine, $^{14}CO_2$ appears in the patient's blood and is expired on passage through the lungs.

(a) Fast the patient overnight.

(b) Note the patient's weight.

(c) Obtain 0.4 MBq of ^{14}C-glycocholic acid in 10 ml of 10% ethanol.

(d) Administer dose orally, followed by a glass of orange juice and breakfast.

(e) Collect breath samples at 2, 4, and 6 h post-administration.

(f) Samples and standards are counted as described in Section 4.5 above.

(g) Express results as %dose/mmol CO_2, multiplied by the weight in kg.

The upper limit of $^{14}CO_2$ expiration is 0.05, 0.14, and 0.32 kg%dose/mmol at 2, 4, and 6 h respectively. Patients with bacterial colonization exhale greater quantities of $^{14}CO_2$. Results should be interpreted with caution since false negative results are not uncommon; false positive results occur also but at a much lower frequency.

4.6.2 ^{14}C-Glycerol Palmitate and ^{14}C-Palmitic Acid Breath Tests

Malabsorption of fat (steatorrhea) in the gastrointestinal tract can be investigated using ^{14}C-labeled fat (glycerol tripalmitate) and ^{14}C-labeled fatty acid (palmitic acid). An end product of the normal fat absorption process is CO_2, which is almost completely expired. Since the first stage in the absorption of fat is breakdown to fatty acid by a pancreatic enzyme (lipase), it is possible to determine whether malabsorption is due to pancreatic insufficiency by repeating the test with labeled fatty acid. An improved result would suggest pancreatic steatorrhea.

(a) Fast the patient overnight.

(b) Note the patient's weight.

(c) Obtain 0.4 MBq of ^{14}C-glycerol tripalmitate in 1 ml/kg bodyweight of corn oil flavored with orange.

(d) Administer dose orally and continue to fast the patient for a further 4 h, keeping the patient at rest.

(e) Collect breath samples at hourly intervals for 6 h.

(f) Count samples and standards as in Section 4.5.

(g) Express results as %dose × 100/mmol CO_2, multiplied by the patient's weight in kg.

In normal subjects, the peak ^{14}C level in breath is greater than 18 units. Results in the range 14–18 are equivocal, with a value of less than 14 indicating steatorrhea. When an abnormal value is obtained, the test is repeated one week later using a test dose of 0.4 MBq ^{14}C-palmitic acid and following exactly the same procedure. If the peak level of ^{14}C in breath increases by a factor of 2 or more, pancreatic steatorrhea is indicated. An improvement by 1.4–2.0 is equivocal, while a ratio of less than 1.4 indicates that the steatorrhea is not due to pancreatic insufficiency.

The test should be interpreted with caution, since some conditions (liver disease, chronic respiratory disorders, diabetes mellitus, obesity) can invalidate the result.

4.7 Red Cell Studies

Red cell survival studies are undertaken to establish the presence, and assess the severity, of hemolytic anemia. It is possible also to determine the sites of red cell destruction by body counting – sequestration studies. It is common practice to estimate red cell volume (see Section 4.4.2) in the course of these studies.

4.7.1 Red Cell Survival

(a) No patient preparation is necessary, but note height (m) and weight (kg). Determine whether any other radionuclides have been administered recently and, if so, obtain a background blood sample. Refer to local Standard Operating

Instructions for patients with HIV, hepatitis B or C.

(b) Establish whether the patient is likely to require a blood transfusion during the period of study. This should be delayed as long as possible to establish a true survival pattern.

(c) Obtain 2 MBq ^{51}Cr-sodium chromate in 1 ml (in 30 ml vial).

(d) Label patient's red cells as in Section 4.4.2 (d)–(i).

(e) Reinject red cells, note time and date of administration and take a 10 ml blood sample into a heparinized tube at 10 min for volume estimation (see Section 4.4.2).

(f) Take 10 ml blood samples into a heparinized tube at 24 h post-administration and every 48 h thereafter for 14 days.

(g) Perform a PCV estimation on each sample, lyze the remainder with saponin and transfer 2.5 ml into a counting tube.

(h) After the first few samples have been collected, obtain rough counts on each to determine whether the half-life has been reached.

(i) Count all samples in a single batch (avoiding the need for decay corrections) and express net cpm in each sample as a percentage of that in the 24 h sample.

(j) Plot data against time on a linear plot. In almost every case, the result will be a straight line; the half-time may be read directly or obtained from a linear regression on the data.

If the PCV changes over the course of the study, express counts as cpm per milliliter of red cells and plot values as percentages of that in the first sample.

In normal subjects, the half-time is greater than 24 days. Lower values indicate abnormal destruction of red cells.

4.7.2 Sequestration Studies

In this case, an activity of 4 MBq of ^{51}Cr-sodium chromate is used. The same procedure as above (see Section 4.7.1) is followed except that external counting over three sites is carried out also:

- heart – third intercostal space near sternal border with patient supine;
- liver – mid-clavicular line about 2–4 cm above right costal margin with patient supine;
- spleen – mid-axillary line at tenth intercostal space with patient in right lateral position.

A typical counting system will employ a 5 cm diameter sodium iodide crystal, fitted with a cylindrical collimator of 5 cm diameter and 12 cm depth.

(a) Mark counting sites in indelible ink.

(b) Commence counting at 30 min post-administration and repeat at 24 h and every 48 h thereafter, taking care to reposition the counter accurately.

(c) Correct counts obtained for room background. A 500 ml water-filled bottle containing 1 MBq of ^{51}Cr-sodium chromate may be used as a standard on each occasion to correct for any instability.

(d) Calculate spleen/heart, liver/heart and spleen/liver ratios and plot against time from administration.

In normal subjects, counts over liver and spleen should fall at the same rate as the heart count, with the spleen/liver ratio at the half-time of the cells being less than 2. An increasing spleen/liver ratio with a value greater than 2.3 at the half-time is indicative of significant splenic sequestration.

4.8 Gastrointestinal Blood and Protein Loss

Loss of blood or protein from the gastrointestinal tract can be detected and quantified by the use of ^{51}Cr red cells or ^{51}Cr chromic chloride respectively. It should be noted that these tests require complete fecal collection over several days.

4.8.1 Blood Loss

(a) Proceed as in Section 4.7.1 (a)–(f), except utilize an activity of 4 MBq of ^{51}Cr sodium chromate and collect blood samples for only 7 days.

(b) Commencing at 08.00h on the day following administration, collect 24 h fecal samples for 5 days. Request the patient to try to avoid urine contamination.

(c) To each fecal collection, add 15 g Actizyme and make up volume to 500 ml with water. Mix well and leave the sample for 24 h to homogenize before counting.

(d) Withdraw 2 × 2.5 ml aliquots from the standard flask to use as standards for the blood assay and a further 50 ml into an empty fecal collection bucket as a standard for the fecal assay. Make up the latter volume to 500 ml with water.

Net counts from the fecal samples are expressed as %dose. The net counts from the blood samples (%dose per ml whole blood) are plotted against time to provide an estimate of the ^{51}Cr activity in the blood over each fecal sampling period. From this, the volume of blood in each collection is estimated.

In normal subjects, the rate of blood loss is less than 1.5 ml per day.

4.8.2 Protein Loss

(a) No special patient preparation is necessary.

(b) Obtain 6 MBq of ^{51}Cr chromic chloride in 6 ml saline.

(c) Prepare the standard solution by withdrawing 1 ml into a flask and make up to 100 ml with water.

(d) Administer 4 ml of the dose to the patient and begin 24 h fecal collections for a period of 5 days. Request the patient to attempt to avoid urine contamination.

(e) To each fecal collection, add 15 g Actizyme and make up volume to 500 ml with water. Mix well and leave the sample for 24 h to homogenize before counting.

(f) Prepare standard by withdrawing 10 ml of the standard solution into a sample bucket and make up to 500 ml with water.

Net counts from the samples are expressed as %injected dose. In normal subjects, the total %dose excreted in the 5-day period is typically less than 0.7%. Excretion of more than 2% in five days is indicative of significant protein loss.

4.9 Schilling Test

Labeled vitamin B_{12} – ^{57}Co cyanocobalamin – is of considerable use in the investigation of patients with megaloblastic anemia. It is absorbed in the ileum after forming a complex with intrinsic factor, a component of gastric juice.

In normal subjects, 50–90% of an oral dose of 1 µg of vitamin B_{12} is absorbed, whereas there are varying degrees of decreased absorption in the megaloblastic anemias. In pernicious anemia, absorption is enhanced greatly if intrinsic factor is administered at the same time as the vitamin B_{12}. In the Schilling test, a flushing dose of 1 mg of unlabeled vitamin B_{12} given intramuscularly is used to flush out (in the urine) the tracer vitamin B_{12}, which has been absorbed through the ileum.

(a) Obtain 0.02 MBq of ^{57}Co-cyanocobalamin for a Part I test: for a Part II test (undertaken if Part I absorption is low), a 1 USNF hog intrinsic factor capsule is required also.

(b) Fast the patient from 21.00 the day previous to the test (or for a minimum of 12 h) until the unlabeled vitamin B_{12} has been injected.

(c) Request the patient to empty his/her bladder.

(d) Administer the labeled vitamin B_{12} orally (together with intrinsic factor capsule if Part II test). If the B_{12} is in liquid form, the vial is rinsed twice with water and this is drunk also: if the B_{12} is in capsule form, the patient should be given a glass of water after swallowing it.

(e) Start a 26 h urine collection, stressing the importance of obtaining a complete collection to the patient.

(f) Two hours after the oral dose, administer intramuscular injection of 1 mg of Cytamen (cyanocobalamin) to inhibit hepatic uptake of the absorbed oral dose. The absorbed dose is then excreted in the urine over the following 24 h.

(g) Read off volume of urine excreted; if less than 150 ml, make up to 150 ml with water. Remove 150 ml aliquot into a counting container.

(h) Prepare standard by diluting 0.02 MBq of labeled vitamin B_{12} to 150 ml in water. If the dose is in capsule form, dissolve in warm water and rinse out the container.

(i) Calculate % dose excreted, D_e, from:

$$D_e = \text{(net urine counts} \times \text{urine volume} \times 100)/(150 \times \text{net standard counts).}$$

Note that if the urine volume is <150 ml, then set to 150 ml in the above equation. The results are interpreted as follows:

D_e > 10%: normal result;

D_e 5–10%: result equivocal (in Part I);

D_e <5%: pernicious anemia or malabsorption (in Part I).

In Part II, malabsorption will still yield a value <5% while, in pernicious anemia, excretion should be at least double the Part I value and be in the normal range (>10%).

4.10 Ferrokinetics

Iron is essential for erythropoiesis. Iron is absorbed through the small intestine and transported in the bloodstream bound to transferrin. It is taken up by erythropoietic tissue and incorporated into red cell hemoglobin. At the end of their lifespan, red cells are broken down and the iron released is recycled. The study of ferrokinetics is useful in the diagnosis of several hematological disorders where the rate of plasma iron disappearance, proportion of iron incorporated into red cells or sites of uptake may be abnormal. Red cell survival studies (see Section 4.7.1) will be carried out in parallel.

If the patient's plasma iron is within the normal range (11–31 μmol/l), ^{59}Fe ferric citrate is administered directly. If the plasma iron is elevated, the labeled ferric citrate requires to be incubated in vitro with plasma from a normal donor, obtained via the hematology department.

(a) Mark the patient's heart, liver and spleen with an indelible marker as in

Section 4.7.2. Identify the sacrum (patient prone) by palpation and mark this area.

(b) Obtain 0.6 MBq of ^{59}Fe ferric citrate in 6 ml sodium citrate dihydrate/saline solution or, for in vitro labeling, 0.6 MBq in 2 ml in a 30 ml vial. Note that the diluent is not saline in order to prevent precipitation of iron.

(c) (i) If the patient's plasma iron is normal, inject 4 ml (0.4 MBq) of ^{59}Fe ferric citrate solution intravenously. (ii) If the patient's plasma iron is elevated, add 15 ml of screened plasma to the 30 ml vial, working in a laminar flow cabinet and using a bleed needle to equalize pressure. Incubate the mixture for 45 min at 37°C. Inject 10 ml of the labeled plasma intravenously.

(d) Prepare a standard solution by adding 1 ml of the dose residue to a partially filled 100 ml flask. The diluent should be a solution containing 5.9 mg sodium chloride and 10 mg sodium citrate dihydrate per milliliter or, if using labeled plasma, water with a few milliliters of unlabeled plasma to minimize sticking. Make up volume to 100 ml and shake well.

(e) Withdraw 10 ml blood samples into a heparinized tube at 10, 20, 30, 60, 90, 120, and 240 min and 24 h postinjection. Withdraw further samples every other day until the activity in the sample reaches a maximum (at 7–10 days).

(f) Using an external probe, obtain 100 s counts over the heart, liver, spleen, and sacrum within the first 10 min and at 1, 3, 5, and 24 h post-injection. Repeat every other day until the blood count reaches a maximum.

(g) Correct counts for room background and radioactive decay.

(h) Generate a linear plot of counts from each site against time.

(i) From each blood sample, take an aliquot for PCV estimation (see Section 4.4) and a 3 ml aliquot of whole blood into a counting tube and hemolyze with saponin. Spin the remainder at 1500g for 10 min and withdraw 3 ml plasma into a counting tube (note that plasma counting is required only for samples up to 240 min).

(j) Count all samples as a single batch with two background samples and two aliquots from the standard solution (one of each at the beginning and end of the batch).

(k) Calculate plasma iron turnover by plotting the plasma counts (up to 240 min) against time on a semi-logarithmic graph. Draw a straight line through the data points and read off the time taken for the counts to fall to 50% of the initial value (the clearance half-time). It is conventional to express plasma iron turnover in terms of μmol per liter of blood per day:

$$\text{Plasma iron turnover} = \frac{\text{plasma iron}\,(\mu\text{mol l}^{-1}) \times 1440 \times 0.693 \times (100 - \text{PCV}_{\text{corr}})}{\text{clearance half-time (min)} \times 100}.$$

(l) Calculate iron utilization by plotting whole blood counts against time on a linear graph. These will reduce initially as ^{59}Fe is cleared from the plasma but will increase to a maximum around 10–14 days as red cells containing ^{59}Fe enter the circulation. At the time of maximum incorporation into the circulation,

Iron utilization =
(total activity in blood × 100)/
total activity administered.

The total activity in blood is the product of the concentration of ^{59}Fe in blood and the blood volume, the latter being obtained by direct measurement or by estimation from height and weight. In normal subjects, the half-time for plasma iron clearance is 60–120 min, while normal values for iron utilization at 10–14 days lie in the range 70–80%. Normal plasma iron turnover is in the range 70–140 μmol/l per day. In hemolytic anemia there is an increase in the rate of plasma iron clearance, an increase in plasma iron turnover, an increase in iron utilization and increased marrow uptake of iron. Myelofibrosis is characterized by reduced marrow uptake but increased uptake by the spleen. Aplastic anemia is accompanied by a prolonged plasma iron clearance and decreased iron utiliza-

tion. There is also reduced marrow uptake but increased accumulation of iron in the liver.

4.11 Renal Studies

Measurement of renal function may utilize ^{125}I-hippuran, which is virtually cleared from the blood on first passage through the kidneys and is a measure of effective renal plasma flow (ERPF), or $^{51}\text{Cr-EDTA}$, which is cleared by glomerular filtration and measures glomerular filtration rate (GFR). In the protocols given here, three blood samples are required for GFR investigations, but only one for ERPF determination.

(a) Obtain 2 MBq of $^{51}\text{Cr-EDTA}$ in 5 ml saline (for GFR) and 2 MBq of ^{125}I-hippuran in 5 ml saline (for ERPF).

(b) The patient should have only a light breakfast or light lunch prior to the test and should have nothing to eat or drink during the test.

(c) Note the patient's height (m) and weight (kg) and obtain body surface area from standard tables.

(d) The patient should be kept lying down for 10–15 min prior to starting the test and kept at rest – lying or sitting – during the test.

(e) Insert a cannula into one arm and withdraw a 10 ml blood sample into a heparin tube and mix well. If a cannula is used which requires to be flushed with heparin after each sample, then 2 ml of blood should be withdrawn and discarded immediately prior to each timed sample.

(f) Withdraw 4 ml from the dose vial and inject through a 19-gauge butterfly into the opposite arm, flushing with 10 ml saline. Care must be taken to ensure injection of the whole 4 ml dose.

(g) Withdraw 10 ml blood samples into heparin tubes at 2 h, 3 h, and 4 h after dose administration for GFR estimation or at 45 min for ERPF measurement. Note that these timings are critical.

(h) Spin all blood samples at 1500g for 10 min and withdraw 3 ml plasma into counting tubes.

(i) Prepare standards by withdrawing 0.5 ml from each dose vial into a flask, adding one or two pellets of sodium hydroxide and diluting to 500 ml with water. Mix well and withdraw 2 × 3 ml aliquots into counting tubes.

(j) Count each sample for 10 min in an automatic gamma counter.

ERPF is calculated from

$$ERPF = F(1 - \exp(-a(V - V_e)))$$

where F = 1131.5 ml/min, a = 0.0078 l^{-1}, V_e = 7.68 l and V = volume of distribution at sampling time. This value must be normalized to a body surface area of 1.73 m^2, following which the normal range is 556 ± 46 ml/min.

In order to calculate GFR, the best-fit straight line through the logarithm of the net sample counts at 2, 3, and 4 h is found by the method of least squares. This enables determination of the decay constant, k (min^{-1}), of the blood disappearance curve. The intercept on the y-axis yields the activity concentration at time zero, permitting calculation of the volume of distribution, V (ml). Then

$$GFR = 0.93 \times k \times V$$

where 0.93 is a factor to correct for the overestimation of GFR by this particular method. The result is normalized to a body surface area of 1.73 m^2. Normal GFR values are 129 ± 23 ml/min in adult males and 111 ± 17 ml/min in adult females.

GFR measurements can also be made using ^{99m}Tc-DTPA instead of ^{51}Cr-EDTA [4]. Some centers find this useful as it can be combined with renography (see Section 11.5.2).

4.12 Thyroid Uptake

The 20 min thyroid uptake measurement provides a rapid indication of thyroid status before, during, and after therapy. Counter and thyroid phantom should comply with the IAEA guidance [5]. A typical uptake counter will consist of a sodium iodide detector, 5 cm in diameter and 5 cm thick, fitted with a tapering lead collimator and connected to a computer-based MCA. The latter will have an internal diameter of 5 cm at the detector face, increasing to a final diameter of 11 cm; the wall thickness will be 1 cm and the depth 18.5 cm. The neck and thyroid phantom will be a water-filled Perspex container 15 cm in diameter and 15 cm thick with a cylindrical insertion 0.5 cm from the edge capable of holding a 30 ml water-filled plastic vial.

(a) Obtain 2 × 2 MBq of ^{123}I sodium iodide in 1 ml saline.

(b) Divide one dose between two glass bottles and place in thyroid phantom.

(c) Collect a room background count for 1 min.

(d) Place the phantom on the counter axis, the front face of the phantom being 10 cm from the front end of the detector collimator, and collect a 1 min standard count. A 10 cm long Perspex rod is useful for accurate positioning. Calculate the net standard count.

(e) Remove the standard and position the patient so that the edge of the collimator is 10 cm from the patient's neck, centered between the sternal notch and chin. Collect a 1 min patient background count.

(f) Inject the dose, noting the time.

(g) At 2 and 20 min post-administration, collect 1 min patient counts.

(h) Express the net patient count, U_n, as % injected dose by comparison with the net standard count. This has two components, true thyroid uptake and extrathyroidal activity (ETA). The latter is estimated by making measurements in patients with no thyroid uptake and will be found to be approximately 5% of the injected dose.

(i) Calculate thyroid uptake (% injected dose), U_{thy}, from:

$$U_{thy} = (U_n - ETA)/(1 - (ETA/100)).$$

The more useful uptake is that at 20 min, when the euthyroid value lies in the range 2–8%. Values in excess of this are found in hyperthyroidism and in patients with an organification defect or iodine deficiency. In acute thyroiditis, the result will be zero.

4.13 Bile Acid Malabsorption

Malabsorption of bile acid can be investigated using ^{75}Se-labeled tauroselchoic acid (SeHCAT), which is an analogue of the naturally-occurring bile acid conjugate taurocholic acid. In normal subjects, bile acids are produced and excreted into the duodenum by the hepatobiliary system and are reabsorbed by the distal ileum. If the functional integrity of the ileum is impaired, bile acids entering the colon reduce the reabsorption of water, resulting in chronic diarrhea. The SeHCAT test, involving measurement of the 7-day retention of an oral dose of the radiopharmaceutical, is useful in the investigation of diarrhea of unknown origin. Retention can be measured using a gamma camera, either uncollimated or fitted with a high sensitivity collimator, or a whole body counter. A gamma camera method is described:

(a) Fast the patient overnight.

(b) Obtain a 370 kBq SeHCAT capsule.

(c) Give the patient at least 15 ml of water to drink, followed by the SeHCAT capsule and a further drink of at least 15 ml of water.

(d) Wait 3 h before the first measurement to allow dissolution of the capsule and a satisfactory distribution of the Se-HCAT.

(e) Set the gamma camera energy analyzer window to 265 keV ± 10%. If a dual energy analyzer is available and the room background is sufficiently low, a second window of 136 keV ± 10% can be used also.

(f) Position the camera at its highest position above the patient couch and count room background for 300 s.

(g) Place the patient supine on the couch, with the xiphisternum-umbilicus region directly below the camera and obtain a 300 s count.

(h) Repeat (g) with the patient prone.

(i) Obtain another background count and calculate the mean.

(j) Calculate the geometric mean of the net AP and PA counts.

(k) Repeat (e)–(j) after 7 days and calculate the percentage retention.

The 7-day retention in normal subjects is greater than 10%. Values below this are consistent with bile malabsorption.

4.14 Isolated Perfusion Measurements

A number of cytotoxic drugs are available which have severe systemic side effects at concentrations that are toxic to the target cells. In some cases, it may be possible to isolate the blood supply to the target organ from the systemic circulation, which permits the addition of a therapeutic concentration of drug to the isolated circuit while not compromising the systemic circulation. It is crucial to monitor the amount of drug "leaking" into the systemic circulation and to terminate the procedure should a significant quantity be detected. As an example, the following procedure is suitable for use in isolated limb perfusion in melanoma: in this case, a 10% leakage into the central circulation is deemed the maximum acceptable before the procedure would be terminated. The relative amounts of radioactivity added to the central circulation and perfusate mean that such a leakage would cause a doubling of the count rate from the probe and would be readily detectable with high statistical validity.

(a) Reconstitute a vial of pyrophosphate with 10 ml saline and administer 6 ml to the patient approximately 15 minutes before the surgeon effects limb blood flow isolation.

(b) Add the remaining 4 ml to the perfusate prepared for the limb circulation.

(c) Position a collimated cadmium telluride probe over the left ventricle.

(d) Immediately after limb isolation, administer 10 MBq ^{99m}Tc pertechnetate to the patient and take 20 s counts until a stable reading is obtained (within 2–3 minutes).

(e) Add 100 MBq ^{99m}Tc pertechnetate to the limb perfusate.

(f) Obtain further 20 s counts for 2–3 minutes and, if no increase is detected, administer cytotoxic drug(s) to the perfusate.

(g) Continue to acquire 20 s counts for the duration of the procedure, correcting for radioactive decay.

(h) Determine any increase in count and calculate corresponding leakage into central circulation.

(i) Advise surgeon if agreed limit is approached.

4.15 Radioimmunoassay

This technique was developed by Berson and Yalow and by Ekins in the 1950s. It was in widespread use in the 1960s–1980s, but has generally been superseded by methods (e.g. fluorescence assays) that do not require the use of radioactive materials. The radionuclide used most commonly is ^{125}I, the samples being counted in an automatic gamma counter.

The concentration of an unknown unlabeled antigen in a sample is measured by comparison of its inhibitory effect on the binding of radiolabeled antigen to specific antibody with that of standards of known concentration. While it is vital that the immunological behavior of the antigens in the sample and standards is identical, it is not necessary for them to exhibit the same chemical or biological properties.

In order to set up a standard curve, a constant amount of antibody is added to several counting tubes. Increasing (and known) amounts of antigen are added to successive tubes and, after a suitable incubation period, bound complexes will be formed. In the tubes with low quantities of antigen, less bound complex will be formed and, in tubes with more antigen, more bound complexes will be formed. The amount of antigen present can thus be measured by assaying the amount of bound complex formed.

Radioimmunoassay utilizes radiolabeled antigen in the measurement. A constant amount is added to the antibody in the counting tubes together with the varying amounts of unlabeled antigen. Labeled and unlabeled antigen thus "compete" to form bound complex – the greater the quantity of unlabeled antigen present, the lower the amount of labeled bound complex formed. The bound complex is separated and assayed.

In the case of immunometric assays, the amount of complex is measured directly by adding a constant (excess) amount of a second radiolabeled antibody, which is targeted to a binding site on the antigen different to that identified by the first antibody. The labeled bound complex is then separated and the activity assayed. In both cases, it is usual to create a calibration curve from a minimum of eight known concentrations. The concentrations in unknown samples are then obtained by interpolation.

Concentrations in the nanomolar range are measured readily and, with care, this can be extended into picomolar concentrations. It is important to carry out adequate quality control, both internally and by membership of external schemes; it is usual to run low, medium, and high concentration standards at the beginning and end of each analysis run.

4.16 Sentinel Node Detection

This is usually carried out as an imaging investigation in the first instance and so is described in Section 16.10.1. The intraoperative segment of the procedure utilizes a shielded cadmium telluride probe.

References

1. Eldridge JS, Crowther P. Absolute determination of I-125. Nucleonics 1964; 22:6–62.
2. Hall R, Malia RG. Medical Laboratory Haematology. London: Butterworths; 1984.
3. International Committee for Standardization in Haematology. Recommended methods for radioisotope red cell survival studies. Br J Haematol 1980; 45:659–666.
4. Fleming JS, Zivanovic MA, Blake GM, et al. Guidelines for the measurement of glomerular filtration rate using plasma sampling. Nucl Med Commun 2004; 25:759–769.
5. IAEA. Special report No. 7. Thyroid uptake measurements. Report of a panel convened by the International Atomic Energy Agency, 1971. Br J Radiol 1973; 46:58–63.

5

Quality Assurance

Alex T. Elliott

5.1 Introduction

Quality assurance (QA) is the archetypal topic "more honored in the breach than the observance". Nevertheless, it is of vital importance if the best possible patient service is to be provided and should form part of the routine of every department. The aims are to ensure that the equipment meets (and preferably surpasses) specification and to keep it operating at peak performance. The two most important facets of a QA program are to produce objective (usually, quantitative) data and to keep adequate records, both of those results and of equipment faults. Guidance on QA is offered in the publications of the Institute of Physical Sciences in Medicine [1], Institute of Physics and Engineering in Medicine [2], American Association of Physicists in Medicine [3], World Health Organization [4], the US Department of Health and Human Services [5–7], and the British Standards Institution [8].

Quality assurance should begin at the time of placing an order for equipment, when a detailed performance specification should be drawn up and form part of the order. For gamma cameras, data to assist in this may be obtained from the series of reports published by the Department of Health and Social Security/Scottish Home and Health Department [9–12] or from manufacturers' data measured according to the National Electrical Manufacturers' Association (NEMA) protocol [13,14]. The DHSS/SHHD reports utilize mainly the tests specified by the International Electrotechnical Commission (IEC) [15–17] and

British Standards Institution (BSI) Standards [18], which are carried out in the presence of scatter and thus reflect more closely the camera's clinical performance. The NEMA tests are carried out largely in air and are designed to allow a manufacturer to assure himself of consistency of production. For a computer system, an operational requirement document should be prepared, outlining the major items of hardware and detailing the functions to be carried out by the software. This will usually suffice at the tender stage, but a more detailed specification will be required at the time of ordering. This should include benchmark data against which the installed system can be assessed. A general discussion of points to be considered when ordering camera/computer systems can be found in papers by Wells and Buxton-Thomas [19] and Tindale [20].

The British Nuclear Medicine Society has published a document which may be used for tendering purposes. This was first published in 1996 and is now at Version 3.1 [21].

Following hand-over (which may be some time after installation), the user should obtain a written statement from the supplier that the equipment complies with the specification and should then undertake comprehensive testing to verify this. With the equipment in regular clinical use, simple but regular quality control checks should be made to ensure that it continues to perform within specification. Some of these checks should be made daily, while others need be made only on a weekly or 3-monthly basis. All quantitative data should be archived carefully and, where appropriate, subjected to trend analysis.

5.2 Gamma Cameras

Immediately after installation, a close physical inspection of the mechanical and electrical safety aspects of the equipment should be made. It is worthwhile arranging to X-ray a camera's collimators on delivery to check for defects in construction, particularly if they are assembled by gluing strips of lead foil.

5.2.1 Performance Parameters

The performance of a gamma camera is characterized by six parameters, spatial resolution, nonuniformity, spatial distortion, sensitivity, count rate characteristic, and energy resolution. Most of these are interrelated; some 60% of nonuniformity, for example, is due to spatial distortion, while energy resolution affects the system spatial resolution.

Spatial Resolution

The spatial resolution is related to the smallest separation between two point sources which will permit them to be distinguished as two distinct sources and is measured by imaging a point or, more usually, line source. The line spread function, L(x), is the graph of count rate as a function of the x-coordinate when the line source is placed parallel to the y-axis in a plane parallel to the collimator face and at a given distance from it. The measured quantities are the full width at half maximum (FWHM) and full width at tenth maximum (FWTM) of the resulting curve (Figure 5.1). The detector system itself has an intrinsic spatial resolution (R_i), due to the electronics, and the collimator has a geometric resolution (R_c). The system (overall) resolution (R_s) is given, to a good approximation, by

$$(R_s)^2 = (R_i)^2 + (R_c)^2.$$

It is usual to measure both the intrinsic and system resolution.

The modulation transfer function (MTF) is an index often used to convey the ability of a gamma camera to yield an image corresponding exactly with the physical distribution of the radionuclide. Consider a source distribution that varies

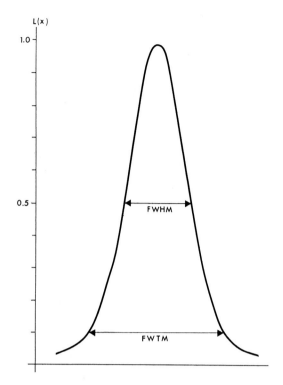

Figure 5.1. Line spread function, L(x), showing full width at half maximum (FWHM) and full width at tenth maximum (FWTM). FWHM is the figure usually quoted as a measure of resolution.

sinusoidally in the x-direction with a frequency ν (Figure 5.2). The modulation of this distribution, m_i, is defined as the amplitude (peak-to-peak) of the curve divided by twice the mean value. The source distribution recorded by the gamma camera will also have a modulation, m_o. The modulation transfer function is given by m_o/m_i and is a function of the frequency. A perfect imaging system would have an MTF of unity at all frequencies.

For a symmetrical line spread function, the MTF may be obtained as a normalized Fourier transform:

$$MTF(\nu) = \int L(x) \cos(2\pi\nu x) dx / \int L(x) dx.$$

In practice, although treated mathematically as a continuous function, the line spread function data are in a discrete form, being the count rates L_i within the ith pixel; if we consider each pixel to have a width dx, then, for any arbitrary value of ν, the MTF can be calculated as:

$$MTF(\nu) = \Sigma_i L_i \cos(2\pi i \nu \Delta x) / \Sigma_i L_i.$$

QUALITY ASSURANCE

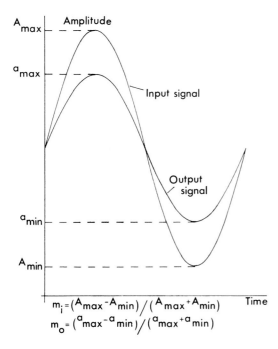

Figure 5.2. Response of an imaging system to a sinusoidal input. The input (m_i) and output (m_o) modulations are given by the formulae shown.

There will be an MTF curve for each set of operating conditions, i.e. collimators, distance from collimator face to source, presence or absence of scatter etc. Typical MTF curves are shown in Figure 5.3.

Non-uniformity

The non-uniformity is a measure of the slightly different response of different areas of the detector to irradiation by a uniform source. This may be measured also with or without the collimator. Although an image obtained on photographic film is adequate for daily assessment, quantitative data from a digital (computer) image are necessary for comparison purposes. In the latter case, it is the variation in pixel count values which is analyzed.

It is usual to carry out the calculations for both the geometrical field of view (GFOV) – the whole usable field of view – and the central field of view (CFOV); the CFOV is defined as an area, centered on the GFOV, having linear dimensions of the GFOV scaled by a factor of 0.75. In practice, for ease of calculation, the CFOV is defined as a circle having a radius 75% of the largest circle that it is possible to inscribe within the GFOV.

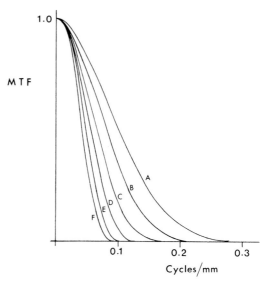

Figure 5.3. Modulation transfer curves for a modern gamma camera at 10 mm (A), 50 mm (B), 100 mm (C), 150 mm (D), 200 mm (E), and 250 mm (F) from the collimator face in scatter.

For both the GFOV and CFOV, the mean and standard deviation (SD) of the pixel counts are calculated. The coefficient of variation (CoV) of the pixel counts is given by $CoV = 100*(SD/C_m)$ where C_m is the mean pixel count. The integral non-uniformity, a measure of the range of pixel values, is given by

$$U(+) = 100(C_{max} - C_m)/C_m\%$$
$$U(-) = 100(C_{min} - C_m)/C_m\%$$

where C_{max} and C_{min} are the maximum and minimum pixel counts respectively. The differential non-uniformity, measuring the rate of change of pixel count values, is defined by

$$U_d = 100(C/M)\%$$

where C is the maximum difference in counts between two adjacent pixels and M is the larger of the two counts.

Spatial Distortion

The coordinates calculated by the detector for any event are subject to both random and systematic errors, the result being that events are plotted at the wrong location in the image. This effect is known as spatial distortion, occasionally (and incorrectly) termed linearity. It is measured by imaging a set of equispaced parallel line sources or a grid.

Integral spatial distortion is assessed by calculating the variation in distances between adjacent pairs of line source images, while differential spatial distortion measures the maximum "ripple" in adjacent segments of any one line image.

Sensitivity

Sensitivity may be regarded as the detection efficiency of the camera. It is defined as the counting-rate obtained per unit radioactivity in a standard source geometry. It is affected primarily by the choice of collimator and deteriorates as resolution improves for a given camera. It is a function also of the energy window chosen.

The geometric efficiency of a collimator is often quoted by manufacturers. This is the ratio of the number of photons entering the collimator to the number emitted per unit area by the source. It is related to sensitivity by the intrinsic efficiency.

Count Rate Characteristic

A gamma camera has a pulse processing time associated with each event and so, as the counting rate increases, a region is reached in which the response of the camera (observed count rate) is no longer linear with increasing source radioactivity (true count rate). A typical curve is shown in Figure 5.4. The theoretical linear response is obtained by extrapolation of the data points corresponding to count rates below 10 000 counts per second, it being assumed that no data loss occurs below this rate.

The point at which the data loss is, say, 10% can be defined in one of two ways. It could be the point at which the observed count rate is 90% of the corresponding true count rate or where the true count rate is 10% greater than the observed count rate. The first definition has been adopted and it is usual to quote the observed count rates at which the data loss is 10, 20, and 30% (i.e. at which the observed count rate is 90, 80, and 70% of the corresponding true count rate). When data loss becomes significant, quantitative studies may be compromised and it is good practice not to operate a gamma camera at counting rates beyond that at which 10% of the data are lost.

Note that some cameras offer a "fast count rate" mode for dynamic studies. Although this raises the count rate at which 10% data loss occurs, it is important to establish whether spatial resolution deteriorates as a consequence and, if so, whether it remains within acceptable limits.

Energy Resolution

The energy analyzer of the camera is where events associated with scattered photons are rejected. The ability of the analyzer to accomplish this is dependent upon the width of the photopeak in the energy spectrum, usually expressed in terms of the FWHM. This is an important parameter for emission tomography, where better discrimination against scattered photons leads to improved tomographic uniformity.

5.2.2 General Test Conditions

In the case of multi-headed systems, the following tests should be carried out for each detector. All measurements should be carried out at counting rates below 20 000 counts per second (cps) as specified in the standards; it is advisable to check the count rate performance (see Section 5.2.8) to ensure that the 10% loss rate exceeds this value prior to conducting other tests. It is good practice to cover the detector with a sheet of plastic in case of any leaks from phantoms and to enclose active phantoms in a further plastic bag.

1. Since modern cameras have an energy resolution of approximately 10% full width at half maximum (FWHM) for ^{99m}Tc, set the energy analyzer window at 15% (i.e. ±7.5%), centered on 141 keV.
2. Remove the collimator and position a point source of 100 MBq (3 mCi) of ^{99m}Tc at a distance of more than 2 m from the detector, on the central axis.
3. Carefully peak the camera (i.e. check that the photopeak is correctly positioned within the window), according to the manufacturer's instructions.
4. Carry out any calibration procedures required by the manufacturer (e.g. flood field acquisition) immediately prior to QA measurements.

5.2.3 Intrinsic Resolution

The intrinsic resolution should be measured using a transmission phantom such as that described by NEMA [14], but having slits of 0.5 mm thickness rather than the 1 mm specified, since the latter is some 25% of the FWHM of modern cameras and will lead to distortion of the results. The phantom (Figure 5.5) must be aligned carefully with

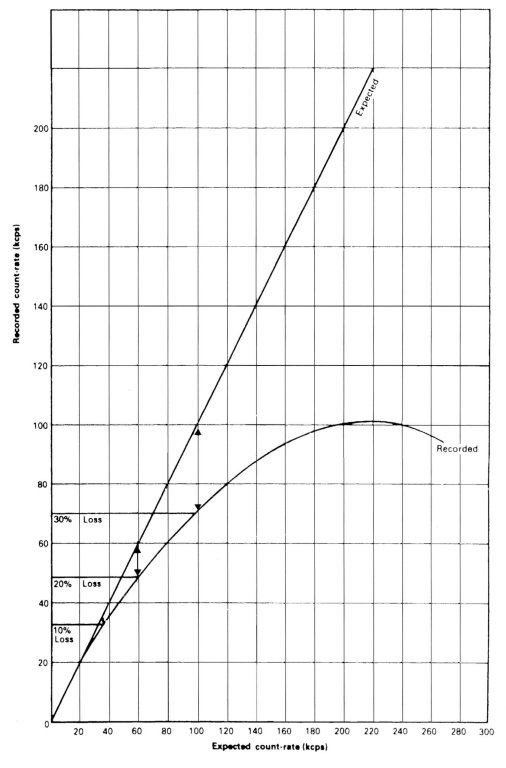

Figure 5.4. Typical count rate performance curve for an Anger-type gamma camera.

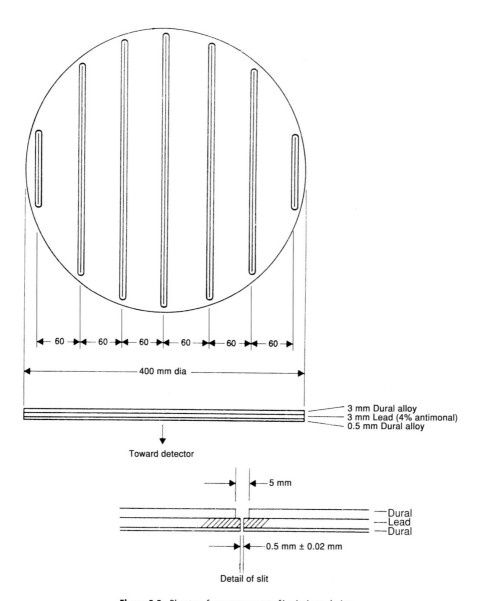

Figure 5.5. Phantom for measurement of intrinsic resolution.

the camera's x (or y) electronic axes, with one of the slits being positioned as closely as possible to the center-line of the field of view (FoV), it being usual to assume that the minimum spatial distortion will occur on the central axes of the FoV.

In order to achieve the requirement of 10 channels per FWHM, it is necessary to collect data from a 400 mm FoV into a 2048 resolution matrix, well beyond the capabilities of most nuclear medicine computer systems even using any "zoom" facility. In cases where the analogue to digital converter

(ADC) gains are readily accessible, it may be possible to achieve the desired resolution by increasing the gain of one axis at a time and imaging a portion of the FoV. If this is not feasible, the highest resolution matrix offered by the system should be employed.

1. Remove the collimator.
2. Place the phantom centrally on the camera face (if the electronic axis is marked, align the central slit of the phantom with this by eye)

3. Mask the area outside the FoV with lead sheeting of a minimum 3 mm thickness.

4. Place an uncollimated source containing some 750 MBq (20 mCi) of ^{99m}Tc vertically above the center of the FoV at a distance of more than five times the FoV in order to give approximately parallel beam conditions (i.e. uniform irradiation across the FoV).

5. Acquire a test image containing 2 000 000 counts.

6. If, say, the intrinsic x-resolution is being measured, reformat the image data to give 16 profiles parallel to the x-axis.

7. For each peak in each of the top, bottom, and center profiles, establish the centroid. This may be accomplished either by fitting a Gaussian function or by other peak fitting routines.

8. Check that the centroids of the peaks corresponding to the central slit occur in the same channel (to an error of less than 1%); if not, realign the phantom and repeat from step 5.

9. Acquire the image for analysis. In acquiring the data, a peak channel count of 10 000 should be attained in the profiles for definitive performance measurements. Since the standard deviation of the count may be approximated by its square root (100), this value will give a 1% standard deviation, statistically highly accurate. Thus, if the y-axis resolution of the acquisition matrix is 256, a peak pixel count of approximately 700 (10 000/16) should be obtained. Waddington et al. [22] have shown that, for routine QA, a peak channel count exceeding 1000 is satisfactory, provided a Gaussian peak-fitting routine is employed.

10. For each peak image in each profile, establish the centroid, and FWHM and FWTM in channels.

11. Calculate the calibration factor required to convert channels to millimeters (mm) by measuring the distance (in channels) between the centroids of adjacent peaks and calculating a grand mean, which can be equated to the known separation between the slits in the phantom. Use this to express FWHM and FWTM in mm.

12. If the user does not have access to such a phantom, the measurement can be made with a line source of 30 mm length and 0.5 mm internal diameter (a capillary tube) mounted behind two lead blocks 50 mm thick and spaced 0.5 mm apart (Figure 5.6). The source should contain approximately 70 MBq (2 mCi) of ^{99m}Tc.

13. Remove the collimator.

14. Place the blocks and source in the center of the FoV and align the source parallel to the y-axis.

15. Mask the remainder of the FoV with lead sheeting of a minimum 3 mm thickness.

16. Acquire an image as in step 9 above.

17. Repeat with the blocks displaced a measured distance along the x-axis.

18. Calculate the calibration factor required to convert channels to millimeters by measuring the distance in channels between the centroids of the peaks from these two acquisitions and equating this to their known separation.

19. Repeat steps 14 and 15 for at least four other random positions within the FoV, the source being aligned parallel to the y-axis in each case.

20. Repeat steps 2 to 7 with the source aligned parallel to the x-axis.

21. Calculate the FWHM and FWTM for each peak.

The data that should be logged are the means, coefficients of variation (CoV), and ranges of FWHM and FWTM for both x- and y-axes. The CoV for both measurements should be less than 5% for a well-adjusted camera and there should be no significant difference between axes.

5.2.4 System Resolution

This is the resolution obtained with the collimator in place and, in line with the IEC/BSI recommendations, should be measured in the presence of scatter to give clinically meaningful results. The phantom used (Figure 5.7) comprises parallel line sources filled with a uniform solution of ^{99m}Tc. In order to ensure that the diameter of the source does not affect the result, the internal diameter of the line source should be no more than 1 mm

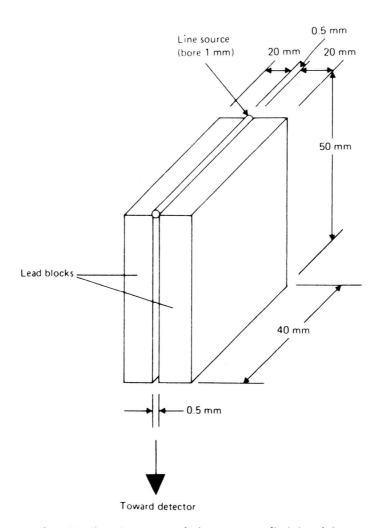

Figure 5.6. Alternative arrangement for the measurement of intrinsic resolution.

and, preferably, 0.5 mm. The line source should extend beyond the FoV and should be checked for straightness. A minimum of two line sources, placed 60 mm apart to avoid overlap of images at depth, should be employed; this permits a check to be made on the pixel size calibration at each depth.

1. Fill the line sources with a solution of ^{99m}Tc having a concentration of 700 MBq ml^{-1} (20 mCi ml^{-1}).

2. Place the phantom on the collimator surface (the line source centers at 10 mm from the surface) and align the sources as closely as possible with the camera's electronic axis.

3. Place sheets of Perspex on top of the phantom to give an overall depth of 200 mm.

4. Carry out data acquisition and analysis as in Section 5.2.3, steps 5 to 11.

5. Repeat the measurement with the line sources at distances of 50, 100, and 150 mm from the collimator surface, placing sheets of Perspex in front of and behind the phantom to maintain an overall depth of 200 mm.

6. Repeat the measurement with the phantom placed on the collimator surface (line source centers at 10 mm depth) and the sources aligned with the other electronic axis.

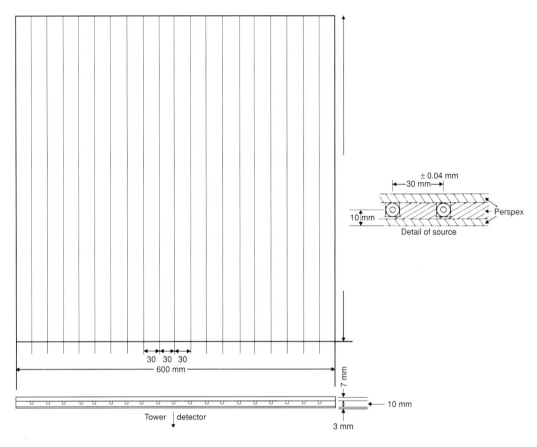

Figure 5.7. Line source phantom for the measurement of system resolution. When filling this phantom the radioactive solution should be colored with a little dye or ink so that complete filling of each line source can be checked readily.

7. Repeat the measurements for each low-energy collimator. The results should be compared with the manufacturer's data and checked to ensure that there is no difference between the 10 mm results for the two axes – if there is, there is a flaw in the collimator (such as a split in one of glued foil construction) and it should be returned to the manufacturer.

5.2.5 Sensitivity

Plane sensitivity is determined for each collimator using the source shown in Figure 5.8.

1. Fill the phantom with a solution containing a known quantity (approximately 70 MBq (2 mCi)) of ^{99m}Tc and mix well. Note the time of preparation.

2. Obtain a count for 300 seconds without the source present.

3. Position the source, in air, 100 mm above the collimator surface in the center of the FoV.

4. Record the total counts obtained in a 100 s acquisition.

5. Correct the count for background and for radioactive decay since the preparation of the phantom to obtain the sensitivity in counts per second per MBq.

6. Repeat steps 2 to 5 for all low-energy collimators.

5.2.6 Non-uniformity

System

It is the system non-uniformity (i.e. with the collimator fitted) that is the more important in clinical

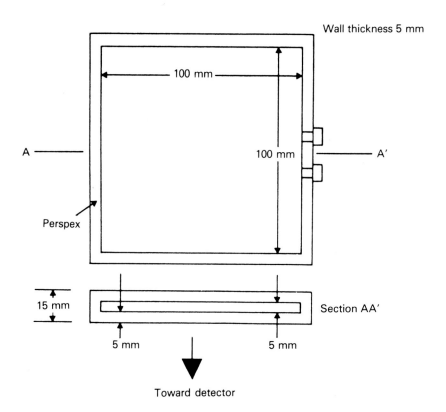

Figure 5.8. Source used for measurement of plane sensitivity.

use, particularly in emission tomography. All users should be familiar with the best flood field image that is possible with their camera so that any deterioration is recognized. The uniform (flood field) source (Figure 5.9) should be larger than the camera's FoV and should be well mixed; since the performance of modern cameras can vary between 122 and 141 keV, it is preferable to use a ^{99m}Tc flood source rather than a solid ^{57}Co source. Also, the uniformity of solid sources (comprising a layer of radioactive material sealed into a plastic disk) is now approximately the same, if not worse, than that of the camera itself.

1. Add a known quantity (approximately 200 MBq or 6 mCi) of ^{99m}Tc to the phantom and note the time.

2. Mix well and, if possible, leave for at least one hour to equilibrate. A possible alternative is to use an automated system to fill the phantom with a pre-mixed radioactive solution.

3. Place the highest resolution, low-energy collimator available on the camera.

4. Place the flood source on the collimator surface.

5. For daily QA, acquire both analogue and digital images containing not less than 3 000 000 counts; the digital image should be collected into a 64 × 64 matrix. Note the acquisition time.

6. Calculate and note an index of sensitivity by dividing the counting rate by the corrected activity in the source. The most likely cause for discrepancy in this figure is inaccuracy in setting the energy window.

7. Examine the analogue image for intensity, inspect the dot size and shape and make a visual assessment of the uniformity of the image. Log any adjustments to camera or display settings. Examine the digital image for any gross abnormality.

In addition to the daily test, a flood field image containing at least 30 000 000 counts should

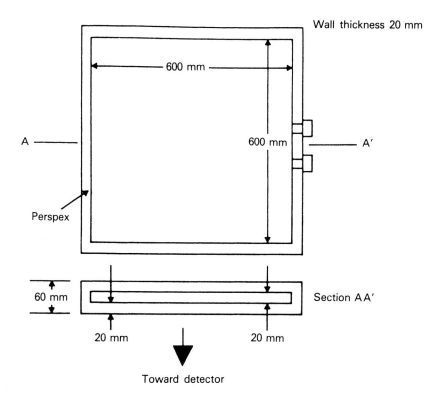

Figure 5.9. Source used for measurement of system non-uniformity (flood source).

be acquired into the computer system once per week; it is convenient to carry out this acquisition overnight or, if scheduling permits, over a lunch break – at an initial count rate of 20 000 counts per second (see Section 5.2.2), the acquisition will take approximately half an hour.

1. Prepare the flood source as above.

2. Acquire a 30 000 000 image into a 64 × 64 matrix.

3. Define regions of interest (ROIs) encompassing the geometrical and central fields of view.

4. Process the data within the GFOV and CFOV separately to yield values for mean pixel count and CoV.

5. Prepare a histogram showing the number of pixels containing values up to 15% from the mean in 2.5% steps. For a current generation camera, no pixels should be more than 10% from the mean.

6. Calculate the integral non-uniformity according to Section 5.2.1.

7. Calculate the differential non-uniformity according to Section 5.2.1.

8. Log the results obtained from steps 4 to 7.

A typical set of data is shown in Figure 5.10. The data should be subjected to trend analysis to detect the onset of any drift in the system. The pixel value histogram is more sensitive to changes in performance than the global uniformity figures. It is advisable to archive these flood field images.

Intrinsic

This requires the availability of a 3 mm thick lead masking ring to limit the FoV to that defined by the collimators. If this is unavailable, the edges of the crystal should be masked to eliminate edge effects and acquisition carried out using a FoV larger than the collimator exit field. The intrinsic non-uniformity is a simpler test to carry out than the system measurement, particularly if studies are undertaken at different energies, obviating the need to fill a flood source and ensure mixing.

```
NO     JE PIXELS = 2559.0     MEAN  COUNT    =    8396.2
RANGE    = +    8.2 PERCENT   TO    -     7.5  PERCENT
SD    =   152.8   COUNTS      COV   =   1.8  PERCENT
MAX    COUNT    =  9087.0    MIN  COUNT  =  7768.0
DIFF   UNIF   =   10.53  PERCENT  AT   5, 28  AND   4, 29
```

% OF MEAN	NO OF PIXELS	% OF PIXELS
80	0.0	0.0
81	0.0	0.0
82	0.0	0.0
83	0.0	0.0
84	0.0	0.0
85	0.0	0.0
86	0.0	0.0
87	0.0	0.0
88	0.0	0.0
89	0.0	0.0
90	0.0	0.0
91	0.0	0.0
92	1.0	.0
93	2.0	.1
94	9.0	.4
95	47.0	1.8
96	117.0	4.6
97	250.0	9.8
98	408.0	15.9
99	458.0	17.9
100	488.0	19.1
101	345.0	13.5
102	248.0	9.7
103	112.0	4.4
104	43.0	1.7
105	23.0	.9
106	4.0	.2
107	3.0	.1
108	1.0	.0
109	0.0	0.0
110	0.0	0.0
111	0.0	0.0
112	0.0	0.0
113	0.0	0.0
114	0.0	0.0
115	0.0	0.0
116	0.0	0.0
117	0.0	0.0
118	0.0	0.0
119	0.0	0.0
120	0.0	0.0

```
%  PIXELS  WITHIN  1%  OF  MEAN  =  37.0
%  PIXELS  WITHIN  2%  OF  MEAN  =  66.0
%  PIXELS  WITHIN  3%  OF  MEAN  =  85.9
%  PIXELS  WITHIN  4%  OF  MEAN  =  94.8
%  PIXELS  WITHIN  5%  OF  MEAN  =  98.3
%  PIXELS  WITHIN  6%  OF  MEAN  =  99.6
%  PIXELS  WITHIN  7%  OF  MEAN  =  99.8
%  PIXELS  WITHIN  8%  OF  MEAN  = 100.0
%  PIXELS  WITHIN  9%  OF  MEAN  = 100.0
%  PIXELS  WITHIN  10% OF  MEAN  = 100.0
```

Figure 5.10. Sample printout of analysis of data from non-uniformity measurement.

1. Remove the collimator and position the masking ring or shield the crystal edges with 3 mm thick lead.
2. Place an uncollimated source of approximately 100 MBq (3 mCi) of ^{99m}Tc axially with the center of the FoV at a distance not less than five times the GFOV.
3. Acquire a 30 000 000 count image.
4. Carry out the data analysis as for the system non-uniformity, using the same ROIs as for the latter.

5. Repeat this test for one high-energy (e.g. ^{131}I) and one low-energy (e.g. ^{201}Tl or ^{133}Xe) radionuclide.

It is vital to ensure that there are no artifacts due to nearby radioactive sources or to radiation scattered from nearby structures.

5.2.7 Spatial Distortion

This test utilizes the data obtained for both x- and y-axes when measuring the intrinsic resolution using the NEMA phantom (Section 5.2.3).

1. For each line image, average the peak centroid positions in the profiles to give the mean channel corresponding to the position of the line.
2. For each line image, calculate the absolute magnitudes of the differences between the mean channel for that line and the fitted positions for each line segment.
3. Calculate the mean and standard deviation of the deviations in millimeters using the calibration factor obtained above.
4. Express the mean as a percentage of the GFOV diameter.
5. Calculate the maximum difference between fitted peak positions for any line in adjacent profiles. This is a measure of differential spatial distortion [11].

If the NEMA intrinsic resolution phantom is not available, use the system resolution data (Section 5.2.4) for the line sources at a depth of 10 mm on both axes as the input data for this test. This will be an inferior measurement due to the distortions introduced by the collimator.

5.2.8 Count Rate Performance

As detailed above, it is desirable to operate a gamma camera at counting rates at which there is no appreciable data loss. Although measurements can be made more readily in air without the collimator, the clinical situation is more closely approximated by the phantom suggested by the IEC standard [15]. This phantom, however, is suited only to the ideal method of conducting this test, which is to place a fixed amount of radioactivity (several GBq or tens of mCi) in the phantom and take readings of counting rate as the source decays.

QUALITY ASSURANCE

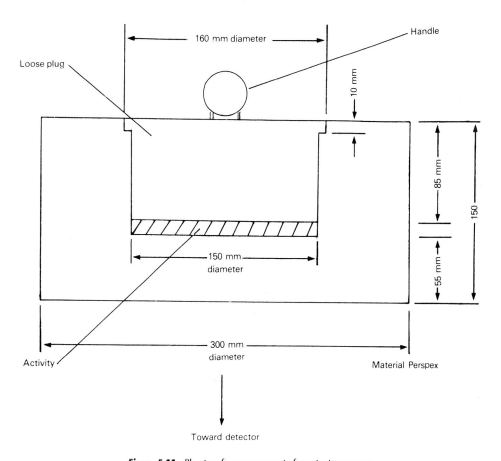

Figure 5.11. Phantom for measurement of count rate response.

This will take some 10 half-lives and is usually impractical. An alternative phantom (Figure 5.11) and method is described [12].

1. Prepare three solutions of ^{99m}Tc of known concentrations, approximately 20 MBq ml^{-1}, 200 MBq ml^{-1}, and 2000 MBq ml^{-1} (0.5 mCi ml^{-1}, 5 mCi ml^{-1}, and 50 mCi ml^{-1}). Note the times at which the activity was assayed.

2. Place the phantom in the center of the FoV and record a background count for 300 seconds.

3. Add 0.5 ml of the lowest concentration solution to the active volume of the phantom and record the total counts acquired over 50 seconds. Record the time at which the count started and the total amount of radioactivity in the phantom.

4. Repeat step 3 until the lowest concentration solution is exhausted, then add the medium concentration solution and, finally, the highest concentration solution.

5. Continue to add to the active volume until the observed counting rate begins to decrease, as evidenced by three consecutive decreasing readings.

6. For each data point, correct the observed counting rate for background count rate and for radioactive decay from the start of the test.

7. Graph the corrected counting rate against the amount of radioactivity present.

8. Making the assumption that there are no data losses at counting rates less than 10 000 counts per second (cps), derive the theoretical linear response function

by applying a linear regression to data points below this rate.

9. Superimpose the derived response on the graph and determine the observed counting rate at which the observed curve shows losses of 10, 20, and 30% with respect to the theoretical linear response.

5.2.9 Energy Resolution

In modern cameras, the energy signal has already been modified by passage through the energy signal correction circuits, but it is usually possible to obtain the unmodified signals.

1. Place a ^{99m}Tc flood source on the surface of the highest resolution low-energy collimator available as in Section 5.2.6.

2. Input the unmodified energy signals to a multichannel analyzer, adjusting the gain so that there are at least 10 channels within the FWHM of the photopeak.

3. Accumulate the spectrum until there are at least 10 000 counts in the peak channel.

4. Apply a Gaussian peak-fitting routine to the spectrum to obtain the centroid (C_{Tc}) and FWHM of the photopeak.

5. Replace the ^{99m}Tc flood source with a ^{57}Co source and accumulate a second spectrum until there are 10 000 counts in the peak channel.

6. Apply the Gaussian peak-fitting routine to obtain the centroid of the photopeak (C_{Co}).

7. Using the centroids of the two photopeaks, calculate the keV/channel calibration factor as; $F = 19/(C_{Tc} - C_{Co})$.

8. Calculate the energy resolution (E) as; $E = FWHM \times F/141 \times 100\%$.

A less rigorous measure of energy resolution may be made using the camera itself.

1. Set up the camera's energy analyzer as detailed in Section 5.2.2.

2. Reset the window width to 1 keV.

3. Note the number of counts acquired in 30 seconds and calculate the count rate.

4. Calculate the counting period necessary to accumulate 10 000 counts and use this as the count time for subsequent acquisitions.

5. Set the window center-line (photopeak position) to 120 keV.

6. Record the number of counts acquired in the calculated count period.

7. Increase the window center-line setting by 1 keV.

8. Repeat steps 3 and 4 until the window center-line has reached 160 keV.

9. Draw a graph of counts versus window center-line setting.

10. Measure the FWHM in keV directly from the graph and express as a percentage of 141 keV.

Note that this technique assumes that the camera's electronics do not retune (i.e. alter the peak setting) during the measurement. If the window width is expressed as a percentage, a 1% window can be used but an additional error is introduced (the measurement window varies from 1.2 to 1.6 keV). It is still possible to use the result for comparative purposes.

5.2.10 Whole Body Scanning

There are two approaches to achieving this – the continuous motion and step-and-shoot methods. In the latter case, the performance is the same as in conventional static mode and it is necessary merely to ascertain that there is no overlap in the display. For continuous motion, the spatial resolution may deteriorate in the direction of motion and the scanning speed may vary.

Scanning Speed

1. Place a point source containing approximately 20 MBq (0.5 mCi) of ^{99m}Tc on the face of the collimator. Check that the count rate is between 5000 and 20 000 cps.

2. Acquire a whole body image into the standard matrix (usually 1024×256) at the slowest continuous speed that will be used clinically.

3. Repeat the acquisition at the fastest continuous speed that will be used clinically.

4. For both sets of data, obtain a profile along the direction of motion, the width being approximately the FWTM at 10 mm established in Section 5.2.4.

5. Calculate the mean channel count and standard deviation.

6. Any deviation from the mean greater than that due to statistical fluctuation (i.e. two standard deviations) indicates non-uniformity of scanning speed.

Spatial Resolution

1. Fill the line sources of the system resolution phantom (Figure 5.7) with a solution of ^{99m}Tc having a concentration of 700 MBq ml^{-1} (20 mCi ml^{-1}).

2. Place sheets of Perspex on the patient table above and below the phantom so that the centers of the line sources are at a depth of 100 mm.

3. Align the phantom so that the lines are perpendicular to the direction of motion.

4. Adjust the detector height so that it will scan over the phantom as closely as possible (within 10 mm).

5. Acquire a whole body image into the standard matrix (usually 1024 × 256) at the slowest continuous speed that will be used clinically.

6. Repeat the acquisition at the fastest continuous speed that will be used clinically.

7. Carry out data analysis as in Section 5.2.3.

8. Compare the resulting data with that obtained in Section 5.2.4 for the 100 mm depth.

Misregistration

1. Set the energy analyzer to ^{57}Co.

2. Attach a solid flood source of ^{57}Co to the detector.

3. Ensure that the count rate lies within the range 5000–20 000 cps.

4. Acquire a whole body image in step-and-shoot mode into the standard matrix (usually 1024 × 256), with a dwell time chosen to give at least 6 000 000 counts in the total image.

5. Obtain a profile along the direction of motion, the width being that of the FoV.

6. Calculate the mean channel count and standard deviation.

7. Any deviation from the mean greater than that due to statistical fluctuation (i.e. two standard deviations) is indicative of misalignment of adjacent parts of the image, either overlap or gap.

For a multi-headed system, the values of all of the above parameters should not differ by more than 10% between detectors, with any variation in sensitivity being less than 5%.

5.3 Emission Tomographs

Since few centers possess positron emission tomography (PET) facilities, this section is restricted to rotating camera single photon devices. Test methods for PET systems are given in IEC Document 61675–1 [23], NEMA Document NU2–2001 [24], and IPEM Report 86 [2]; they are detailed in Chapter 3.

5.3.1 Gantry Checks

1. Place a spirit level on the collimator with the detector in the 0° and 180° positions. If the gantry is vertical, the reading will be the same in both positions. If not, adjust the leveling.

2. Check that there is no play in the detector.

3. Ensure that the system returns "home" accurately.

4. Time the interval taken to rotate from 0° to 180° and from 180° to 360°. If these intervals are not identical, the rotational speed differs and should be rectified.

5. With the detector in the 90° and 270° positions, measure the distances from the detector to the bed. These should differ by less than 10 mm. Repeat this measurement with the bed at the extremes of its travel.

6. Using a point source of 50 MBq (1.5 mCi) of ^{99m}Tc, suspended approximately 1 m above the detector, ensure that the absorption caused by the bed does not exceed 5%.

5.3.2 Pixel Size Calibration

1. Prepare two point sources containing 20 MBq (0.5 mCi) of ^{99m}Tc.
2. Place the sources on the collimator surface, on the x-axis, approximately 50 mm from opposite edges of the FoV.
3. Acquire a 1 00 000 count planar image into a 128 × 128 matrix.
4. Repeat steps 2 and 3 with the sources on the y-axis.
5. Calculate the center of gravity of the point sources for each image as

$$CoG(x) = \Sigma_i.\Sigma_j i.M(i, j)/\Sigma_i.\Sigma_j M(i, j)$$
$$CoG(y) = \Sigma_i.\Sigma_j j.M(i, j)/\Sigma_i.\Sigma_j M(i, j)$$

where i and j are the indices in the x- and y-directions and M(i,j) is the pixel count at (i,j). The limits define a box, approximately 20 mm square centered on the point source image.
6. Obtain the calibration factors by dividing the actual distances in mm between the point sources by the distances calculated in pixels.
7. If the values differ by more than 5%, take remedial action and repeat.

The value of pixel size should be less than 4 mm. If it is not, it is necessary to repeat the test using a 256 × 256 matrix and to use this matrix size for all other tests.

5.3.3 Center of Rotation

The most critical parameter for a rotating camera SPECT system, apart from the performance of the detector head itself, is the center of rotation (CoR) offset. When an axially rotating detector device (such as a rotating camera) is used, the axis of rotation is taken as the origin of the tomographic plane. The center of each projection should therefore be aligned with the same axis. The actual center of rotation has to be measured as a matrix position and the difference between this and the center of the matrix (the CoR offset) input to the computer so that the projections can be shifted to align the centers prior to reconstruction.

1. Place a point source containing 200 MBq (6 mCi) of ^{99m}Tc in air, within 20 mm of the axis of rotation and within 20 mm of the center of the FoV.
2. Using a 200 mm radius of rotation, perform a 32-angle tomographic acquisition into a 128 × 128 matrix, collecting a minimum of 10 000 counts at each angle.
3. Repeat step 2 with the point source placed 100 mm radially from the center of rotation.
4. Calculate CoG(x) and CoG(y), as in Section 5.3.2 step 5, for each image.
5. Plot CoG(x) as a function of angle over the total angle of rotation.
6. Fit a sine function $(A + B. \sin(\theta + \phi))$ where θ is the angle of rotation and A, B, and ϕ are constants.
7. The CoR offset is given by the magnitude of the difference between the expected center of the matrix (64.5) and the constant A.
8. If the CoR offset is greater than 1 mm, take corrective action and repeat. The CoR offsets estimated at the center and edge of the FoV should be within 2 mm of each other.

If the CoR offset is not independent of the position of the point source within the FoV, it may be an indication that the y-axis is not aligned with the axis of rotation. Note that the value obtained is valid only for the collimator tested.

5.3.4 Tomographic Resolution

1. Prepare a point source containing 200 MBq (6 mCi) of ^{99m}Tc.
2. Place the point source in air within 10 mm of the CoR, near the center of the FoV.
3. Select a 15 cm radius of rotation.
4. Perform a tomographic acquisition into a 128 × 128 matrix, collecting not less than 10 000 counts per view at each of 128 angles.
5. Reconstruct the data using a ramp or sharp filter (see Section 2.2.2).
6. Repeat steps 3 to 5 with the point source positioned 80 mm off-axis.
7. Draw profiles through the image of the point source in the reconstructed images

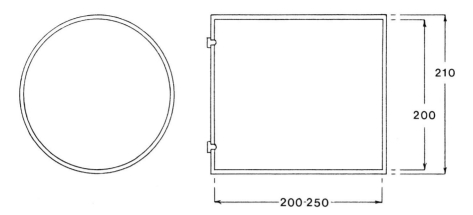

Figure 5.12. Phantom used to measure tomographic uniformity. Measurements are in mm.

and measure the FWHM in both the horizontal and vertical directions.

8. Measure the corresponding FWHMs on one of the projection views.

9. If the tomographic FWHM is more than 15% worse than the planar, check the CoR correction and repeat; if still poor, check the system for vibration.

5.3.5 Tomographic Uniformity

1. Fill the tomographic uniformity phantom (Figure 5.12) with a solution containing 350–700 MBq (10–20 mCi) of ^{99m}Tc.

2. Fit the low-energy, all-purpose collimator.

3. Position the phantom so that its axis is parallel with the axis of rotation and its center is not more than 20 mm from the CoR.

4. Select a 64 angle acquisition, collecting data into a 64 × 64 matrix.

5. Perform a tomographic study, collecting 500 000 counts per planar view.

6. Reconstruct the data with a ramp or sharp filter, having carried out uniformity correction if necessary. Whether it is appropriate will depend on the non-uniformity measured in Section 5.2.6; if the CoV is less than 2–3%, the application of a uniformity correction will introduce a larger error into the projection data than the non-uniformity it-

self. If a correction is applied, it must be based upon a stored flood field image containing at least 30 000 000 counts obtained as in Section 5.2.6.

7. Perform attenuation and scatter correction, if available.

8. Place a profile 5 pixels wide through the center of the image.

9. Identify the minimum or maximum value corresponding to the location of any ring artifact seen on the reconstructed image (see Section 2.4.1); record this value ($C_{min/max}$).

10. Record the two values, C1 and C2, along the profile just beyond the edges of the artifact.

11. Calculate $C_{ave} = (C1 + C2)/2$.

12. Estimate the contrast as:

$$(C_{min/max} - C_{ave})/(C_{min/max} + C_{ave})$$

13. Repeat steps 8 to 12 for all other transaxial sections and determine the maximum absolute value of contrast. This should not exceed 10% [25].

14. For a central slice, place 5 × 5 pixel ROIs over the center and edge of the image. The difference between these should not exceed 10% [25].

5.3.6 System Performance Check

1. Fill a total performance (Jaszczak) phantom with a solution containing 700 MBq (20 mCi) of ^{99m}Tc.

2. Fit the highest resolution, low-energy collimator available.

3. Align the phantom parallel to the axis of rotation, displaced approximately 20 mm from the CoR.

4. Check the counting rate and calculate the acquisition time per planar view to collect a total of not less than 100 000 000 counts for the whole study.

5. Acquire a tomogram into a 128×128 matrix, using a 15 cm radius of rotation.

6. Reconstruct the tomogram using a ramp or sharp filter.

7. Place a profile 5 pixels wide through the center of the image of the uniform region of the phantom and measure the ratio of counts at the center to counts at the edge. Measure the amplitude in percent of any artifacts as described in Section 5.3.5.

8. Note the number of spherical lesions that are detected successfully and, by using appropriate profiles or ROIs, measure the contrast of these lesions.

5.4 Computer System

5.4.1 Analogue to Digital Converters

These are the most important components of the system and are often neglected. Other than utilizing a precision ramp generator, the tests that can be carried out are limited, as is the degree of user adjustment.

1. Prepare and position a point source as for the measurement of intrinsic uniformity described in Section 5.2.6.

2. Remove the collimator.

3. Acquire a 120 000 000 count image into the largest matrix offered by the acquisition software.

4. Create a profile in the x-direction, centered on the x-axis and 10 pixels wide.

5. Create an equivalent profile for the y-direction.

6. For each profile, fit a linear regression to the data and record the slope. The slope of the regression is a measure of the integral non-linearity and should be zero if the ADC is perfectly linear over its range.

7. For each data point in the profile, calculate the difference ($d(i)$) between the actual value ($a(i)$) and that expected from the regression ($c(i)$).

8. For each pair of adjacent points, calculate the absolute magnitude of $d(i) - d(i + 1)$. The largest value obtained is a measure of the differential non-linearity.

For SPECT imaging, differential non-linearity is the more important parameter and a more sensitive test has been described by Gillen and Elliott [26]. This employs the normalized Fourier transform of the profile, in which the value of the zero spatial frequency component should be one, with all other components zero. Any bit giving rise to differential non-linearity will give rise to a non-zero value at the corresponding frequency.

5.4.2 Hardware Tests

In addition to the following, run the disk and memory tests which should be provided by the supplier.

Timing Test

Assuming that the software accesses the clock correctly, the timing functions of the computer are determined by the accuracy of the clock itself.

1. Place a source of 100 MBq (3 mCi) of ^{99m}Tc in the center of the camera's FoV.

2. Set up a static acquisition, into a 64×64 matrix, for a preset time of 300 seconds.

3. Start the data collection and a reliable stopwatch simultaneously.

4. Record the stopwatch reading at the end of data collection and check the acquisition time recorded by the computer.

5. Compare the time recorded on the stopwatch with the requested and recorded acquisition times. All three values should be identical.

System Count Rate Performance

This may be assessed at the same time as the camera's count rate performance (Section 5.2.8).

1. Prior to the phantom being placed on the camera, acquire a 50 second background frame.

2. At each data point, acquire a 50 second static frame into a 64×64 matrix.

3. Correct the total counts in each frame for background and for radioactive decay from the start of the test.

4. Analyze the data as for the camera test.

In frame mode, the count rate capability of the computer should exceed that of the gamma camera and so the curves generated from the analogue and digital data should be essentially identical. If there is a difference of more than 5% in recorded counting rate, the computer system's performance is unsatisfactory.

Where a multi-headed camera is connected, this test should be carried out for each detector operating alone and with all detectors acquiring simultaneously in order to ensure that there are no additional losses in the latter case. If the computer is capable of multi-tasking, the test should be repeated while any function thought to make a high processor demand (e.g. printing out a compressed image) is being carried out simultaneously.

Framing Rate Test

When a dynamic study is carried out, there may be data losses and/or timing errors between frames. These may become considerable at high counting and framing rates.

1. Place a source of ^{99m}Tc on the collimator surface to yield a counting rate of approximately 20 000 cps.

2. Note the total number of counts obtained in a 20 second period, using the camera's control console in order to calculate the counting rate accurately.

3. Set up a dynamic study as follows:
   framing rate – maximum accepted by the software
   matrix size – smallest offered by the software
   number of frames – selected to give total acquisition time of 30 seconds.

4. Start the study and a reliable stopwatch simultaneously.

5. Note the recorded time at the end of the study.

6. Calculate the apparent acquisition time for each frame by dividing the total counts in the frame by the known counting rate obtained in step 3.

7. Sum the apparent frame times and compare with the elapsed time recorded by the stopwatch and the 30 seconds requested. If there are significant discrepancies between any of these figures, remedial action should be taken.

8. If disk space permits, repeat the test for the largest matrix size offered by the software.

9. If the system permits acquisition at more than one terminal, repeat steps 3 to 7 with each terminal acquiring data simultaneously.

5.4.3 Software Tests

One of the first QA requirements, and the most important, for computer software, is the provision by the supplier of an adequate set of manuals. These must be clearly laid out, well indexed and contain adequate information on how to run each program. The latter may be provided by means of an online "help" facility. Less than adequate manuals may be indicative of the quality of the software itself. It is impossible to test all aspects of software, but the following investigate the more obvious facets of the system.

1. Write a user program to create a bar pattern, e.g. for a 64×64 matrix, write 16s into the first four rows, 32s into the next four rows etc.

2. Use this matrix to establish the display orientation (i.e. where is the point $(1,1)$ etc.) and that the programs controlling image rotation, display threshold, and saturation levels function correctly.

3. Define a one pixel width profile across the bars and check that the profile data are correct; repeat for multi-pixel width profiles, ensuring that the multiple of the original equals the specified pixel width.

4. Select a dynamic study and define three rectangular ROIs, one large and two dividing the large one in half. Note the number of pixels included in the ROIs.

5. Print out the area of each ROI and the number of counts within it for the frame on which they were defined; ensure that

the areas are correct and that the counts are summed correctly.

6. Generate the activity–time curves for each ROI, add the results from the smaller areas and ensure that the resulting curve is identical to that from the large area.

5.4.4 Software Audit

It is difficult to check on the absolute performance of the many programs within the suite offered on modern systems. It is good practice, however, to maintain a library of raw data which can be used as input to check that a new system gives the same results as that which it is replacing (or that a software update has not introduced any errors). While a difference in output does not necessarily indicate that the problem lies with the new system, it does demonstrate that further investigation is required.

The Institute of Physics and Engineering in Medicine has a Software Group which conducts audits across the UK and publishes the anonymized data; one example is that of renal data analysis [27]. Participation in such exercises is to be recommended.

5.5 Dose Calibrators

Other than battery failure, radionuclide dose calibrators are generally trouble-free in the short and medium term. Some long-term drift may occur, but is readily detected by a simple daily check. Centralized radiopharmaceutical production facilities, where the calibrator performance is more critical, normally carry out double checking of doses prior to dispatch on different calibrators; this in itself is a useful QA procedure for the calibrators.

The dose calibrator should be positioned in the area of the laboratory where the background radiation level may be expected to be at its lowest. In order to minimize the effect of transient background increase due to exposed sources, it is good practice to enclose the calibrator chamber in a lead shield. Note that shielding may affect the operation of a calibrator; all tests must be carried out in the working configuration.

The tests detailed in Sections 5.5.1, 5.5.2, 5.5.3, and 5.5.4 are required by the US Nuclear Regula-

tory Commission [28], while the IPSM has published guidance [29] and the IEC Standard [30] sets out the information to be provided by manufacturers.

5.5.1 Absolute Calibration Check

On delivery, the calibration certificate should be examined to ensure that the calibrator's performance is satisfactory and that the measurements on which it is based can be traced back to national standards of radioactivity.

External Standard Assay

1. Obtain sealed sources (preferably vial-type) of radionuclides emitting a range of gamma energies; the activities should be in the range 4–40 MBq (0.1–1 mCi). Suitable sources would be ^{133}Ba, ^{57}Co, ^{137}Cs, and ^{60}Co. These should be certified to an accuracy of better than 2% by a national or secondary standard laboratory.

2. Assay each source using the appropriate calibration factor and ensure that the result is within 2% of that stated; if not, take remedial action.

This is the primary test method laid out by the IEC for a "reference device" and should be used for at least one calibrator within a department. Further calibrators ("individual", or "field", devices) may utilize the secondary test method, whereby comparative measurements may be made against the reference device. The secondary test method may be employed usefully in a QA program organized by a central radiopharmacy.

Reproducibility Test

1. Prepare four vial sources of 10 ml solutions of ^{99m}Tc containing approximately 4, 40, 400, and 4000 MBq (0.1, 1, 10, and 100 mCi) of activity.

2. Assay each source and note the result.

3. Repeat step 2 ten times.

4. Calculate the standard deviations (SD) of the measurements for each source.

5. If any SD exceeds 1%, take remedial action.

5.5.2 Routine Calibration Test

It is sufficient to use a single long-lived source (e.g. ^{137}Cs or ^{226}Ra) for daily measurements, unless an error is detected, in which case a limited absolute re-calibration should be carried out.

1. Obtain a sealed source of ^{137}Cs (approximately 15 MBq) or ^{226}Ra (approximately 5 MBq), certified to an accuracy of 2–5%.

2. Assay the source at the time of the absolute calibration measurements, ensuring that the reading obtained is within the accuracy of the chamber, and record the result.

3. The source should be assayed at the start of each working day, using both the calibration settings for the radionuclide in use and for 141 keV, and the results recorded.

4. If the result is in error, take remedial action.

5.5.3 Geometrical Dependence

Even so-called "invariant response" chambers will yield slightly, sometimes markedly, different readings dependent on the geometry (i.e. volume and container) of the source being assayed. This is particularly so for low-energy gamma-cmitters such as ^{125}I and for beta-emitters such as ^{32}P, but should be much less of a problem for ^{99m}Tc.

1. Prepare a solution of ^{125}I at a concentration of approximately 20 MBq ml^{-1} (0.5 mCi ml^{-1}) from a solution of a known concentration.

2. Select the manufacturer's standard setting for ^{125}I on the calibrator.

3. Draw up a typical volume of the prepared solution into an appropriate syringe and assay.

4. Calculate the true activity in the source and compare with the assay result.

5. If these values differ, select the manual range (if appropriate) and adjust the calibration factor until the desired reading is obtained. Note the calibration factor.

6. Dispense the desired volume of the prepared solution into a typical container and assay.

7. Compare the assay result with the calculated source activity and, if different, proceed as in step 5.

8. Repeat steps 3 to 7 for all volumes and containers used routinely.

9. Repeat the above for other radionuclides such as ^{32}P.

This test should be repeated whenever the containers (or suppliers) are changed.

5.5.4 Saturation Level

The maximum activity that can be assayed in a dose calibrator is limited by the saturation characteristics of the chamber. As the rate of ion pair production increases, there is an increased space charge effect and a higher recombination probability. The chamber thus underestimates the true reading. Note that, since the current generated in the chamber per unit activity varies according to energy, saturation will occur at different levels for different radionuclides.

It is likely, however, that the only radionuclides for which the effect is of practical importance are ^{99m}Tc and ^{131}I, the latter only if high activity therapy doses are prepared.

1. Ascertain the saturation activity for ^{99m}Tc claimed by the manufacturer.

2. Prepare a solution containing approximately 125% of this activity. If such a quantity of activity will never be used in the facility, start the test with the maximum activity encountered in practice. The start activity can be calculated, to an acceptable accuracy, from the yield data of a Tc generator.

3. Assay the source and record the result.

4. Remove 5% of the activity from the vial, assay the quantity removed and re-assay the vial. Note the reading and the amount of activity remaining.

5. Repeat step 4 until only 5% of the original activity remains in the vial.

6. Use the data to construct a graph of the ratio of measured to true activity against true activity (Figure 5.13).

7. From the graph, determine the amount of activity at which the ratio has fallen to 0.95. This represents the maximum

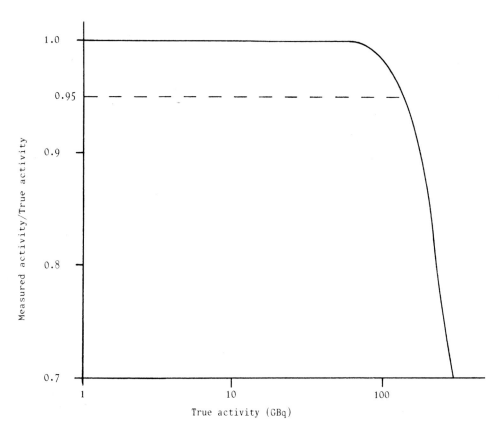

Figure 5.13. Saturation curve for a dose calibrator. Assuming a 5% error to be acceptable, the maximum activity capable of being assayed is approximately 300 GBq.

activity that the chamber can reliably assay.

5.6 Automatic Counters

Performance is most likely be affected by electronic drift (e.g. high voltage supply, amplifier) and by contamination. The testing of these (and manual counting systems) is described in a BSI/IEC document [31].

1. Within each counting run, include one of each of the standard and background samples at the beginning and end of each batch. Check that the background values are within normal limits for the energy window in use.

2. Check long-term stability of gamma counters by assaying standard sources (few kBq) of (for example) ^{133}Ba and/or ^{137}Cs.

3. In the case of liquid scintillation counters, monitor sensitivity by assaying an unquenched ^{14}C source.

4. For both types of counter, ensure that the expected count obtained from the standards is within statistical limits. Sensitivity variations > 2% are unacceptable.

5. The counting precision of the system should be tested by counting a standard 10 times for a fixed period to give at least 10 000 counts. Calculate χ^2 from

$$\chi^2 = \sum_i (N_i - M)^2 / M$$

where N_i ($i = 1$–10) are the individual counts obtained and M is the mean count. The resultant χ^2 value should lie within the range 3.3–16.9.

QUALITY ASSURANCE

5.7 Radiation Monitors

1. Check the probe for physical damage.
2. Check the battery level.
3. Inspect the calibration curve supplied with the instrument and ensure its accuracy over the stated range.
4. If a calibration source is supplied, check that the expected reading is obtained.

5.8 Acceptance Testing Schedule

At acceptance, all the tests specified above should be carried out and the results logged. Any parameter which does not comply with either the manufacturer's specification or the tender/contract document should be notified to the supplier, who should take immediate action to rectify the deficiency. A proportion of the purchase price (typically 5–10%) should be withheld until the acceptance tests yield satisfactory results.

5.9 Routine Quality Control Schedule

5.9.1 Daily Checks

Gamma Camera

1. Peak the camera for ^{99m}Tc (Section 5.2.2).
2. Carry out any calibration procedures specified by the manufacturer.
3. Collect and assess a 3 000 000 flood field image (Section 5.2.6).
4. Check for damage to the detector head, collimator surfaces, and mountings and collimator carts.

Emission Tomographs

SPECT – check the center of rotation offset (Section 5.3.3).

Dose Calibrators

Check the display and the zero adjustment and background suppression settings. The latter

should be investigated with and without any chamber liner or source-holder to ascertain any contamination. Obtain and log the reading obtained with the standard source (Section 5.5.2).

5.9.2 Weekly Checks

In addition to being carried out weekly, these tests should be carried out immediately following any preventative maintenance.

Gamma Camera

1. Collect and assess a 30 000 000 count flood field image (Section 5.2.6).
2. On a modern system, resolution is unlikely to deteriorate rapidly and so a qualitative test is sufficient. An image of a modified Anger phantom such as an "Anger + 3" [11] or of an ortho-hole phantom [32] should be scrutinized visually for evidence of worsening resolution. Of these, the ortho-hole phantom is superior since it also permits evaluation of spatial distortion. Both phantoms measure the intrinsic performance of the camera (i.e. without the collimator). For qualitative evaluation of system resolution and contrast, Murray et al. [33] have described a suitable phantom; an improved version is described in reference 12.

Emission Tomographs

SPECT – acquire and assess images of the total performance (Jaszczak) phantom (Section 5.3.6). This permits assessment of tomographic uniformity and resolution.

PET – collect and assess uniformity images

Computer System

1. Assess the ADC performance (Section 5.4.1).
2. Run disk and memory tests.

Radiation Monitors

1. Check the probe for physical damage.
2. Check the battery level.
3. Obtain and record the reading from the standard source.

5.9.3 Three-monthly Checks

The following parameters should be assessed every 3 months, or following modification or major servicing.

Gamma Cameras

1. Uniformity – acquire and assess a 30 000 000 count flood field image (Section 5.2.6).
2. Intrinsic resolution – measure for both x- and y-axes (Section 5.2.3).
3. Spatial distortion – obtain from the same raw data as the intrinsic resolution measurement, processing data as in Section 5.2.7.
4. Energy resolution – measure as specified for ^{99m}Tc (Section 5.2.9).
5. System resolution – only a single measurement of overall system resolution need be made as specified above (Section 5.2.4), using a given collimator at a depth of 100 mm in scatter and compared to the value obtained at installation.

Emission Tomograph

SPECT:

1. Carry out gantry checks (Section 5.3.1).
2. Measure pixel size (Section 5.3.2).
3. Check center of rotation offset (Section 5.3.3).
4. Assess tomographic resolution (Section 5.3.4).
5. Assess tomographic uniformity (Section 5.3.5).

PET:

1. Assess system sensitivity.
2. Assess system spatial resolution.

Computer System

1. Assess ADC performance (Section 5.4.1).
2. If hardware/software modifications have been made, run appropriate tests from Sections 5.4.2 and 5.4.3 in addition.

Dose Calibrator and Radiation Monitors

1. Wipe test the long-lived calibrator check source.

2. The calibration required under the Ionising Radiations Regulations or, in the USA, by the Nuclear Regulatory Commission should be carried out annually by an approved laboratory and a certificate of calibration obtained.

5.10 Implementation

5.10.1 Assessing the Data

It is important not only to make the QA measurements, but also to maintain a fault log for each machine. The latter should detail the fault manifested, the circumstances surrounding it (what was the machine doing at the time, any error messages output, etc.), the action taken to remedy the fault and, if appropriate, the response time of the service engineer.

In order to utilize the data, one member of the department should have the clear responsibility for supervising the QA program. This person should review the measurements weekly, although it must be impressed on all staff that any abnormal result must be notified to the supervisor immediately.

As emphasized above, the most powerful technique in QA is trend analysis; in its simplest and most effective form, this consists of simple graphs of numerical data against time. Faults in equipment may be detected as they begin to develop, hopefully before their effects are noticed practically. An example is the lowering of the percentage of pixels within 2.5 and 5% of the mean in a flood field image; gradual deterioration will be apparent in this figure before any visual change is noticed.

5.10.2 Servicing Arrangements

In general, gamma cameras and computer systems should be placed on a maintenance contract with the supplier. Other equipment may be repaired in-house or by return to the supplier. All service reports should be filed carefully and inspected for evidence of recurring failures. For equipment on contract, it is difficult to define situations in which manufacturers' service personnel should be called out. Clearly, if the performance of a piece of equipment deteriorates to the point where it no longer meets specification, action should be taken. The purpose of a QA program, however, is not just to ensure that performance is within specification but that it is kept at as high a level as possible, i.e. the best the equipment is capable of. Once a fault or deterioration in performance has been identified, remedial action should be instituted; the difference between such a case and a breakdown should be the response time, not whether there is a response.

References

1. Institute of Physical Sciences in Medicine. Report No. 44: An introduction to emission computed tomography. London: Institute of Physical Sciences in Medicine, 1985.
2. Institute of Physics and Engineering in Medicine. Report No. 86: Quality control of gamma camera systems. York: Institute of Physics and Engineering in Medicine; 2003.
3. American Association of Physicists in Medicine. AAPM Report No. 9: Computer aided scintillation camera acceptance testing. Chicago: American Association of Physicists in Medicine; 1982.
4. World Health Organization. Quality assurance in nuclear medicine. Geneva: World Health Organization; 1982.
5. US Department of Health and Human Services. HHS Publication FDA83-8209: Joint NCDRH and state quality assurance surveys in nuclear medicine; phase 1 – scintillation cameras and dose calibrators. Washington: US Government Printing Office; 1983.
6. US Department of Health and Human Services. HHS Publication FDA84-8224: Quality assurance in nuclear medicine: Proceedings of an international symposium and workshop Washington 1981. Washington: US Government Printing Office; 1984.
7. US Department of Health and Human Services. HHS Publication FDA85-8227: Recommendations for quality assurance programs in nuclear medicine facilities. Washington: US Government Printing Office; 1984.
8. British Standards Institution. Nuclear Medicine Instrumentation – Routine tests – Part 2: Scintillation cameras and single photon emission computed tomography equipment, PD IEC/TR 61948-2. London: British Standards Institution; 2001.
9. Department of Health and Social Security. Report STB/11/80: Performance assessment of gamma cameras – part I. London: Department of Health and Social Security; 1980.
10. Department of Health and Social Security. Report STB/13/82: Performance assessment of gamma cameras – part II. London: Department of Health and Social Security; 1982.
11. Department of Health and Social Security. Report STB6D/85/6: Performance assessment of gamma cameras – part III. London: Department of Health and Social Security; 1985.
12. Department of Health and Social Security. Report STB/86/9: Performance assessment of gamma cameras – part IV. London: Department of Health and Social Security; 1986.
13. National Electrical Manufacturers' Association. Standards for performance measurements of scintillation cameras. Washington: National Electrical Manufacturers' Association; 1981.
14. National Electrical Manufacturers' Association. Publication NEMA NU1-1986: Performance measurements of scintillation cameras. Washington: National Electrical Manufacturers' Association; 1986.
15. International Electrotechnical Commission. Publication 789: Characteristics and test conditions of radionuclide imaging devices; Anger type gamma cameras. Geneva: International Electrotechnical Commission; 1992.
16. International Electrotechnical Commission. Publication IEC61675-2: Characteristics and test conditions of radionuclide imaging devices Part 2: single photon emission computed tomographs. Geneva: International Electrotechnical Commission; 1995.
17. International Electrotechnical Commission. Publication IEC61675-3: Characteristics and test conditions of radionuclide imaging devices Part 3: gamma camera based wholebody imaging systems. Geneva: International Electrotechnical Commission; 1995.
18. British Standards Institution. British Standard 6609: Methods of test for radionuclide imaging devices. London: British Standards Institution; 1985.
19. Wells CP, Buxton-Thomas M. Gamma camera purchasing. Nucl Med Commun 1995; 16:168–185.
20. Tindale WB. Specifying dual detector gamma cameras and associated computer systems. Nucl Med Commun 1995; 16:534–538.
21. British Nuclear Medicine Society. Gamma camera and data processor system tender questionnaire (version 3.1). www.bnms.org.uk; 2003.
22. Waddington WA, Clarke GA, Barnes KJ, et al. A reappraisal of current methods for the assessment of planar gamma camera performance. Nucl Med Commun 1995; 16:186–195.
23. International Electrotechnical Commission. Publication IEC61675-1: Characteristics and test conditions of radionuclide imaging devices. Part 1: positron emission tomographs. Geneva: International Electrotechnical Commission; 1995.
24. National Electrical Manufacturers Association. NEMA Standards Publication NU 2-2001: Performance measurements of positron emission tomographs. Rosslyn: National Electrical Manufacturers Association; 2001.
25. International Atomic Energy Agency. Single photon emission computed tomographic (SPECT) systems using rotating scintillation cameras, Chapter 8, TECDOC-317. Vienna: IAEA; 1987.
26. Gillen GJ, Elliott AT. Quality control of analogue to digital conversion circuitry for artefact-free SPECT imaging. Phys Med Biol 1992; 37:2175–2188.
27. Houston AS, Whalley DR, Skrypnuik JV, et al. UK audit and analysis of quantitative parameters obtained from gamma camera renography. Nucl Med Commun 2001; 22:559–566.
28. US Nuclear Regulatory Commission. NRC Regulatory Guide 10.8 Revision 1: Guide for the preparation of applications for medical programs: Appendix D – methods for calibration of dose calibrators. Washington: Nuclear Regulatory Commission; 1980.
29. Institute of Physical Sciences in Medicine. Report 65: Protocol for establishing and maintaining the calibration of medical radionuclide calibrators and their quality

control. York: Institute of Physical Sciences in Medicine; 1992.

30. International Electrotechnical Commission. Publication IEC1303: Medical electrical equipment: particular methods for declaring the performance of radionuclide calibrators. Geneva: International Electrotechnical Commission; 1994.

31. British Standards Institution. PD IEC/TR 61948-1: Nuclear Medicine Instrumentation – Routine tests – Part 1: Radiation counting systems. London: British Standards Institution; 2001.

32. Paras P, Hine GJ, Adams R. BRH test pattern for the evaluation of gamma camera performance. J Nucl Med 1981; 22:468–470.

33. Murray KJ, Elliott AT, Wadsworth J. A new phantom for the assessment of nuclear medicine imaging equipment. Phys Med Biol 1979; 24:188–192.

Notes

(a) DoH (DHSS) Reports may be obtained from Medicines and Healthcare products Regulatory Agency, Hannibal House, Elephant and Castle, London SE1 6QT.

(b) BSI documents may be obtained from British Standards Institution, 389 Chiswick High Road, London W4 4AL.

(c) IEC Documents may be obtained from Bureau Central de la Commission Electrotechnique Internationale, 3 rue de Varembe, Geneva, Switzerland.

(d) NEMA Documents may be obtained from National Electrical Manufacturers' Association, 2101 L Street, NW, Washington, DC 20037, USA.

(e) US Dept of Health & Human Services Documents may be obtained from Superintendent of Documents, US Government Printing Office, Washington, DC 20402, USA.

6

Radiation Protection

Philip P. Dendy, Karen E. Goldstone,
Adrian Parkin, and Robert W. Barber

6.1 Introduction

This chapter deals with a problem that has direct implications for every other chapter in the book – namely that ionizing radiation, even at very low doses, is potentially capable of causing serious and lasting biological damage. If this were not so, the stringent measures that have to be taken to limit the amount of radioactivity administered to the patient, and thereby the radiation dose, would be unnecessary. Indeed they would be undesirable since the key factor limiting radionuclide image quality is the very low count density that results from the strict protocols of dose limitation.

Since such great care is taken to control the amount of radioactivity administered to the patient, it is clearly essential that no avoidable irradiation of either staff or patients should occur. Thus the purpose of this chapter is three-fold. First, we offer some general background information, drawn primarily from radiobiology, to illustrate how sound radiation protection principles are established. Then, some essential practical advice, generally set out in the form of basic "do" and "don't", is given. Finally, we revert to a more discursive style to deal with some legal aspects of radiation protection. Since it is not possible to cover in detail the legislation in every country where this book will be read, only the principles involved, together with one or two specific examples of their implementation, will be considered.

6.2 Fundamentals of Radiation Biology

6.2.1 Radiation Sensitivity of Biological Materials

Ionizing radiation may be defined as any form of radiation that has sufficient energy to release one or more electrons from the atomic nucleus to which the electrons are normally bound. The secondary electrons released when X- or gamma rays interact with matter generally have sufficient energy to travel short distances and cause further ionizations along their tracks. The creation of one ion pair results in an energy deposition of about 35 eV and ion pairs tend to occur in clusters such that the average energy deposition per ion cluster is about 100 eV. These clusters may occupy a volume of 1–5 μm^3 and thus at the subcellular level the deposition of energy is highly non-uniform with amounts of energy that are very large by biochemical standards being deposited in very small volumes. This explains the extreme sensitivity of biological tissues to ionizing radiation. The dose of acute whole body gamma radiation that would be lethal to a human contains so little energy that it could raise the body temperature by no more than 10^{-3} K. However, if this energy is packaged and deposited in large quantities close to particularly sensitive biological sites, for example strands of DNA, the damage caused is quite out of proportion to the energy involved. The limits that must be set on doses have to be chosen with this exceptional sensitivity in mind.

6.2.2 Important Dosimetric Concepts: the Gray, LET, RBE, and Sievert

The unit of radiation absorbed dose is the gray (Gy) and 1 Gy is defined as the deposition of 1 joule of energy as ionizing radiation in one kilogram of matter. Thus if total energy E is absorbed in a mass m the dose $D = E/m$. Doses measured in gray give the total energy deposition and make no allowance for any effects of the spatial distribution of ionization. However, the ionization density is very variable from one type of radiation to another, being sparse for, say X- and gamma rays but dense for alpha particles. A useful concept that expresses the density of ionization along the track of a particle is the linear energy transfer (LET). The LET of a radiation is defined as the mean energy loss per unit track length and values can range from about 0.3 keV/μm for energetic gamma rays to 50 keV/μm for 5 MeV alpha particles. For a detailed consideration of LET, see Report No. 16 of the International Commission on Radiation Units and Measurements [1]. The spatial distribution of ionizations has an important effect on biological sensitivity. If cells growing either in vitro or in vivo are exposed to doses from different types of radiation and the proportion of cells that retain reproductive integrity is scored (the classical cell survival curve experiment) results such as those shown in Figure 6.1 are obtained. From such curves, it is possible to derive the relative biological effectiveness (RBE) of a given radiation as the inverse of the ratio of the doses of two types of radiation to produce the same biological effect under the same conditions.

Comparing the two curves vertically shows that, at a given dose, the surviving fractions are different and thus the purely physical concept of dose is inadequate to describe fully the biological effect.

Reported values of RBE for a given radiation vary considerably from one experiment to another, being very dependent on the dose, dose rate, and the nature of the biological endpoint chosen. Therefore, for the purposes of practical radiation protection, a fixed value is selected for each type of radiation to be representative of values of the RBE of that radiation at low doses. This is called the radiation weighting factor w_R

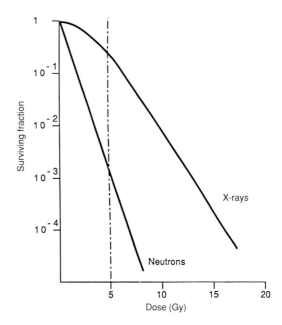

Figure 6.1. Typical survival curves for cells exposed to X-rays and neutrons.

and currently recommended values of w_R [2] are shown in Table 6.1. A reappraisal of the relationship between RBE and w_R is given in ICRP Publication 92 [3]. Values of w_R are then used to calculate the weighted absorbed dose averaged over a tissue or organ according to the equation

$$H_T = \sum_R w_R \cdot D_{T,R}$$

where $D_{T,R}$ is the absorbed dose averaged over the tissue or organ T due to radiation R. H_T is called the equivalent dose and is measured in sieverts (Sv).

Table 6.1. Current recommended values for the radiation weighting factor w_R

Radiation type and energy range	Weighting factor w_R
Photons (all energies)	1
Electrons (all energies)[a]	1
Neutrons (variable with energy)	5–20
Protons other than recoil protons, energy >2 MeV	5
Alpha particles, fission fragments, heavy nuclei	20

[a] Note that Auger electrons emitted from nuclei bound to DNA present a special problem because it is not realistic to average the absorbed dose over the whole mass of DNA as required by the current definition.

RADIATION PROTECTION

6.2.3 Biological Effects of Radiation

A number of important biological effects of radiation must be considered in any review of radiation protection procedures.

Cell Killing

Extensive studies have been made of cell killing by radiation both in vitro and in vivo for a variety of reasons, and in particular to try to establish a dose–effect relationship. Since DNA is thought to be the target for both cell killing and long-term harmful effects of radiation, a similar dose–effect relationship is likely to apply.

The balance of radiological evidence supports the view that, for doses of low LET, radiation up to a few gray delivered at high dose rate, say 1 Gy per minute, the response can be represented by a linear quadratic expression of the form

$$F = aD + bD^2$$

where F is the average frequency of lethal events, D the dose, and a and b are constants.

At lower doses and lower dose rates the value of b is less and the quadratic term is of diminishing importance. This has been interpreted to mean that some lethal events are caused by the cell accumulating a certain number of damage events within a short time such that the cumulative effect results in a lethal event. If time elapses between exposures and hence damage events, repair of sublethal damage can occur and the lethal event will be prevented. For further discussion on this point see Hall [4].

Within the range of absorbed doses to both patients and staff usually encountered in nuclear medicine, it is reasonable to assume a linear relationship without threshold between the dose and the probability of cell killing or analogous effects (see Section 6.3.2). The International Commission on Radiological Protection (ICRP) [2] has, however, concluded that in extrapolating from observed effects at high doses and dose rate to radiation protection levels, the quadratic effect will be important and predicted risks should be reduced by a dose and dose rate effectiveness factor of 2 to allow for this.

One consequence of the linear model is that the risk will be the same if relatively large doses are given to a small number of persons or smaller doses are given to a larger number of persons provided the collective dose – the product of the number of persons multiplied by the dose (man Sv) – is the same.

Cell killing is generally unimportant in nuclear medicine investigations because the doses are small and the number of cells in the body is large. However, during fetal development the number of cells will be small and the problem requires more careful consideration. At a very early stage of pregnancy there are so few cells that damage is likely to result in cell death. A little later there may be sufficient cells overall for the embryo to survive but only small numbers are performing any one specialized function so radiation causes abnormal development [5].

Otake et al [6] re-evaluated the information on mental retardation following in utero exposure to atomic bomb radiation in Japan and found evidence for a clear maximum in the incidence of radiation damage to the brain if exposure was between the 8th and 16th week after fertilization. Extrapolation from animal experiments suggests that doses as low as 120 mGy at critical stages during pregnancy may cause abnormalities and the evidence for a threshold for these effects is equivocal. For a review of the effect of ionizing radiation on the developing human brain see Schull [7].

Chromosomal Aberrations

Direct evidence that ionizing radiation can damage DNA comes from well-documented information on chromosomal aberrations. When samples of human peripheral blood are cultured in such a way that the lymphocytes are stimulated into cell division and chromosome spreads are prepared during mitosis, a variety of abnormalities are observed if the blood has been irradiated either in vivo or in vitro. Amongst the most common observations are chromosomes with a shortened chromatid arm and acentric fragments (single break in one chromosome), ring structures (two breaks in the same chromosome and faulty rejoining) and chromosomes with two centromeres (dicentrics) resulting from two breaks in different chromosomes and faulty rejoining. For a good account of radiation-induced chromosomal aberrations see Steel [8]. The induction of chromosomal changes in human lymphocytes by radiation has been studied at doses below 100 mGy [9].

Long-term Effects

Work with high doses of radiation delivered at high dose rates to animals suggests non-specific life shortening by approximately 5% per Gy of radiation but direct evidence on humans is equivocal. At doses encountered in nuclear medicine – generally no more than 10 mGy – any effect of life shortening will be minimal. Ionizing radiation may also cause long-term effects at specific sites in the body. Probably the most important is cataract formation resulting from direct radiation damage to the cells that comprise the lens. The time interval for the appearance of opacities is very variable and may be anything from 6 months to 30 years. There are also well-documented cases of severe radiation damage to the hands of radiation workers, e.g. veterinary radiologists, as a result of excessive radiation exposures. Most sources used in nuclear medicine are capable of delivering high doses to the fingers. For example, the dose rate to the fingers in contact with an unshielded syringe containing 400 MBq ^{99m}Tc or ^{18}F is 140 mGy h^{-1} and 1150 mGy h^{-1}·respectively [10]. However, for reasons to be explained in Section 6.3.2, the main concerns in nuclear medicine are carcinogenesis and mutagenesis. Evidence that radiation causes cancer in human comes from many sources. For example, occupational exposure results in an increased incidence of lung cancer in uranium miners and there is well-documented evidence on the "radium dial painters". They were mainly young women employed to paint the dials on clocks and watches with luminous paint in about the 1920s. It was their custom to draw the brush into a fine point by licking it. In so doing the workers ingested substantial quantities of ^{226}Ra which traveled via the bloodstream to the skeleton. Years later a number of tumors, especially relatively rare osteogenic sarcomas, were reported.

Additional evidence comes from careful follow-up of the historical use of radiation for approved medical procedures including radiotherapy to the spine to treat ankylosing spondylitis, the use of Thorotrast, which contains the alpha-emitter ^{232}Th, as a contrast medium in diagnostic radiology and regular chest X-rays to monitor tuberculosis. In each instance a number of excess cancers was subsequently recorded in the relevant target organs.

Finally there are the well-documented data gathered from survivors of the Japanese atomic bombs. This work has confirmed the long latency period for many types of radiation-induced cancer and that the carcinogenic effect, considered without regard to type and measured in terms of relative risk, is highest amongst those under 10 years of age at the time of exposure.

The circumstantial evidence that ionizing radiation will have a mutagenic effect in humans is overwhelming. For example, there is extensive direct evidence of mutation in flies and mice, the learning ability of rats and mice can be impaired by irradiating the parents and extensive chromosome damage is known to occur. Although researchers have so far failed to demonstrate convincing statistical evidence for hereditary or genetic change in humans as a result of radiation, due allowance is made for mutagenesis in all calculations of risk.

6.3 Dose Limits for Staff and Patients

6.3.1 Calculation of Dose

With the possible exception of staff in the radiopharmacy who may receive quite large radiation doses to the hands, dose estimates to staff in the nuclear medicine department from sources that are external to the body can be based on whole body personal dosimetry.

Dose rates can be measured directly with an ionization chamber; typical figures 30 cm and 1 m from a patient who has just been injected with 500 MBq of ^{99m}Tc are 6.5 μGy h^{-1} and 2 μGy h^{-1} respectively. Although the dose rate does not decrease in accordance with the inverse square law because the patient is an extended source, the importance of distance as a factor in radiation protection is apparent from these figures.

All technical and nursing staff will be issued with personal monitors. The two standard methods of personal monitoring are by film badges or thermoluminescent dosimetry (TLD). For further details see Wilks [11]. If simple precautions are taken (see Section 6.5) effective doses to staff should not exceed 0.2–0.4 mSv per month even in large departments. With the use of aerosols, care must be taken to ensure that staff do not ingest significant quantities of activity. If a whole body monitoring facility is available, occasional monitoring may be useful, although for ^{99m}Tc this must obviously be done shortly after the diagnostic test.

Calculation of the dose to the patient (or staff) from internally deposited radionuclides is much more difficult because the activity will be distributed to, and cleared from, the various organs in the body quite differently. Furthermore, since the radiation risk varies for different parts of the body (see Section 6.3.2) the dose to each organ from all parts of the body must be calculated.

Only the main features of a typical dose calculation will be summarized. Let the organ containing the activity be called the source organ (S) and the organ for which the dose is being calculated the target organ (T).

The decay scheme and the types of radiation emitted must be known. For non-penetrating radiations such as beta particles from ^{14}C most of the energy will be deposited in S. For more penetrating gamma rays, say from ^{99m}Tc, the fraction of emitted energy that is absorbed in T, say ϕ, will depend on the relative sizes of S and T and their separation. In many cases, for example ^{131}I, the radionuclide will emit mixed radiations and separate calculations will be required for the beta and gamma doses.

The type of radiation and the decay scheme will also allow the total energy emitted by the radionuclide (Δ) measured in kg.Gy kBq^{-1} h^{-1} to be calculated. If values are assumed for the masses of the organs (see, for example, references [12] and [13]), ϕ and Δ may be used to draw up a table of the dose from one organ to any other organ for unit deposited radioactivity and unit time. A small extract from such a table for ^{99m}Tc is shown in Table 6.2. For further details on methods for calculating doses from internal emitters see the Medical Internal Radiation Dose Committee (MIRD) primer [14]. Useful websites are also available [15] and comprehensive lists of radiation doses from radiopharmaceuticals are published by ICRP [12].

Finally the variation of activity in the organ with time must be known. The rate of clearance is nor-mally assumed to be exponential with an effective half-life T_e determined by the physical half-life T_p and the biological half-life T_b according to

$$1/T_e = 1/T_p + 1/T_b.$$

The area under the curve measured in MBq h^{-1} provides a basis for dose calculation using source to target factors.

Note that the concept of an absorbed dose to the whole body has little meaning in nuclear medicine since the doses to individual organs will, in general, be very different.

6.3.2 Assessment of Risk

Deterministic and Stochastic Effects

The long-term radiation effects described in Section 6.2.3 are basically of two types. Deterministic effects (Figure 6.2a) show a well-defined threshold, above which the severity of the effect increases non-linearly with dose, e.g. cataract formation. For deterministic effects radiation protection principles are straightforward. All doses must be kept well below any threshold at which such effects might occur.

Stochastic effects, of which carcinogenesis and mutagenesis are the most important, are assumed to show no threshold and a linear increase in the probability of an effect from the level of natural incidence at zero dose (Figure 6.2b). There is no "safe" level of radiation so all doses to both staff and patients must be as low as reasonably achievable and, with specific reference to patients, the radiation risk must be assessed against the quality of information likely to be gained from the examination.

Table 6.2. Value of dose to one organ (the target) from another organ (the source) for unit deposited radioactivity (Tc-99m) in unit time. These are known as S values and are given here in mGy MBq^{-1} h^{-1}

Target organs	Source organs		
	Liver	Spleen	Bone marrow
Liver	1.2×10^{-2}	2.6×10^{-4}	2.5×10^{-4}
Spleen	2.5×10^{-4}	8.9×10^{-2}	2.5×10^{-4}
Bone marrow	4.3×10^{-4}	4.6×10^{-4}	8.4×10^{-3}
Gonads	1.2×10^{-4}	1.1×10^{-4}	8.6×10^{-4}
Lung	6.7×10^{-4}	6.2×10^{-4}	3.2×10^{-4}
Rest of body	2.7×10^{-4}	3.8×10^{-4}	4.3×10^{-4}
Total body	5.9×10^{-4}	5.9×10^{-4}	5.9×10^{-4}

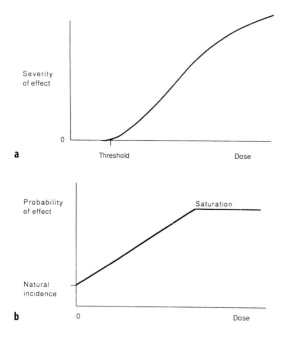

Figure 6.2. Dose – response curves for **a** deterministic effects and **b** stochastic effects of radiation.

Table 6.3. Risk factors and tissue weighting factors (w_T) for different organs in the body for the whole population

Tissue or organ	Probability of fatal cancer 10^{-2} Sv^{-1}	Tissue weighting factor w_T
Bladder	0.30	0.05
Bone marrow	0.50	0.12
Bone surface	0.05	0.01
Breast	0.20	0.05
Colon	0.85	0.12
Liver	0.15	0.05
Lung	0.85	0.12
Esophagus	0.30	0.05
Ovary	0.10	a
Skin	0.02	0.01
Stomach	1.10	0.12
Thyroid	0.08	0.05
Remainder^b	0.50	0.05
Total	5.00	0.80

^{a} A tissue weighting factor of 0.2 is assigned to the gonads – this allows for both hereditary effects and malignancy and brings the total value of w_T to 1.0 as required.

^{b} For the purpose of calculation the remainder is composed of a number of additional tissues and organs, e.g. kidney, pancreas, some of which are known to be susceptible to radiation.

Relative Organ Sensitivities and Weighting Factors

Sufficient direct evidence on the long-term effects of radiation on humans is now available to demonstrate convincingly that different organs are not equally at risk. The risk of fatal cancer varies greatly with age and usually with sex. Risk factors for different organs are summarized in Table 6.3. The summed risk over all organs is estimated at 5×10^{-2} Sv^{-1} and a further 1×10^{-2} Sv^{-1} is added to allow for the detrimental effects of non-fatal cancer.

Two possible effects of gonadal irradiation are impairment of fertility in the irradiated individual and hereditary effects in descendants. The former effect is much more likely in the rapidly dividing, very radiosensitive spermatogonia in the male than in the more differentiated oocytes of the female (law of Bergonié and Tribondeau [16]). Doses of a few tenths of a gray to the male gonads will induce temporary sterility. As mentioned previously, the evidence for mutagenic effects of radiation in humans, although circumstantial, is very strong. The total risk over many generations is difficult to estimate because of lack of information on the genetic stability of radiation-induced recessive mutations. The current best estimate is about 1.3×10^{-2} Sv^{-1}, giving a total stochastic risk of 7.3×10^{-2} Sv^{-1} or 7.3 cases per 100 man Sv.

In situations where the dose to different parts of the body is highly non-uniform (as is usual in nuclear medicine) allowance must be made for the different risks to different organs in calculating the overall risk. This is done by assigning a tissue weighting factor to each tissue as shown in Table 6.3.

Provided H_T, the equivalent dose to each tissue, is known, the effective dose, $\Sigma w_T H_T$, summed over all tissues can be calculated and the risk assessed. A worked example is shown in Table 6.4. Note that values of w_T were revised by ICRP in 1990 [2], so recent values of effective doses arising from different administered radiopharmaceuticals [12, 13] will differ from earlier estimates.

6.3.3 The Concept of Comparative Risk

There are two ways in which radiation risk can be assessed. First, we are all exposed continuously to background radiation from cosmic rays, radioactive potassium in the body, radon gas, and gamma radiation from terrestrial rocks. A typical average figure is 2 mSv per annum but variations of a factor of two in different parts of the world are

RADIATION PROTECTION

Table 6.4. Calculation of effective dose for a hypothetical radiopharmaceutical with a simple biodistribution

Suppose that 75 MBq of a compound labeled with ^{99m}Tc is administered and rapidly distributes to the liver (80%), spleen (15%), and bone marrow (5%). Assume the biological half-life is equal to the physical half-life in each organ.

Stage 1: calculate the time integral of the activity A in each organ, i.e. the area under the activity – time curve. If localization is rapid and $T_b = T_p$ the curve will be a simple exponential decay with half-life 3 h (equation 1).

$A_{liver} = 0.8 \times 75 \times 3/\ln 2 = 260$ MBq.h

Similarly,

$A_{spleen} = 48$ MBq.h and $A_{bm} = 16$ MBq.h

Stage 2:
1. Use the S values in Table 6.2 to calculate the dose in mGy to each target organ from each source organ.
2. Find the total dose to each target organ by adding the three contributions (column 1 below).
3. Convert to H_T by multiplying the w_R of 1.0 for gamma rays (column 2).
4. Calculate $w_T H_T$ (column 4).
5. Sum to find the effective dose equivalent.
6. Estimate risk.

Target organ	Total dose (mGy)	H_T(mSv)	w_T	$w_T H_T$ (mSv)
Liver	3.1	3.1	0.05	0.16
Spleen	4.4	4.4	0.05	0.22
Bone marrow	0.3	0.3	0.12	0.04
Gonads	0.05	0.05	0.20	0.01
Lung	0.2	0.2	0.12	0.02
Rest of body	0.1	0.1	0.46	0.05
			$\Sigma w_T H_T =$	0.50

Hence the effective dose from this administration is 0.5 mSv and assuming 7.3 cases of serious radiation detriment per 100 man Sv the risk is about 4×10^{-5}.

not uncommon, with occasionally much higher values. Occupational exposures that are comparable with background radiation are generally considered acceptable and if monthly effective doses for staff in nuclear medicine departments are in the range 0.2–0.4 mSv, the annual effective dose is quite comparable to background.

Second, the figure of 7.3 cases of severe radiation harm per 100 man Sv given earlier may be used to work out the risk associated with a given dose of radiation. For example, this implies that the risk associated with 1 mSv of radiation is about 7×10^{-5} and is about equivalent to the risk associated with travelling 4000 miles by car.

ICRP [2] has used the risk factors to establish recommended dose limits (Table 6.5). For occupational exposures a level of dose has been chosen above which the consequences for the individual would be widely regarded as unacceptable. In deciding dose limits on public exposure, a similar approach has been taken but in addition consideration has been given to known variations in background radiation.

Table 6.5. Recommended annual dose limits

	Dose limit/mSv	
Application	Occupational	Public
Effective dose (averaged over a number of years)	20^a *	1
Equivalent dose to:		
lens of eye	150	15
skin	500	50

^{a} No special dose limit applies to occupational exposure of women who may be of childbearing age. However, once a pregnancy has been declared the dose to the surface of the abdomen during the remainder of the pregnancy should be limited to 2 mSv and intakes of radionuclides should be limited to one-twentieth of the ALI.

By making calculations similar to those outlined in Section 6.3.1, dose coefficients for intakes of radionuclides by workers can be worked out [13]. These may be used to calculate annual limits on intake (ALI) such that dose limits are not exceeded from radioactivity within the body [17]. For nuclear medicine staff the combined dose from internal and external sources should be well limit if proper procedures are ~~llowed.~~

Most diagnostic examinations in nuclear medicine involve effective doses of less than 10 mSv so the long-term risk for the patient is also acceptably low, provided the test is justified and all unnecessary exposures are avoided, especially when set against the natural incidence of cancer, which is almost 1 in 3.

In recognition of the assumption that there is no safe threshold for long-term deleterious effects, an earlier ICRP publication [18] reinforced in ICRP 60 [2] laid down three basic principles of dose limitation:

1. Justification – no practice shall be adopted unless its introduction produces a positive net benefit.
2. Optimization – all exposures should be kept as low as reasonably achievable, economic and social factors being taken into consideration (this is usually abbreviated to ALARA).
3. Limitation – the dose equivalent to individuals should not exceed the limits recommended for the appropriate circumstances by the Commission.

These principles still apply and the sections that follow give practical advice on the measures to be taken in a nuclear medicine department to ensure compliance with them.

6.4 Design of Facilities

The layout, construction, and finish of the building housing the nuclear medicine department are all influenced by radiation protection considerations. In nuclear medicine work risks arise from the radioactive materials used, the patients who have received radiopharmaceuticals, and the radioactive waste produced. The hazards to personnel are due to external exposure, surface contamination, and ingestion.

6.4.1 Buildings

All rooms where radioactivity is present must show the familiar radiation warning sign. A system of designation of areas with restrictions on who may enter will usually be a legal requirement. The largest activities are handled during the prepa-

ration of the radiopharmaceuticals, and detailed consideration of radiopharmacy design is given in Chapter 7. Separate areas for the administration of radiopharmaceuticals and the performance of in vivo tests (imaging rooms and other patient counting facilities), and possibly laboratories for in vitro tests, are needed. Waiting areas with designated toilets should be provided for radioactive patients. Space for the safe storage of radioactive waste will also be needed. Careful consideration should be given to layout in order to reduce the movement of radioactivity within the department. All materials used should allow for easy decontamination should inadvertent dispersal of radioactive liquids occur. The use of radioactive gases or aerosols presents an additional hazard, and suitable extraction or forced ventilation should be provided. Hand washing facilities must be provided in areas where unsealed radioactive materials are handled.

Advice on the design of equipment and facilities has been given in ICRP 25 [19].

6.4.2 Equipment

Equipment for the safe handling and monitoring of unsealed radioactive materials should be provided, and staff properly trained in its use.

Any nuclear medicine department needs a method of measuring activity accurately before radiopharmaceuticals are administered. The principal instrument used is a well-type ionization chamber. The sensitivity of such a radionuclide calibrator must be traceable to a national standard for all the nuclides used in the department. The Institute of Physical Sciences in Medicine (IPSM) (now The Institute of Physics and Engineering in Medicine (IPEM)) and the National Physical Laboratory (NPL) have published a protocol for the acceptance testing and subsequent quality control of radionuclide calibrators [20].

All equipment used for patient studies must be carefully selected and maintained, and must be suitable for the procedure intended. The choice of gamma camera collimator will depend on the radionuclide used, and the compromise between sensitivity and resolution must be fully considered to limit the activity used while obtaining adequate information from the study.

All equipment must have regular checks and records of quality control measurements must be kept, in order that any deterioration in performance can be readily identified and corrected.

IPSM Report No. 65 [21] contains information on all aspects of quality in nuclear medicine.

It should be emphasized that a well-designed department and well-maintained equipment do not guarantee good radiation protection. They are only effective when combined with a safety conscious attitude derived from education and understanding on the part of the staff.

6.5 Safety of Staff

The procedure for justifying any radiation exposure involves balancing the gain from the procedure against the harm from the radiation and it is essential that there should be prior evaluation to identify the nature and magnitude of the radiological risk to exposed workers. Staff working in the nuclear medicine department should have no difficulty in complying with recommended dose limits (see Table 6.5). Therefore the ALARA principle is, in practice, the overriding one.

6.5.1 Staff Training and Local Rules

The first requirement is to provide adequate training which must be both practical and theoretical. Staff must be advised of the basic physical principles by which their radiation dose can be reduced, namely time, distance, and shielding, as well as the need for containment when handling unsealed radioactive materials.

Advice on protection should be formulated in the local departmental rules and procedures. New members of staff should be handed a copy and given the opportunity for discussion and clarification, and should sign to indicate they have read and understood the contents. Records should be kept of staff training. Copies of relevant rules and regulations should also be on display in the department.

6.5.2 Physical Factors in Radiation Protection

Time

Time spent in the vicinity of radioactive sources must be minimized, so sitting, reading, or holding conversations in a radiation environment should be avoided. Patients to whom radioactive materials have been administered are radioactive sources, albeit temporarily, and therefore all patient in-terviews, documentation, examination, and any anatomical marking should be carried out before the administration. All sources should be quickly returned to shielded containers, and all contaminated items and radioactive waste removed to a safe place. Skill acquired in the techniques of handling radioactive materials will reduce the time spent on procedures.

Distance

Gamma radiation obeys the inverse square law; for example, doubling the distance from a point source reduces the dose rate by a factor of four. The distance between the radioactive sources and the operator should be maximized. Use should be made of carrying boxes, handling tools and forceps. Straight forceps are not very convenient for holding small bottles or vials; shaping the tips makes handling easier and safer. The volume of radioactivity in a syringe should not normally exceed 50% of the syringe capacity; the use of a large syringe size increases the source to finger distance.

Unobtrusive methods can be used to ensure an adequate distance between radioactive patients and other people. Positioning furniture, flower tubs, and ornaments in the right places is preferable to advisory notices. Discretion should be used in maintaining distance from radioactive patients without alarming or upsetting them.

Shielding

Appropriate shielding will depend on the type and energy of the radiations emitted by a source. ^{99m}Tc is easily shielded; a few millimeters of lead are usually sufficient. ^{99}Mo emits much higher energy gamma rays, and thus radioactive generators should be stored behind lead walls. The bench surface should be shielded to avoid exposure to the lower body. Lead or a lead/glass screen should be used when manipulating gamma-emitting radioactive material. Stock solutions should be kept in lead pots. When dispensing from a stock solution, it may be found convenient to use the stock vial inverted in a lead pot with a hole drilled in the bottom of the pot. This allows the safe transfer of radioactive liquids without undue dose to the fingers. Syringe shields should be used when injecting radiopharmaceuticals. A range of shielding devices are available commercially; when working with beta-emitting nuclides, Perspex shielding of an appropriate thickness is more suitable.

Sometime a compromise is needed. Shielding and distance may be counterproductive if they make a procedure more cumbersome, thereby increasing the time spent on it.

6.5.3 Contamination

When unsealed radioactive materials are used it is necessary to protect against both external radiation and the possibility of contamination. To minimize the risk of ingestion staff should be forbidden to eat, drink, or smoke in areas where unsealed sources are handled. Chewing of pens and licking of labels should be forbidden. Gloves and a protective uniform should be worn. For some procedures a plastic apron is advisable. Since gloves may become contaminated, instrument switches should not be touched directly, but disposable paper should be used. If it is necessary to use a calculator, it should be put into a clear polythene bag. All working areas should be clear and uncluttered, and paperwork kept away from radioactive areas. Taps, having elbow or foot controls, serving laboratory sinks should be fitted with tubing to reduce splashing, particularly if the sinks are used for the disposal of radioactive liquid waste. At the end of any procedure involving unsealed sources the hands should be washed and monitored.

6.5.4 Monitoring

Radiation levels in a nuclear medicine department will be above background. Monitoring of the environment both for external radiation and for contamination, and of staff for internal and external radiation is necessary to assess the extent of this increase and ensure it is kept as low as reasonably achievable. National regulations and local rules and procedures may specify the extent of monitoring, and the nature of the record-keeping required.

Areas

In the radiopharmacy or high activity laboratory a measurement of dose rate is required. A detector set to sound an audible alarm is a useful warning to staff of the presence of unusually high radiation levels. A portable dose-rate meter can be used to identify different designated areas in the department and to check on the adequacy of shielding during working procedures. In clinical areas dose rates fluctuate with the pattern of work so an in-

tegrating device such as a film badge or thermoluminescent dosimeter (TLD) is needed to assess the overall dose. To get a representative reading, monitoring points must be chosen carefully. Results have to be scaled in the ratio of working hours/total hours of exposure.

Staff

Depending on legal requirements some or all staff may need to wear personal dosimeters (film or TLD), usually changed monthly. Radiopharmacists, dispensing technicians and staff who administer radiopharmaceuticals regularly should have their finger doses measured. Thin TLD dosimeters do not unduly impede the work and should be used for this purpose. Solid state monitors are now available both for measuring whole body dose and for assessing finger doses in real time.

Monitors should be available near handbasins to check possible contamination on gloves, hands, and coats. The monitors should be mains operated and permanently switched on so that it is not necessary to touch any controls. Geiger Muller counters are suitable since they are sensitive enough to indicate contamination that may require attention without going off scale when radioactive patients are nearby.

The personal dosimeters worn by staff to detect external exposure are not sensitive enough to measure body contamination at low levels. The emphasis must be on prevention of ingestion or inhalation, so staff should be encouraged to monitor hands, skin, and clothing frequently. Monitoring (including that of the feet) should also be carried out when leaving designated areas to minimize the risk of spreading contamination. There should be spot checks by radiation protection supervisors and measurements on staff after the introduction of new procedures. If available, whole body monitoring with a sensitive instrument should be performed once or twice a year.

For work with beta-emitters, a system of excreta monitoring may be necessary, depending on the use and activity handled.

Contamination

A more sensitive, portable scintillation monitor or proportional counter should be available to search for splashes, the extent of spills, the effectiveness of decontamination, and for measuring surface contamination. Such a monitor may also be used for checking that radioactive waste is within allowed disposal limits. It is sensible to cover the radiation detector with plastic or cling film to prevent contamination. Except for low-energy beta-emitters, e.g. ^{14}C, the covering will not excessively reduce the monitor reading.

In laboratories where radioactive sources are kept, direct measurements of low level contamination may be impossible because of the high background. Surfaces of known area should be wiped with a swab moistened with alcohol and the activity on the swab measured in a non-radioactive room. The proportion of contamination that can be removed depends on the surface. For varnished wood it is typically 60%, for Perspex and stainless steel it is around 80%. A mask cut out of film (an area 10 cm by 10 cm is suitable) is useful for quantifying this indirect monitoring. Syringe shields, handling tools, and the outside of lead pots should be checked for contamination before reuse. IAEA transport regulations [22] require that the outside of all packaging be free of contamination.

If radioactive gases or aerosols are used, measurement of air concentrations may be necessary. Gases can be measured using monitors which draw air at a known rate through or in front of detectors. Iodine vapor can be trapped by chemically treated filters. Aerosols are deposited on filters such as Whatman GF/A. Air flow can be regulated by inserting a small aperture in the pumping line. Aerosol particles also settle under gravity so their presence can be detected as surface contamination.

All monitors should be calibrated with traceability to national standards. Their performance should be checked yearly or after repairs. For portable monitors it is useful to have sensitivity figures for surface measurements, for special applications such as thyroid monitoring and for approximate dose rate estimations.

6.5.5 Incidents

Even in well-organized departments mishaps occur from time to time. In the event of any accident involving unsealed radioactive materials, the principal requirements are first to ensure the safety of all individuals, and then to avoid the spread of radioactivity. The seriousness of any spill will depend on the activity released, the radionuclide toxicity, and whether personnel or equipment are contaminated.

The general procedure for dealing with an incident involving radioactivity is to:

1. stop work;
2. notify a supervisor and summon assistance;
3. treat any injuries;
4. decontaminate personnel;
5. decontaminate the room;
6. prepare a report.

6.5.6 Decontamination of Persons

Should contamination of personnel be suspected, every effort should be made to prevent external contamination entering the body through damaged skin or by ingestion. Suitable procedures should be followed, repeatedly if necessary, until the contamination is below the acceptable levels specified locally.

Contaminated clothing should be removed as soon as possible, taking care not to spread the contamination. Clothing, if highly radioactive, should be put into a polythene bag and stored behind shielding.

Affected areas should be cleaned locally before bathing or showering. Contaminated hands should be washed repeatedly with large quantities of soap and running water, paying particular attention to the nails. Should this treatment fail to remove the contamination, 2% DECON solution or other purpose-made solution should be tried. Care should be taken not to damage the skin, and that the skin does not react to decontamination soaps or other chemicals.

Contaminated hair should be washed with soap and water and if necessary, 2% DECON. Other chemicals should not be used.

Damp swabs soaked with soap and water can be used to clean the face, taking care to ensure that the active liquid does not touch the lips or enter the eyes. Lips and mouth should be washed with water or 0.9% saline solution. Contamination should be cleaned from the skin surrounding the eyes before irrigating with sterile 0.9% saline solution. Other chemicals should not be used near the eyes.

If the skin is broken or cut in the area of contamination, the wound should be opened and irrigated immediately with tap water. Bleeding, to a reasonable extent, should be encouraged.

6.5.7 Decontamination of Room

Minor spills (less than one-tenth of an ALI released) present no great hazard and are easily dealt with. Plastic gloves should be worn. Paper towels can be used to soak up liquid. Care should be taken not to spread any contamination. The area of contamination should be determined by monitoring and marked. The area should be scrubbed with detergent. All contaminated paper towels, swabs, and brushes should be placed in a polythene bag, the bag labeled and taken to the radioactive waste store. Monitoring and cleaning should continue until the activity is below acceptable levels as specified in national legislation and codes of practice. Typical figures for ^{99m}Tc are 300 Bq cm^{-2} in the radiopharmacy and 30 Bq cm^{-2} for areas accessible to the public. All persons and equipment involved in the cleaning should be monitored afterwards.

In the event of a major spill the room should be vacated, leaving contaminated articles behind. The room should be closed and warning signs posted. The treatment of contaminated personnel should begin immediately. The equipment necessary for cleaning the room should be obtained from the spill kit, and a plan of action decided. It may be easier in the case of a short-lived nuclide to seal off the room and allow physical decay to reduce the activity.

If it is necessary to clean the room, overshoes, gloves, and plastic aprons should be worn. A dose-rate monitor should be used to estimate the external hazard, and in cases of high dose rates an electronic personal dosimeter should be worn. A survey of the room using contamination monitors should be carried out, marking any spots of contamination with a felt tip pen. Contamination monitors should be protected with plastic covers. The procedure then is as for a minor spill, but paper towels and swabs should be handled with forceps. If there is no external dose-rate hazard after initial cleaning, the spread of contamination can be prevented by covering the affected area with polythene. Contamination by short-lived nuclides can be reduced by allowing the activity to decay. Restrictions on access may be necessary.

If long-lived contamination persists, the following cleaning materials may be effective: paintwork – paint remover or carbon tetrachloride; plastics – organic solvents; wood – steel wool or sandpaper. If such drastic treatment is necessary, face masks should be used and good ventilation ensured. Should contamination remain above the levels specified locally, equipment must be taken out of use and access to affected areas controlled.

It is essential to have an emergency spill kit available with brief instructions printed on a plastic-covered card. The contents may vary with the radioactive materials handled, but the kit should include all the items needed for the decontamination of people and of surfaces (e.g. plastic gloves, overshoes, apron, tissues, plastic bags, forceps, warning labels, nail brush, liquid soap).

6.6 Safety of Patients

The European Directive on the protection of those medically exposed (which includes research) [23] requires all medical exposures to be effected under the clinical responsibility of a practitioner. Practical aspects of the exposure may be delegated by the practitioner to other individuals (in the UK known as operators). Practitioners and those to whom responsibilities are delegated must be adequately trained. Training should include a theoretical "core of knowledge" as well as practical experience in relevant techniques. Staff must be experienced, knowledgeable, and able to recognize unusual features as the investigation proceeds. The reporting should be competent and timely and the transmission of results prompt. Duplicate records of investigations should be kept so tests are not repeated in the event of lost results. Tests should only be repeated for clinical reasons not for administrative convenience, for example when the patient is transferred to a different clinician, ward, or hospital. Past results should be available on request.

6.6.1 Requirements of the Investigation

Effective doses in diagnostic nuclear medicine investigations are generally low. With the exception of tests involving longer-lived nuclides like ^{75}Se, ^{67}Ga or ^{131}I, effective doses are usually a few mSv or less (see reference 12). Good quality radiopharmaceuticals are needed, and their activity must be assayed accurately. Sensitive, well-maintained equipment should be used. However, all additional radiation exposures carry an additional risk, and it is essential that each investigation should be justified on clinical grounds. The clinical responsibility should be clearly defined. Clinicians may need certification to clinically direct. The scheme operated by the Administration of Radioactive Substances

Advisory Committee in the UK [24] is an example of such a system.

6.6.2 Strategy for Planning Investigations

The test must be fitted into the sequence of investigations within the "diagnostic pathway" in such a way as to obtain the maximum benefit [25]. Alternative tests not involving radiation should be considered. Tests involving higher radiation exposures should only be performed when the diagnosis is incomplete or if lower dose procedures are not available. If more than one test is needed to elucidate a problem the sequencing of the tests must be carefully considered, so that activity remaining from an earlier test does not compromise a later one. The standard activity for normal sized patients (sometimes known as diagnostic reference levels) should be clearly specified in standard operating procedures (see, for example, reference 24, Appendix 1) but they may need to be varied in special circumstances. Although it is important not to give more activity than necessary, it is important not to give too little. Higher activities are needed for dynamic studies or tomographic imaging, and insufficient activity may lead to inadequate or uninterpretable results. The goal should be to answer the clinical question by the most cost-effective route in terms of radiation dose, without over-investigating the patient.

6.6.3 Patient Preparation

The correct preparation of the patient contributes to the success of the test or treatment. Instructions on diet and stopping or starting drugs should be given well in advance. Protective measures should be used where possible to reduce patient dose, for example giving iodide to block the thyroid gland when radioiodinated compounds are used. Encouragement to take fluids, in the absence of contraindications, may help to eliminate radioactivity and reduce dose by encouraging frequent bladder emptying.

6.6.4 Special Considerations

Children

Since absorbed dose depends on the organ mass, an activity suitable for an adult would result in an unacceptably high effective dose if administered

Table 6.6. Scaling factors to be applied to make allowance for a child's age and weight. The activity normally administered to an adult should be multiplied by the appropriate scaling factor

	Scaling factor	
Age	Based on weight	Based on body surface
Newborn	0.06	0.14
1 year	0.17	0.33
5 years	0.30	0.43
10 years	0.50	0.59
15 years	0.90	0.90
18 years	1.00	1.00

to a small child. A reduction in administered activity based on weight or body surface area should be applied (Table 6.6) [26]. Furthermore, greater care is required in the use of radionuclide investigations in children because of the increased risk of carcinogenesis (see Section 6.2.3).

Pregnant Patients

The greatest care must be exercised in the administration of radioactive materials during pregnancy. A dose to the fetus could arise from direct irradiation by the mother, or from activity passing across the placenta [27]. There is evidence of increased leukemia risk when radiation is delivered in utero and the work of Otake et al (6) on mental retardation was discussed in Section 6.2.3. The National Radiological Protection Board (NRPB) in the UK has published a statement giving advice on exposure to ionizing radiation during pregnancy [28]. The objectives of the statement are to minimize the risk of inadvertent exposure before pregnancy is declared, and to prevent unnecessary exposure of the fetus when diagnostic procedures are indicated during pregnancy.

Administrative arrangements within the nuclear medicine department should ensure that it can be established whether or not a patient is pregnant before the examination is performed. It is useful if the pregnancy status is indicated on the request form from the referring (or prescribing) clinician and if notices are prominently displayed in the department. However, a final check should be made before the radiopharmaceutical is administered by interviewing patients, in confidence, before the start of the examination. If there is a possibility of pregnancy the responsible clinician must decide whether the risk to the fetus from any procedure is outweighed by the risk to the patient from failure to diagnose and treat.

Nursing Mothers

Close contact with an infant should be avoided wherever possible following administration of radioactivity. When the patient is a nursing mother this may present problems. It important to be aware of this before any administration of radiopharmaceutical.

Variable amounts of radioactivity appear in breast milk depending on the radiopharmaceutical. Mountford and Coakley [29] have reviewed the available data on secretion of radioactivity in breast milk and recommended a scheme of suspension of breast feeding in certain instances. This applies particularly to ^{99m}Tc pertechnetate and ^{99m}Tc-labeled red cells or macro-aggregated albumin. It is important to check on radionuclidic purity, for example ^{123}I should be free of ^{124}I or ^{125}I contaminants.

Mountford [30] has published data on the surface dose rate from radioactive patients The dose to an infant from a nursing mother is unlikely to exceed 1 mSv for the usual maximum activities of ^{99m}Tc pharmaceuticals, or from ^{67}Ga, ^{113m}In or ^{201}Tl. Higher doses are possible with ^{111}In leukocytes if there is accumulation in the spleen. The administration of ^{131}I in therapeutic quantities will certainly require restrictions on the basis of dose rate. Secretion of ^{131}I in sweat and saliva will also require restrictions to prevent possible contamination and ingestion.

Other Contacts

The risks to other groups exposed following the administration of radiopharmaceuticals should be suitably assessed [31]. In general the hazards to family members, visitors in hospital, other patients and to staff are low following diagnostic procedures. Assuming an activity of 1 GBq ^{99m}Tc (close to the likely maximum), doses to these groups are unlikely to exceed 2–3% of any dose limit. Nevertheless, cross-irradiation of patients should be minimized by scheduling of tests or treatments (separation in time), by segregation in waiting areas (distance), and if necessary, by the use of screens (shielding). Exposure from PET nuclides may present a problem, firstly because shielding is more difficult, and secondly because exposure rates are higher than for other common radionuclides. Care must be taken with the design of facilities [32] and contact with patients following the procedure [33]. Restrictions will be necessary following therapeutic amounts of ^{131}I.

6.6.5 Adverse Reactions

Side effects and reactions to the administration of radiopharmaceuticals should be noted, investigated, and reported. Radioactivity in itself is not the cause of these rare occurrences but some patients may be allergic to the chemical ingredients of the radiopharmaceutical. National registers of these incidents may reveal common causes not apparent to individual departments meeting an isolated problem.

6.7 Transport of Radioactive Materials

During the transport of radioactive materials, members of the public who are not specially trained in handling radionuclides may come into relatively close contact with them. It is therefore most important to ensure that such persons are neither unnecessarily exposed to radiation nor likely to become contaminated. International and national legislation (see Section 6.9) is directed towards the achievement of these objectives.

Transport of radioactive materials can be considered in two categories – transport within the institution where the materials are used, such as a hospital, and transport outside the institution by means of road, rail, air, etc. This latter case is the subject of IAEA [22] regulations which are reflected in national legislation.

6.7.1 Internal Transport

General principles relating to the transport of the material within an institution are as follows:

1. Procedures should be such that it is clear who is responsible for the radioactive material at a particular time. Even if the user is also the transporter of the material adequate records must be made. A prior risk assessment should be carried out to consider the consequences of reasonably foreseeable incidents and how to protect against them.

2. The material must be transported in a suitable container. It should be doubly contained with a rigid outer container designed to prevent leakage should the primary container break. The container

should be lined with absorbent material to soak up any spill that does occur and must also provide adequate shielding from external radiation.

3. Whilst being transported a container of radioactive material must not be left unattended in areas accessible to the public or staff not concerned with its use.

4. Containers should be suitably labeled. The label should give details of the radionuclide being transported. Care should be taken to ensure that labels are removed from empty containers.

5. Local rules should be written for the institution, detailing the procedures to be followed.

6. The local rules should take into account the possibility of any hazardous situation that is likely to arise during transport. In particular, they should describe the action to be taken in the event of damage to the container and/or its contents. Procedures should also be such that they minimize the possibility of losing a source during transit; therefore documentation must be adequate. Instructions should be included as to the action to be taken should a source be lost (or suspected of being lost).

6.7.2 External Transport

Each country has manifold items of legislation concerned with the safe transport of radioactive material but the definitive source document for all these regulations is the IAEA Regulations for the Safe Transport of Radioactive Material [22] and the supporting safety guide [34].

The aim of these Regulations is to "provide an acceptable level of control of the radiation hazards to persons, property and the environment that are associated with the transport of radioactive material". A major principle underlying the regulations is that safety is built into the package. One of the functions of the Competent Authority, which the Regulations require to be appointed, is the approval of package designs.

Confidence that the controls applied to the transport of radioactive materials are working is demonstrated by satisfactory quality assurance and compliance assurance programs. The former

involves actions by package designers and manufacturers, consignors, carriers, and Competent Authorities; the latter involves reviews and inspections by the users.

If it is necessary to transport radioactive materials, say to outlying hospitals, reference must be made to detailed national legislation. If such procedures are frequent, local procedures should be set down in consultation with the Radiation Protection Adviser (RPA).

The steps to be taken when organizing transport are:

1. Identify the radionuclide and its maximum activity.

2. Establish the type of packaging required. It has to be suitable for both the type, form and activity of the source and the mode of transport. IAEA lay down rigorous type test procedures for the package, e.g. drop test, water spray test.

3. Pack the material in a legally acceptable way. Measure the dose rate on the surface of the package and at one meter from it. The transport index (TI) is defined as this latter quantity measured in $mSv\ h^{-1}$ multiplied by 100. The TI and surface dose rate must be within the limits set by the IAEA.

4. Label the package with the correct international transport labels. The labels must show the radionuclide, the activity, and the transport index.

5. As consignor, fill in transport documents – the details to be included are given in the appropriate national legislation.

6. Follow any specified quality assurance protocols.

UK readers should note that the requirements for transport by post are very stringent [35], so this is not a method to be recommended.

6.8 Disposal of Waste

6.8.1 General Principles

The clinical use of radioactive materials will inevitably result in radioactive waste. This arises from three main sources:

1. excreta from patients undergoing medical procedures;
2. syringes, swabs etc. used during preparation and administration of radioactive materials;
3. waste from spills and resulting decontamination.

If not dealt with satisfactorily, waste will constitute a hazard to staff, patients, and members of the public. Note the waste arising from some sources may have hazards other than its radioactivity associated with it The disposal of waste is subject to legislation, which varies from country to country. The advice that follows may only be implemented provided prior approval has been obtained under the appropriate legislation for both the method of disposal and the types of radionuclide and quantities involved. This section is written with the UK system in mind but other countries have comparable legislation, as indicated in Section 6.9.

Waste may be dealt with in two main ways. It may either be stored until it has decayed to levels where it may easily be dealt with by disposal, or it may be dispersed into the environment, for example through the drainage system, in a suitably controlled manner so that doses of radiation received by persons who may subsequently come into contact with the waste are insignificant. In either case the aim must be to minimize the radiological impact of the waste disposal on the public and the environment, whilst not endangering staff.

The second method is generally most convenient for short half-life ^{99m}Tc, although a short storage time is useful for articles such as syringes.

6.8.2 Liquid and Solid Waste

Liquid

The majority of waste disposed of from a nuclear medicine department comes into the category of liquid waste, the major part of it arising from the excreta of patients. For ease of accounting it is assumed that a certain proportion of the administered radionuclide eventually becomes waste. The generally agreed factors are given in Table 6.7. Obviously some of this waste will not be discharged from the nuclear medicine department itself but from the place to which the patient returns after the procedure. However, the waste is recorded in the nuclear medicine records.

Table 6.7. Generally agreed factors for the proportions of radioactivity that become waste after administration to patients

^{131}I	Ablation therapy	100%
	Thyrotoxicosis treatment	50% for inpatients
		30% for outpatients
^{99m}Tc	Overall figure for the usual broad range of scans	30%
^{32}P		30%
^{67}Ga		30%
^{201}Tl		30%
^{123}I	as MIBG	60%
	as any other compound	100%
Others	(e.g. ^{111}In, ^{75}Se, ^{51}Cr)	100%

Other aqueous radioactivity for disposal may arise from out-of-date stock solutions, unused dispensed activities, spills etc., and may all be disposed of to the drain. The sink used for disposal of radioactive waste should be clearly identified and after disposals the tap should be allowed to run to flush through the waste thoroughly. Pipes carrying radioactive waste should be identified so that they can be checked before any maintenance work is carried out on them.

Water immiscible solvents from liquid scintillation counting should not be disposed of to the drainage system, not because of the radioactivity involved (usually very low concentrations of ^{14}C or ^{3}H), but because of the organic material, e.g. toluene, in the scintillant. Such materials can be collected and incinerated by an authorized contractor.

Solid Waste

Solid waste from the nuclear medicine department will mainly consist of contaminated swabs and syringes etc., used during the preparation and administration of radiopharmaceuticals. As well as being radioactive waste it will also be clinical waste. Since the majority of activity involved will be due to the short half-life ^{99m}Tc, it may be stored for a relatively short time until it is of negligible activity and then discarded with ordinary inactive clinical waste. It is helpful to keep two active waste containers labeled "^{99m}Tc" and "other" to allow for different appropriate storage times.

Solid clinical waste that remains radioactive is likely to be disposed of via an incinerator. Depending on the chemical composition of the activity, the material may be dispersed in the air, e.g. iodine, or may appear in the ash. The ash should be disposed of as very low level waste subject to limitations on the amount of activity allowed in a particular volume. The waste must not contain any alpha-emitters or strontium-90. The waste may be transported off site for incineration elsewhere; if so it must comply with the relevant transport regulations.

Incinerators used for disposal of radioactive waste should be of good design, particularly with respect to the discharge of effluent gases and ash handling. The stack height should be sufficiently above that of surrounding buildings to give efficient dispersal of any radioactive gases emitted. This should be borne in mind when new building developments are planned in the vicinity of incinerator chimneys.

Possible alternative methods of disposal for non-clinical waste are special burial (i.e. in a marked site at a specified depth), or via a special disposal organization, but prior permission to use a particular disposal route must be sought from the Environment Agency (EA – England and Wales) or Scottish Environment Protection Agency (SEPA – Scotland).

6.8.3 Storage and Transport of Waste

Storage

Waste awaiting disposal should be stored in closed containers. In general in the UK, the storage period should not exceed 2 weeks. Longer-lived materials, e.g. iodine-131, may require longer storage before disposal by a convenient method is possible and application should be made to extend the storage period.

Each hospital should have at least one storage area for radioactive waste. The area must be lockable to prevent unauthorized access and should be clearly marked with a radiation warning symbol. It must be adequately shielded and must not contain flammable materials. All items awaiting disposal must be clearly marked and it is a good idea to allocate areas in the store to particular types of waste and radionuclides.

Transport

In theory, radioactive waste is subject to the legislation that applies to the transport of radioactive substances generally and requires proper packaging, labeling, and documentation. However, the waste arising from hospitals is normally of very low activity and, subject to certain constraints, is exempt from the majority of the transport

regulations. Persons wishing to transport waste should therefore refer to the relevant legislation.

6.8.4 Waste Records

It is essential that comprehensive records are kept for all radioactive materials, including their disposal as radioactive waste. The waste record should indicate the radionuclide, its activity (estimated by some suitable means), the disposal route, and the date on which the disposal was made. In order to confirm at a glance that all waste authorization limits are being complied with, a central record should be kept in terms of the time limits given by the authorization, e.g. a monthly summary may be appropriate.

6.9 Legal Requirements

For many years radiation and radioactive materials have been subject to various codes of practice, guidance documents, and more recently legislation. The foremost body dealing with matters of radiation protection is the ICRP. This was established in 1928 under its former name of the International X-ray and Radium Protection Commission. Through the work of its specialist committees the ICRP continues to issue recommendations on many aspects of radiation safety, and to a large extent it is these recommendations that are embodied in the radiation protection legislation of individual countries.

In the UK the major pieces of legislation affecting the use of radionuclides in nuclear medicine are, the Radioactive Substance Act 1993 [36], various regulations relating to transport, the Medicines Radioactive Substances Order 1978 [37], which is an extension of the Medicines Act 1968 [38], the Health and Safety at Work Act 1974 [39], the Ionising Radiations Regulations 1999 [40], and the Ionising Radiation (Medical Exposure) Regulations 2000 [41]. A helpful review of legislation particularly relevant in hospitals is given in the Joint Health & Safety Executive and Health Departments' Guidance [42].

6.9.1 The Radioactive Substances Act 1993

The Radioactive Substances Act deals with the keeping and use of radioactive material, its disposal, and the accumulation of radioactive waste. In common with other users of radioactive materials, hospitals are required to have a registration certificate indicating the nature and quantities of the radionuclides they are able to keep and use. However, anyone who creates radioactive waste is required to have a waste disposal authorization. Usually such an authorization will cover the disposal of solid, liquid, and possibly gaseous waste. Solid waste is normally disposed of via a hospital incinerator or through the Local Authority or through controlled burial. Liquid waste is usually disposed of down the drain. It is a requirement of the legislation that detailed records showing date of disposal, together with activities, are recorded. Usually the authorization applies to a monthly waste figure or possibly a weekly figure and it is helpful to total the waste disposals over this period. For small amounts of radioactivity The Radioactive Substances (Hospitals) Exemption Order 1990 and amendment [43] applies. However, even if this is complied with it is still necessary to keep accurate records.

6.9.2 Transport

The foremost document internationally regarding transport of radioactive material is the IAEA Regulations for the safe transport of radioactive material 2000 [22, 34]. As far as road transport in the UK is concerned, the Radioactive Material (Road Transport) Regulations 2002 [44] are compatible with the IAEA Regulations. Railways [45] and the Post Office [35] also have rules for the carriage of radioactive materials. There are regulations governing transport by air and sea. In any particular circumstance the reader is advised to go to the authoritative document.

6.9.3 Medical Legislation

In 1978 the Medicines Act [38] was modified by the Medicines (Radioactive Substances) Order 1978 [37] to include radioactive substances. Also in 1978 the Medicines (Administration of Radioactive Substances) Regulations [46] were made. These Regulations require that any persons administering radioactive materials to a patient or volunteer shall be in possession of a certificate authorizing them to do so. Each person requiring a certificate must complete a comprehensive application form and submit it to the Department of Health. The Regulations are now commonly known as the ARSAC regulations after the committee which advises health ministers on the granting of certificates.

A list of routine nuclear medicine procedures indicating maximum activities usually administered and the effective dose equivalent is included with the Guidance Notes issued to aid completion of the application form [24]. There is also allowance for giving non-standard administrations, although dose calculations must be provided in support of such requests (see Section 6.3). Certificates also have to be obtained for research projects. The employing authority must be satisfied that persons administering radioactive substances on its premises have a suitably valid certificate.

6.9.4 Legislation for Protection of Employees

The Health and Safety at Work Act 1974 [39] is concerned with the welfare of all employees and the Ionising Radiations Regulations 1999 [40] were made under it. These regulations are accompanied by an Approved Code of Practice (ACOP) [47] which gives details on compliance with the regulations. Alternative methods of compliance are permitted but the onus is on the employer to convince the Health and Safety Executive that he has fulfilled the regulations in as good, or a better way than indicated by the Approved Code of Practice.

The Ionising Radiations Regulations themselves cover all aspects of work with ionizing radiations and specify certain working practices for the purposes of dose limitation. First, the employer must carry out a prior risk assessment to establish the measures that must be put in place to keep radiation doses as low as reasonably practicable (ALARP). Second, the employer must designate "controlled" and "supervised" areas to which access is restricted and only permitted under certain circumstances. Third, employees who may exceed three-tenths of any dose limit prescribed in the Regulations must be designated as "classified persons". Fourth, the employer must appoint a Radiation Protection Adviser and Radiation Protection Supervisors who assist the employer in ensuring compliance with the regulations. Finally, employers are also required to provide information in the form of training and instruction to their employees and to set down written local rules.

In addition there are detailed regulations for dosimetry and medical surveillance which apply mainly to classified persons. With the possible exception of the radiopharmacist in a busy department it should not be necessary to classify nuclear medicine staff.

The control of radioactive substances by means of adequate accounting is covered and there are regulations relating to their storage and transport. Requirements for washing and changing facilities for employees and for personal protective equipment are also specified.

Adequate monitoring of radiation dose rates and surface contamination must be carried out regularly and the results recorded. There are detailed regulations on what to do in the case of a hazardous situation arising or a person being over exposed. The enforcement of the Health and Safety at Work Act, and therefore the Ionising Radiations Regulations 1999, is the responsibility of the Health and Safety Executive.

6.9.5 Protection of Patients

Protection of the patient is provided for by the Ionising Radiations (Medical Exposure) Regulations 2000 [41]. These regulations cover medical exposures taking place as part of the patient's own treatment or diagnosis, exposures undertaken as part of occupational health surveillance, those undertaken as part of a health screening program, those undertaken for medicolegal purposes, and those undertaken for research. Generally only the first and last categories will be relevant for nuclear medicine. The main aim of the regulations is to ensure that all exposures are justified (as far as the individual receiving the exposure is concerned) and all exposures are optimized. These aims are achieved by a number of provisions. Firstly, procedures leading to exposure of patients to radiation must be carried out under the responsibility of a person (the practitioner) who justifies the exposure. (The ARSAC certificate holder is, by definition, the practitioner.) Secondly, the exposure is authorized and undertaken by an operator (who may be the same individual as the practitioner) who ensures that doses to individual patients are kept as low as reasonably practicable. Thirdly, practitioners and operators must have received adequate training (in part this is already covered by some of the ARSAC requirements). Fourthly, there should be adequate quality control of equipment and procedures and finally the ser-

vices of a Medical Physics Expert should be available to the department (this person may or may not be the Radiation Protection Adviser). The Employer has to draw up "Employer's procedures" as specified in the Regulations to provide a framework in which medical exposures can take place.

6.9.6 Legislation in Other Countries

Although there are differences in detail, many other countries have legislation and Codes of Practice covering the aspects of radiation work described for the UK. Because of UK membership of the European Union most of the recent legislation has been as a direct result of various measures laid down by the Council of the European Communities (CEC). The legislation in other member countries therefore bears a strong similarity to that in the UK.

In the USA there is control of radiation at the Federal, State, and local level. In general the use of radioactive materials and their disposal is more tightly regulated than in the EU. The main Federal Agencies concerned with radiation protection are the Nuclear Regulatory Commission (NRC), The Department of Health Education and Welfare through the Food and Drug Administration (FDA), the Center for Devices in Radiological Health (formerly the Bureau of Radiological Health), the Environmental Protection Agency (EPA), and the Department of Transportation.

Of considerable interest to departments of nuclear medicine is the mechanism by which licenses are granted to persons to administer radioactive materials to patients. This is a more complex procedure in the USA than in the UK. In the USA licenses are issued by the NRC and are of several types. In addition, individual states have set up State Agencies under agreement with the NRC to regulate uses of radiation under state mandated programs. General licenses are issued to individuals for the possession and use of limited quantities of pre-packaged individual doses of radiopharmaceuticals. Before a general license is issued the pharmaceutical must have been shown to be safe for human use, which is the FDA's jurisdiction. The equipment to be used for the procedure must have been shown to be appropriate and effective and the user of pharmaceuticals must be someone whose training and experience in matters of radiation safety and clinical use of radionuclides is adequate. Both general and specific licenses can be issued for possession of specific quantities of materials and limited procedures (e.g. radioimmune assays) by authorized users. Any change in amounts, procedures, or equipment requires a modification to the license before actual implementation.

The broader scope licenses are issued to institutions which allow them a greater degree of flexibility in implementation of radiation protection programs. The licensing agency delegates responsibility to the institution's radiation safety committee. The FDA might also delegate approval of certain unapproved radiopharmaceuticals to the institution's radioactive drug committee.

6.10 Summary and Conclusions

In this chapter the many facets of radiation protection that are applicable to a nuclear medicine department have been considered. The main features may be summarized as follows.

1. Ionizing radiation is potentially harmful, the most important long-term risk being radiation-induced carcinogenesis.

2. The risk associated with larger doses of radiation is reasonably well established. A linear extrapolation with no threshold is assumed for lower doses.

3. All radiation exposures to staff, patients, and members of the public must be as low as reasonably achievable.

4. The safety of both patients and staff must be considered and the importance of staff education and training cannot be overemphasized.

5. Legislation has now been introduced to cover most aspects of work with radioactive materials. Well-informed and careful workers in nuclear medicine should have no difficulty in complying with the various regulations or in restricting doses to themselves and to others to acceptably low levels.

References

1. International Commission on Radiation Units and Measurements. Linear energy transfer ICRU (Publication 16), Bethesda, MD; 1970.
2. International Commission on Radiological Protection. 1990 Recommendations of the International Commission on Radiological Protection (ICRP Publication 60). Ann ICRP 1991; 21: No. 1–3.
3. International Commission on Radiological Protection. Relative Biological Effectiveness (RBE), Quality Factor(Q), and Radiation Weighting Factor (w_R) (ICRP Publication 92) Ann ICRP 2003; 33: No. 4.
4. Hall EJ. Radiobiology for the Radiologist, 5th edn. Baltimore: Lippincott, Williams & Wilkins; 2000.
5. International Commission on Radiological Protection. Biological Effects after Prenatal Irradiation (embryo and fetus) (ICRP Publication 90). Ann ICRP 2003; 33: No. 1–2.
6. Otake M, Schull WJ, Lee S. Threshold for radiation-related severe mental retardation in prenatally exposed A-bomb survivors: a re-analysis. Int J Radiat Biol 1996; 70:755–763.
7. Schull WJ. International Commission on Radiological Protection. Risks Associated with Ionising Radiations. Ann ICRP 1991; 22:95.
8. Steel GG. Basic Clinical Radiobiology. London: Arnold; 2003.
9. Yamada T, Mothersill C, Michael BD, Potten CS, eds. Biological Effects of Low Dose Radiation. Amsterdam and London: Elsevier; 2000.
10. Delacroix D, Guerre J, Leblanc P, Hickman C. Radionuclide and Radiation Protection Data Handbook 2002. Radiation Protection Dosimetry 2002; 98: No. 1.
11. Wilks R. Principles of Radiological Physics, 2nd edn. Edinburgh: Churchill Livingstone; 1987.
12. International Commission on Radiological Protection. Radiation dose to patients from radiopharmaceuticals (Addendum to ICRP 53). Ann ICRP 1998; 28: No. 3.
13. International Commission on Radiological Protection. Dose coefficients for intakes of radionuclides by workers (ICRP Publication 68). Ann ICRP 1994; 24: No. 4.
14. Lovinger R, Budinger TF, Watson EE, et al. MIRD Primer for Absorbed Dose Calculations. New York: Society of Nuclear Medicine; 1991.
15. Radiation Dose Assessment Resource. www.dose-info.com.
16. Bergonié J, Tribondeau L. De quelques résultats de la radiothérpie et essai de fixation d'une technique rationnelle. CR Seances Acad Sci. Radiat Res 1906; 143:983. (English translation: Fletcher GH. Radiat Res 1959; 11:587.)
17. International Commission on Radiological Protection. Annual Limits on Intake of Radionuclides by Workers Based on the 1990 Recommendations (ICRP Publication 61). Ann ICRP 1991; 21: No. 4.
18. International Commission on Radiological Protection. Recommendations of the International Commission on Radiological Protection (ICRP Publication 26). Ann ICRP 1977; 1: No. 3.
19. International Commission on Radiological Protection. The Handling, Storage, Use and Disposal of Unsealed Radionuclides in Hospitals and Medical Research Establishments (ICRP Publication 25). Ann ICRP 1977; 1: No. 2.
20. Parkin A, Sephton JP, Aird EGA, et al. In: Hart GC, Smith AH, eds. Quality Standards in Nuclear Medicine. York: Institute of Physical Sciences in Medicine; 1992: 60–77.
21. Hart GC, Smith AH, eds. Quality standards in nuclear medicine. York: Institute of Physical Sciences in Medicine; 1992.
22. IAEA. Regulations for the Safe Transport of Radioactive Material edition (Revised) (Safety Standards No. TS-R-1). Vienna: IAEA; 2000.

23. The Council of the European Union, Council Directive 97/43. Euratom of 30 June 1997 on Health protection of individuals against the dangers of ionizing radiation in relation to medical exposure. Brussels: CEC; 1997.

24. Administration of Radioactive Substances Advisory Committee. Notes for Guidance on the Clinical Administration of Radiopharmaceuticals and Use of Sealed Radioactive Sources. Nucl Med Comm 1998; 21 (Suppl).

25. European Commission. Referral Guidelines for Imaging. Radiation Protection 118. Luxembourg; 2000.

26. Paediatric Task Group of the European Association of Nuclear Medicine. A radiopharmaceutical schedule for imaging in paediatrics. Eur J Nucl Med 1990; 17:127–129.

27. International Commission on Radiological Protection. Doses to the embryo and fetus from intakes of radionuclides by the mother (ICRP Publication 88). Ann ICRP 2001; 31: No. 1–3.

28. National Radiological Protection Board. Diagnostic Medical Exposures: Advice on Exposure to Ionising Radiation During Pregnancy. Chilton, Didcot: NRPB; 1998.

29. Mountford PJ, Coakley AJ. A review of the secretion of radioactivity in human breast milk: data, quantitative analysis and recommendations. Nucl Med Commun 1989; 10:15–27.

30. Mountford PJ. Estimation of close contact doses to young infants from surface dose rates on radioactive adults. Nucl Med Commun 1987; 8:857–863.

31. Mountford PJ. Risk assessment of the nuclear medicine patient. Br J Radiol 1997; 70:671–684.

32. Methe BM. Shielding design for a PET imaging suite: a case study. Health Phys 2003; 84:3–8.

33. Cronin B, Marsden PK, O'Doherty MJ. Are restrictions to behaviour of patients required following fluorine-18 fluorodeoxyglucose positron emission tomographic studies? Eur J Nucl Med 1999; 26:121–128.

34. Advisory Material for the IAEA Regulations for the Safe Transport of Radioactive Materials Safety Guide. Safety Standards Review No. Ts-G-1.1 (ST-2). Vienna: IAEA; 2002.

35. Post Office Guide. 6.3, 17. London: Post Office; 1999.

36. Radioactive Substances Act 1993. London: HMSO.

37. Medicines (Radioactive Substances) Order 1978 (SI 1978 No. 1004). London: HMSO.

38. Medicines Act 1968. London: HMSO.

39. Health & Safety At Work etc. London: HMSO; 1974.

40. Ionising Radiations Regulations 1999. (SI 1999 No 3232). London: HMSO.

41. Ionising Radiations (Medical Exposure) Regulations 2000 (SI 2000 No. 1059). London: HMSO.

42. Joint Health & Safety Executive and Health Departments' Guidance. The regulatory requirements for medical exposure to ionising radiation – An employer's overview. HSG223. London: HSE Books; 2001.

43. Radioactive Substances (Hospitals) Exemption Order 1990 (SI 1990 No. 2512); Radioactive Substances (Hospitals) Exemption (Amendment) Order 1995 (SI 1995 No. 2395). London: HMSO.

44. Atomic Energy and Radioactive Substances. The Radioactive Material (Road Transport) Regulations 2002 (SI 2002 No. 1093). London: HMSO.

45. Guidance on Dangerous Goods – Rail Carriage Arrangements and Risk Management. Railway Group Guidance Note GO/GN3626. London: Railway Safety; 2002.

46. Medicines (Administration of Radioactive Substances) Regulations 1978. London: HMSO.

47. Health and Safety Commission. Work with Ionising Radiation, Ionising Radiations Regulations 1999, Approved Code of Practice and Guidance. London: HSE Books; 2000.

Further Reading

Connor KJ, McLintock IS. Radiation Protection Handbook for Laboratory Workers. HHSC Handbook No. 14. Leeds: H & H Scientific Consultants; 1994.

International Commission on Radiological Protection. Radiological Protection and Safety in Medicine (ICRP Publication 73). Ann ICRP 1996; 26: No. 2.

Martin CJ, Sutton DG, eds. Practical Radiation Protection In Health Care. Oxford: Oxford University Press, 2002.

Martin CJ, Dendy PP, Corbett RH, eds. Medical Imaging and Radiation Protection for Medical Students and Clinical Staff. London: British Institute of Radiology; 2003.

7

The Radiopharmacy

James Doherty and David Graham

7.1 Introduction

Radiopharmacy has become firmly established as a specialist branch of the hospital pharmaceutical service in the UK, Europe, and the USA. This specialist pharmacy service is an integral part of the multidisciplinary team providing services to nuclear medicine departments. Radiopharmacies have tended to develop in two patterns. One where each nuclear medicine facility has its own radiopharmacy, the other where a number of nuclear medicine facilities are supplied by a centralized radiopharmacy. In the following sections we will describe the principles of radiopharmacy design together with what we believe to be the principles of good radiopharmaceutical practice.

7.2 Radiopharmacy Design

Various factors need to be taken into consideration in the planning and the design of a radiopharmacy. While regulatory constraints must always be the prime consideration, the local situation also plays a major role in shaping the final plan. Bearing these two factors in mind, it is important that the design be primarily concerned with the safe production of radiopharmaceuticals in terms of good manufacturing, aseptic dispensing, and radiation protection practices.

7.2.1 Regulatory Constraints

Pharmaceutical Aspects

In the UK the preparation of diagnostic and therapeutic radiopharmaceuticals falls under the legislative control of the Medicines Act 1968 [1]. The NHS premises in which they are prepared are no longer subject to Crown Exemptions as this was withdrawn with the introduction of the NHS and Community Care Act 1990 (Section 60) [2]. Since 1 April 1991, UK radiopharmacy premises have had two options available to them:

1. Apply for a Manufacturer's Special Licence through the Department of Health's Medicines Healthcare products Regulatory Agency (MHRA) previously the Medicines Control Agency (MCA).
2. Seek exemption under Section 10 of the Medicines Act 1968 [1], which allows medicinal products to be dispensed in a hospital by or under the direct supervision of a pharmacist.

Regardless of the option taken UK radiopharmaceuticals must always be:

1. compounded in a controlled environment subject to the requirements of the Department of Health and Social Security (DHSS) Circular "Premises and the Environment for the Preparation of Radiopharmaceuticals (1982)" [3];

2. manufactured following the guidelines given in "Rules and Guidance to Pharmaceutical Manufacturers and Distributors" (GMP) [4].

In 1971 the then Medicines Inspectorate division of the DHSS published the first edition of the GMP as a practical interpretation of the Medicines Act. This, and its subsequent revisions in 1977 and 1983, became recognized as the basic requirements for the safe manufacturing of medicinal products in the UK. In 1992 with the publication of "The Rules Governing Medicinal Products in the European Communities Vol. IV: Good Manufacturing Practice for Medicinal Products" [5], a guiding standard was created which complements the above regulations and now acts as a guiding standard within the European Community (EC). This was incorporated into the GMP in the 1993 and 1997 revisions as well as the current version – "Rules and Guidance to Pharmaceutical Manufacturers and Distributors" – published in 2002.

Radiation Protection Aspects

Radiopharmaceuticals differ from other sterile pharmaceutical preparations in that it is essential to protect the operator, environment, and other persons from ionizing radiation. The handling, storage, and disposal of such radioactive substances are governed by both the Ionising Radiation Regulations, 1999 [6] and the Radioactive Substances Act 1993 [7]. Practical guidelines can also be found in "Medical and Dental Guidance Notes: A good practice guide on all aspects of ionising radiation protection in the clinical environment" [8]. Further attention must also be paid to the "Work with Ionising Radiation. Approved Code of Practice and practical guidance on the Ionising Radiation Regulations, 1999" [9]. For more detailed information see Chapter 6.

7.2.2   Local Constraints

In order to draw up plans at a local level many factors have to be taken into consideration and perhaps the most important of these are cost, nature and volume of work, and availability of suitable premises.

The location of the radiopharmacy is very important. Ideally it should be in close proximity to the nuclear medicine department, while not creating a radiation hazard to other areas or personnel.

In addition, the radiopharmacy should not only be designed to take the existing service into account, but also allow for future developments.

7.2.3   Design of Hospital Radiopharmacies

In the design structure of any new radiopharmacy consideration should be given for the inclusion of the following areas in the plan:

1. cleanroom suite, comprising cleanrooms and clean support rooms as outlined below;
2. laboratory;
3. radionuclide store;
4. office;
5. cloakroom, shower, and toilet facilities;
6. radioactive materials reception area.

A section of the radiopharmacy premises may have to be defined as a controlled or supervised area under the "Ionising Radiation Regulations, 1999" [6], depending on the type and quantity of the radionuclides being handled (see Chapter 6).

Cleanroom Suite or Facility

It is now widely acknowledged that in order to provide the aseptic conditions necessary for the production of sterile radiopharmaceutical injections, other options are available than the traditional laminar flow cabinet sited in a cleanroom. All aseptic manipulation, however, must be performed in a workstation with a controlled internal environment conforming to Annex 1 of the GMP grade A [10]. The options available for the aseptic production of radiopharmaceuticals are:

1. a laminar flow workstation housed within a conventional cleanroom (GMP grade B);
2. an isolator housed in a dedicated room (minimum GMP grade D).

Regardless of which option is chosen the facilities should produce an environment that satisfies both radiation safety and pharmaceutical quality. The NHS QC Committee has published in the third edition of "Quality Assurance of Aseptic Preparation Services" [11] clear guidelines as to the requirements for both of these systems.

Table 7.1. Summary of the environmental facilities required for radiopharmaceutical production

Product type	Production environment	Workstation requirements	Clothing
Oral or inhalation[a]	Radionuclide laboratory	Hygienic conditions conforming to BS EN 12469 class I for protection for volatile radionuclides	Laboratory coat and disposable hat and gloves Face masks and safety glasses may be necessary for some products
Generator storage and elution	(1) Cleanroom GMP grade B[b]	(1) Laminar flow cabinet GMP grade A[b] and BS EN 12469 class II[c]	Sterilized cleanroom clothing
	(2) Cleanroom GMP grade D[b]	(2) Isolator GMP grade A[b] and BS EN 12469 class III[c]	Dedicated clothing appropriate to this environmental background
Parenteral prepared by closed procedures	(1) Cleanroom GMP grade B[b]	(1) Laminar flow cabinet GMP grade A[b] and BS EN 12469 class II[c]	Sterilized cleanroom clothing
	(2) Cleanroom GMP grade D[b]	(2) Isolator GMP grade A[b] and BS EN 12469 class III[c]	Dedicated clothing appropriate to this environmental background
Parenteral prepared by open procedures	(1) Cleanroom GMP grade B[b]	(1) Laminar flow cabinet GMP grade A[b] and BS EN 12469 class II[c]	Sterilized cleanroom clothing
Long-lived radio-pharmaceuticals prepared by closed or open procedures	(2) Cleanroom GMP grade D[b]	(2) Isolator GMP grade A[b] and BS EN 12469 class III[c]	Dedicated clothing appropriate to this environmental background
Blood component labeling			

[a] Most radiopharmacies make these only occasionally and hence they tend to be produced under the same environmental conditions as parenteral radiopharmaceuticals.
[b] Environmental monitoring is necessary to demonstrate compliance with the ISO 14644 and GMP.
[c] Testing is required to demonstrate compliance with the BS EN 12469.

Conventional Cleanroom with Laminar Flow Workstation

The laminar flow workstation must be situated in a cleanroom that is dedicated to aseptic preparation and its environment must comply with GMP grade B. To achieve this cleanrooms should be supplied with air (Table 7.1) which is terminally filtered by high-efficiency particulate air (HEPA) filters. The cleanrooms should be constructed in accordance with the guidelines given in both GMP [4] and BS/EN/ISO 14644 (1999) [12], which give specification as to the design, construction, and commissioning of such areas.

The guidelines recommend that walls, floors, and ceilings should have a smooth, impervious, and non-shedding surface which should allow sanitation and disinfection. Bare wood and other unsealed surfaces must be avoided and there must be no sinks in the facility. The junction between walls, floors, and ceilings should be coved.

Sanitation and disinfection should be carried out on a regular basis, following a written procedure which includes a written confirmation that the procedure has been carried out. The effectiveness of the cleaning should be validated and monitored by environmental monitoring techniques (Section 7.4).

Entry into and exit from the cleanroom should be through a pre-change zone prior to entering the changing room. In the pre-change zone, personnel firstly change out of outdoor clothing and don cleanroom undergarments. They then progress into the changing room (GMP grade B) where sterile cleanroom clothing is donned. This three-stage changing thereby minimizes the microbial and particulate contamination entering the room.

Cleanrooms should have a positive pressure differential with respect to adjacent unclassified areas and this pressure gradient should be continuously monitored (Section 7.4.8, Table 7.5) with

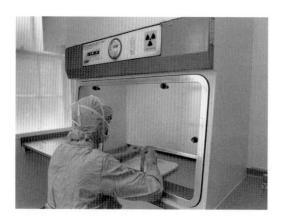

Figure 7.1. Example of a radiopharmaceutical laminar flow safety cabinet, MAT-I-MAT.

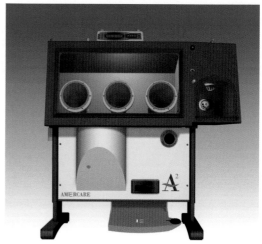

Figure 7.2. Radiopharmaceutical isolator for blood cell labeling. (Reproduced with kind permission of Amercare Ltd.)

an alarm system operating to warn of loss of ventilation. Doors on both sides of a room should be either inter-locked or alarmed to prevent both being open at the same time, thereby ensuring the protective effect of pressure differentials are not lost. Materials may be passed into and out of the cleanroom from a preparation area (GMP grade C) which should lie adjacent to the cleanroom. Access between these areas is provided by a hatch(es) system where the doors are inter-locked to prevent both sides being opened at the same time. A validated and documented transfer procedure should be followed for the movement of materials into and out of cleanrooms.

These cleanrooms must be equipped with laminar flow radiopharmaceutical safety cabinets (Figure 7.1), which offers both operator (BS/EN 12469: 2000) [13] and product (BS/EN/ISO 14644 (1999)) [12] protection.

Isolators with a HEPA-filtered Air Supply

Isolators are contained workstations within which an environment complying with GMP grade A is found. This provides the conditions necessary for aseptically producing sterile injections. It is recommended that isolators used to prepare radiopharmaceuticals are negative pressure with respect to the background environment and be ducted to atmosphere. The design of any such facility should comply with the principles laid out in "Pharmaceutical Isolators: A Guide to their Application, Design and Control" [14]. For aseptic applications, the GMP recommends a minimum background environment of grade D air classification. It may be more practical, however, depending on

overall design, to improve this to grade C or even B. The transfer system is a critical aspect of isolator operation and must be carried out following a fully documented and validated transfer procedure that will not compromise the grade A working environment.

The room in which the isolator is sited should be used only for this purpose and, as with cleanrooms, the dedicated room should have surfaces that are smooth, impervious, and non-shedding, allowing easy cleaning and disinfection. A changing facility must be provided for staff working with the isolator. Dedicated clothing, which is appropriate to the room classification, may have to be worn by operators.

There are many isolators on the market aimed at pharmaceutical manufacturing. One company, Amercare Ltd, provide a range of isolators designed for use in the radiopharmacy (Figure 7.2) which includes technetium dispensing, blood cell labeling, volatile product handling, and heavily shielded PET isolators. These isolators can have included, as an integral part of the enclosure, a lead shielded area for storage and elution of ^{99m}Tc generators, centrifuges for performing blood cell separations, and radionuclide calibrators.

Cleanrooms Versus Isolators

In the two systems described cost, convenience, and containment properties are the major considerations when weighing up the option of

THE RADIOPHARMACY

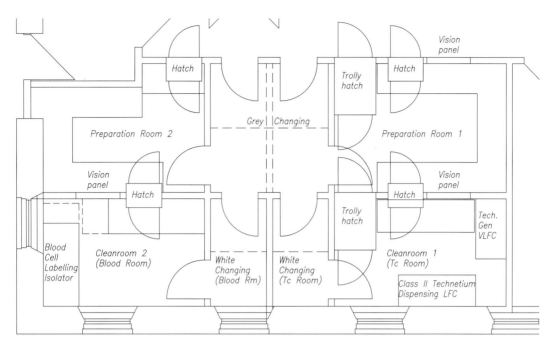

Figure 7.3. Plan of proposed cleanroom suite, Aberdeen Radiopharmacy. (Reproduced with kind permission of Cameron Chisolm Dawson Partnership.)

cleanrooms versus isolators. If the scale of the local requirements for radiophamaceutical production is such that a specialized filter environment is necessary for the siting of an isolator then its major cost advantages may be lost and conventional cleanroom technology may be better.

Figure 7.3 shows a proposed layout of the radiopharmacy cleanrooms in Aberdeen where a conventional cleanroom facility has been proposed in the area shown as "Cleanroom 1 (Tc Room)". This cleanroom (GMP grade B) was included in the design to allow the manufacture of any type of radiopharmaceutical. It is proposed to install two radiopharmaceutical safety cabinets (GMP grade A; BS/EN 12469: 2000) similar to the type shown in Figure 7.1. One will be used to prepare the radiopharmaceutical injection while the other will be used to store and elute ^{99m}Tc generators. Access to and from this room is only through the changing room (GMP grade B) dedicated for this area, since the other cleanroom is reserved exclusively for cell labeling procedures. Consequently the cleanroom reserved for cell labeling must have a separate changing room. Each cleanroom is serviced by its own preparation room (GMP grade C), with a connecting interlocked hatch system as described above. Access for ^{99m}Tc generators is provided by trolley hatches.

"Cleanroom 2 Blood Room" (Figure 7.3) was included in the design for the exclusive handing of blood where different types of blood cells are to be radiolabeled prior to reinjection into patients. It is proposed to house an isolator in this cleanroom, as shown in Figure 7.2, that is equipped with a centrifuge specifically to allow cell separations within the grade A environment. This cleanroom is designed to GMP grade B although it is likely that different clothing will be worn during its operation with the consequence that the room may not be operated at this grade (GMP grade D is the minimum requirement).

Laboratory

A laboratory area is required in which to perform routine quality control procedures (Section 7.4) as well as research and development work. The preparation of oral dose radiopharmaceuticals may also be carried out in such an area. The laboratory should be suitably equipped to perform these functions and would normally be supplied with such services as natural gas, vacuum, and compressed air.

Radionuclide Store

A room that can be securely locked should be part of the design to ensure the safe storage of radioactive stock materials. This room can also act as a decay store, thereby facilitating the safe storage of radioactive residues and other contaminated waste materials.

A feature of such a store may include a shielded facility (i.e. bunker) for the storage of high activity as well as long-lived radionuclides, including ^{99m}Tc generators. A refrigerator and deep freeze may be located here for the storage of radioactive products that require these conditions.

Other Considerations

Space permitting, it is beneficial to include an office in the design of any radiopharmacy. This provides an area for the storage of documents required for radiopharmaceutical production. These are best kept in a location distinct from those areas where radioactive materials are stored or dispensed.

Shower facilities can be provided for decontamination of radiopharmacy personnel in case of accidental spillage. One consequence of the removal of sinks from the cleanroom suite is that hand wash facilities will have to be provided in a suitable location to allow hand washing prior to entry into the cleanroom and preparation areas.

Recently the security of radioactive and other dangerous substances has become an issue. Burglar alarms that communicate to the police should be considered for all areas where radioactive substances are stored. Also consideration should be given to how and when deliveries of radioactive good are made so that these materials are stored securely and their location confirmed to the radiopharmacy concerned.

7.3 Production of Radiopharmaceuticals

As outlined in Chapter 1, the characteristics of ^{99m}Tc make it a nearly ideal radionuclide for imaging purposes. It is therefore not surprising that the majority of investigations use radiopharmaceuticals that are ^{99m}Tc-labeled compounds. In fact many of the new radiophamaceuticals that have recently come on the market are ^{99m}Tc compounds that have replaced radionuclides with less favorable imaging characteristics. For these reasons we shall concentrate mainly on the production processes for ^{99m}Tc radiopharmaceuticals.

7.3.1 Production Facilities

The facilities and environment necessary for radiophamaceutical production are outlined in the GMP [4] and the DHSS circular [3] referred to in Section 7.2. The circular describes the facilities for the production of radiopharmaceuticals as summarized in Table 7.1.

7.3.2 Manufacturing Materials

^{99m}Tc radiopharmaceuticals are produced by combining the radionuclide, as sodium pertechnetate, with a number of non-active sterile compounds contained within a sealed sterile vial (kit). Both of these components are readily available from commercial sources.

Kits

A kit has been defined as a "pre-packed set of sterile ingredients designed for the preparation of a specific radiopharmaceutical" [3]. Most commonly the ingredients are freeze dried, enclosed within a vial under a nitrogen atmosphere, and comprise the following:

1. the compound to be complexed to the ^{99m}Tc. These are known as ligands (e.g. methylene diphosphonate);
2. stannous ions (Sn^{2+}) in various chemical forms (e.g. chloride or fluoride) which are present as a reducing agent;
3. other compounds that act as stabilizers, buffers, antioxidants, or bactericides.

These kits allow the radiopharmacist, in a hospital setting, to transform the pertechnetate, via complex chemical reactions performed within the vial, into the desired radiopharmaceutical. This is achieved usually by the simple addition of pertechnetate into the vial followed by shaking to dissolve the contents. This is then sometimes followed by a short incubation period at room temperature, although heating is necessary with some kits (e.g. ^{99m}Tc-MAG3 and ^{99m}Tc-sestamibi).

Molybdenum/Technetium Generators

Radionuclides with long physical half-lives (e.g. ^{131}I, $t_{1/2} = 8$ days) can be easily transported from production site to the user hospital. With shorter half-life radionuclides (e.g. ^{123}I, $t_{1/2} = 13$ hours) it is more difficult and only centers close to the production site can be supplied. The development of the radionuclide generator has allowed some short half-life radionuclides to be supplied to centers distant from production facilities. All radionuclide generators work on the principle that a relatively long-lived "parent" radionuclide decays to produce a "daughter" radionuclide, where the chemical nature of parent and daughter are quite different. This difference allows separation of the daughter from the parent.

The decay scheme of ^{99}Mo is shown in Figure 7.4. The molybdenum/technetium generator consists of ^{99}Mo absorbed onto an alumina-filled column, the amount of ^{99}Mo being dependent on the activity rating of the generator. The ^{99}Mo is present on the column as ^{99}MoO$_4^{2-}$. ^{99}Mo decays to its daughter radionuclide ^{99m}Tc as pertechnetate, ^{99m}TcO$_4^-$. The amount of ^{99m}TcO$_4^-$ grows as a result of the decay of ^{99}Mo, until a transient equilibrium is reached. At this point the amount of ^{99m}Tc on the column appears to decay with the half-life of ^{99}Mo, as shown in Figure 7.5.

^{99m}Tc is removed from the column as sodium pertechnetate, Na^{99m}TcO$_4$, by drawing a solution of sodium chloride (NaCl) 0.9% $^{w}/_v$ through the column. This process is known as eluting the generator and gives a sterile solution of sodium pertechnetate (the eluate) that may now be used to compound radiophamaceuticals.

The design of a typical generator will be described by reference to the GE Healthcare's generator, Dryrtec. Listed below are the main

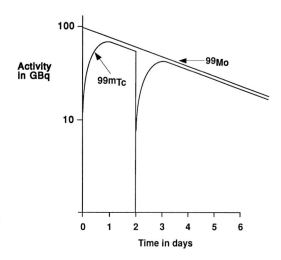

Figure 7.5. Plot of logarithm of ^{99}Mo and ^{99m}Tc activities against time showing transient equilibrium. The generator is eluted on day 2 and the ^{99m}Tc activity grows again until transient equilibrium is reached.

components of this generator:

1. a single spike NaCl inlet;
2. a 0.22 μm air inlet filter;
3. a sterile alumina column to which is bound ^{99}Mo;
4. a replaceable collection elution needle;
5. a terminal 0.22 μm eluate filter.

These components are housed within a compact plastic casing. The alumina column is encased in lead or, in generators with greater than a 30 GBq rating, encased in depleted uranium.

The operating principle is fairly straightforward. The generator is supplied with sterile evacuated vials, one of which is placed in a lead pot designed for the elution process. It is also supplied with vials of NaCl intravenous infusion BP 0.9% $^{w}/_v$ containing either 5 ml, 10 ml, or 20 ml. Firstly a vial of NaCl containing the desired volume is place on the spike on the NaCl inlet. Then a shielded evacuated vial is placed over the elution needle, which draws sterile NaCl Intravenous Infusion BP 0.9% $^{w}/_v$ from the vial through the column and into the shielded evacuated vial. When the volume of eluate has been collected, air enters the elution vial after first passing through the column. The elution vial should not be removed until all the air has bubbled through, thus assuring the column within the generator is dried between

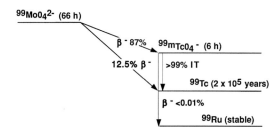

Figure 7.4. Main decay transitions of ^{99}Mo (energy levels not drawn to scale). β, Beta-particle emission; IT, isomeric transition.

elutions. Drying the column is an important process since, if left wet, radiolysis of the water takes place resulting in oxidation of the ^{99m}Tc present on the column, causing a lowering of the ^{99m}Tc activity yield on subsequent elutions.

In Aberdeen we operate a two-generator system where a new generator is delivered each week and is eluted for 2 weeks. We therefore always have two generators, which we call the "NEW" and "WEEK-OLD", being eluted each day. The "NEW" generator is eluted daily to give eluates of approximately 5000–3000 MBq/ml and the "WEEK-OLD" generator to give eluates of approximately 1600–500 MBq/ml. This enables us to produce injections of high and low radioactive concentrations which are manufactured in an accurate and safe manner against the different injection activities we supply. We place a constraint on our production procedures in that all radioactive solutions are transferred using a 2 ml shielded syringe where the volume of liquid never exceeds 1 ml. This gives improved operator protection from ionizing radiation while also ensuring a measurable volume. Where we need to dispense an amount of ^{99m}Tc between 1000 MBq and 4000 MBq then it may be safely and accurately withdrawn from the "NEW" generator eluate, while those between 100 MBq and 1000 MBq may be taken from the "WEEK-OLD" eluate.

Although the generator is a device that is designed and licensed to provide sterile eluates over a period of time, the individual eluates will, however, only be used to manufacture radiopharmaceuticals during the day of elution. The sterility of the eluates is maintained throughout the useful life of the generator by the following means:

1. the eluting solution is terminally sterilized NaCl Intravenous Infusion BP 0.9% $^w/_v$;
2. air entering the system to dry the column passes through a 0.22-μm filter;
3. a terminal 0.22 μm eluate filter is placed between the column and the elution filter;
4. between elutions the NaCl spike and elution needle is protected from the environment by single-use, disposable, sterile guards;
5. the elution of the generator should be carried out in a GMP grade A environment in one of the two systems outlined in Table 7.1.

Some of the factors that should be taken into consideration when deciding which generator is most suitable for local use are:

1. tailoring ^{99m}Tc generator yields to daily and weekly ^{99m}Tc production requirements;
2. a suitable day of delivery in relation to the generator reference dates;
3. radiation hazard;
4. cost.

Any generator system should be chosen and used in a manner to fit the ^{99m}Tc requirements of the user. In Aberdeen we require a minimum of 29 GBq of activity, which is provided by purchasing 40 GBq weekly and using each generator for two weeks.

One disadvantage of this single-generator system is that there is a large amount of unused ^{99m}Tc produced with initial elutions and this waste material must be dealt with. Another strategy for generator purchase would be to buy two smaller generators one at the beginning and the other in the middle of the week (Figure 7.6). This type of system works well but we have found the former to be more economical.

7.3.3 Methods of Production

^{99m}Tc requirements are provided by the daily elution of the ^{99m}Tc-generator(s), giving a sterile solution of sodium pertechnetate that is subdivided to provide the activity component of the radioparmaceutical. Some nuclear medicine investigations use sodium pertechnetate alone as the radiopharmaceutical (Table 7.2). In these cases pertechnetate will need only to be subdivided from the generator eluate with perhaps some dilution with a suitable diluent (sterile injection of NaCl BP 0.9% $^w/_v$). Others, and these are in the majority, use radiopharmaceuticals that involve transformation of the sodium pertechnetate into another radiochemical form. This dispensing activity is performed by adding the sodium pertechnetate to the kit or kit aliquot as described below. The compounding procedures must be carried out within the facilities described in Section 7.3.1 using aseptic technique and carried out as "closed" procedures.

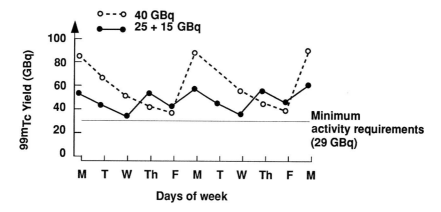

Figure 7.6. Comparison of the ^{99m}Tc yields from a single 40 GBq Amertec II generator with those of a combination of a 25 GBq and 15 GBq Amertec II generator (40 GBq and 25 GBq delivered Saturday, eluted Monday to Friday. 15 GBq delivered Wednesday, eluted Monday to Friday).

Table 7.2. Standardized manufacturing instructions for ^{99m}Tc sodium pertechnetate routinely prepared in the radiopharmacy, adult doses assumed

Study type	Activity administered to patient (MBq)	Activity to be dispensed, decay corrected to time of injection (MBq)	Final volume (ml)
Pertechnetate:			
Thyroid imaging	80	100	2
Sialoscintigram	40	100	2
Meckel's diverticulum	400	500	1
Dacryoscintigram (eye drops)	4	200	2
MUGA (multiple gated acquisition)	800	1100	1
Red cell survival	400	500	1

The Manufacturer's Method

The manufacturers of radiopharmaceutical kits recommend the production method as shown in Figure 7.7. This method involves two simple steps.

1. The freeze-dried kit is reconstituted by aseptically transferring the necessary activity of sodium pertechnetate via sterile syringe and needle. This step may also include a further dilution of the eluate with a suitable diluent. The amount of activity withdrawn for the reconstitution of the kit vial depends on two factors, the number of patient doses to be produced and the amount of activity required at injection time for each of the patient doses.

2. The reconstituted kit is aseptically subdivided to provide each patient dose with sufficient activity to allow proper imaging after administration. As in step 1, a diluent may be added to the final dose to give the desired radioactive concentration.

The "Wet" Method

This method of radiopharmaceutical production is shown in Figure 7.7 and is a three-step process [15].

1. The kit is aseptically reconstituted with a standard volume of diluent (Table 7.3).

2. The kit is then subdivided by aseptically transferring a fixed volume into each of the patient dose vials (Table 7.3).

3. To each of these patient dose vials is added a volume of sterile eluate, the volume used depending upon the activity required for each patient dose. This step may also involve a dilution with suitable diluent to a fixed final volume.

Table 7.3. Standardized manufacturing instructions for ^{99m}Tc radiopharmaceuticals routinely prepared in the radiopharmacy, adult doses assumed

Radiopharma-ceutical	Kit manufacturer	Activity administered to patient (MBq)	Max. permitted activity added to kit (MBq)	Wet labeling method			
				Kit reconstitution volume (ml)	Subdivision volume (ml)	Max. permitted activity added to aliquot (MBq)	Final volume (ml)
MDP	GE Healthcare	600	18 500	10.5	1	1850[a]	2
DTPA	GE Healthcare	800	11 100	6.5	1	2600[a]	2
MAA	Scherring	100	3 700	9.5	1	1000[a]	2
Tin colloid	GE Healthcare	200	3 700	5	1	700[a]	2
Mebrofenin	Scherring	150	3 700	5	1	700[a]	2
Tetrofosmin	GE Healthcare	400	1 200 in 8 ml	9.5	1	2000[a]	2
Sestamibi	Bristol-Myers Squibb	400	11 100	7.5	1	2000[a]	2

[a] Activity capacity and shelf-life validated in-house.

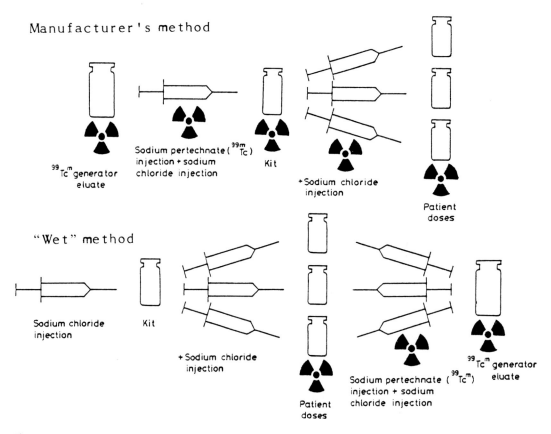

Figure 7.7. Comparison of the manufacturer's and the "wet" method of production. The steps involving the handling of radioactive materials are indicated by trefoil signs. (Reproduced with kind permission of A. Millar (1985). In: A.E. Theobald, ed. Radiopharmacy and Radiopharmaceuticals. Taylor and Francis Ltd, London, 162.)

This method has two main advantages over the manufacturer's method. Firstly, since radioactive material is handled only once, in step 3, the radiation dose to the operator is reduced. Secondly, additional radiopharmaceuticals may be requested outwith the pre-planned production schedule. Catering for these requests, can be performed more economically with the "wet" method as the remains of a non-active kit are still available.

The major drawback with this method is that it lies outwith the manufacturer's recommendations. Before adopting it, extensive quality assurance must be undertaken to determine the pharmaceutical stability as well as the clinical acceptability of the final products. Table 7.3 shows how we have developed this method to meet our requirements and it would have to be adapted to suit other situations. Adoption of this method requires validation of the process and must be carried out to show products manufactured in this manner are equivalent to those produced by following the manufacturer's instructions.

The "wet" method may be more advantageous in larger central radiopharmacies, where two operators work together in the same laminar downflow workstation, one carrying out steps 1 and 2 whilst the other carries out step 3.

7.3.4 Production Procedures

It is essential that ^{99m}Tc radiopharmaceuticals are administered on the day of production, for the following reasons.

1. Sterility – aseptically prepared pharmaceuticals should ideally be administered within a few hours of production, in accordance with GMP [4].
2. Radioactivity – ^{99m}Tc has a half-life of only 6 hours.
3. Radiochemical stability – ^{99m}Tc complexes are generally stable for a period between 4 and 8 hours after production.

Documentation and Labeling

Documentation and labeling are fundamental to good manufacturing practice in all aspects of work within the pharmacy department and the radiopharmacy is no exception. In the section that follows we will show examples of documentation which will be illustrated in conjunction with a description of our production procedure. We rec-

ognize, however, that each hospital department should tailor its production procedures and documentation to suit its own individual requirements.

The purpose of documentation is to describe uniformity and good practice in terms of working procedures, and to record the details of those procedures, in such a way as to illustrate that it has been followed correctly. Such a system of documentation must be in operation so that the history of each preparation may be traced from the receipt of raw materials to the administration of the radiopharmaceutical. A manual of written procedures must be created for all procedures and activities associated with each operation within the radiopharmacy and these must be reviewed at specified intervals (at least every two years). Each document should have its own unique code number and be approved by a second person, usually a quality controller or head of department. Documentation and records kept should include:

1. purchase of raw materials and ingredients and their suppliers;
2. stock levels of radioactive materials;
3. generator operation and elution records;
4. product preparation methods and associated records, including product release;
5. environmental and microbiological controls;
6. cleaning and maintenance of the department;
7. equipment operation, calibration, and maintenance;
8. staff training procedures and records;
9. transport of radioactive materials;
10. commissioning, inspection, and audit.

All radiopharmaceuticals are labeled as described below. Incorporated into the design of each label is a yellow and black radioactive warning trefoil logo. The following information is present on each label:

1. preparation volume;
2. approved name of the preparation and route of administration;
3. radionuclidic activity in Bq;
4. the time and date the radioactive concentration was measured (reference time/date);

5. POM (Prescription Only Medicine);
6. where applicable patient's name, identity number, ward, and hospital;
7. where applicable special license of production unit;
8. batch number and expiry date/time of product;
9. address of manufacturing department;
10. any special storage conditions if applicable;
11. any special storage instructions (e.g. "SHAKE BEFORE USE" for ^{99m}Tc-MAA);
12. name and concentration of any added substances.

It is good manufacturing practice to have all labels checked by more than one member of staff.

Dedicated labeling systems have been developed for use in the radiopharmacy [16]. Those that link the radionuclide calibrator to the labeling processor reduce the risk of transcription errors and produce clear labels both quickly and efficiently.

In Aberdeen we use a radionuclide database system developed on Microsoft Access to generate the information for the labels. This includes software that creates much of the routine documentation describing product preparation. This software also includes radionuclide stock control, solid waste and liquid waste disposal records, all of which are required under the Radioactive Substances Act [7].

Production Scheduling

On the day prior to production individual patient order forms (Figure 7.8), along with a copy of the nuclear medicine patient list, are electronically

ABERDEEN ROYAL INFIRMARY
Department of Nuclear Medicine
Bio - Medical Physics & Bio - Engineering
Central Radioisotope Store

Serial: 13142-1

Issue and Use of Radioactive Materials

A. RADIOISOTOPE DISPENSING

Radio-pharmaceutical	Activity Required	Date & Time
99mTc Methylene Diphosphonate	600MBq	22/06/2004, 09:15

B. PHARMACEUTICAL DISPENSING

Pharmaceutical Form Required:

Dose Activity	Time	Volume	Checked Activity	Time	Approved: Pharmacist	Approved: Physicist

C. USE

Bone

Patient's Full Name	Unit No.	Ward and Hospital	Administered By	Amount Administered
A.N.Other	0649619G	ARI 49 O/P		

Figure 7.8. Specimen order form.

transferred by the nuclear medicine department to the radiopharmacy. Using the order forms and the list, the following day's production schedule is organized as follows.

Firstly, all the materials necessary for the production of one type of injection are collected in a plastic tray which can be easily disinfected. These trays are product specific so as to minimize the possibility of dispensing errors – for example, one tray for all the methylene diphosphonate (MDP) doses.

Next all the relevant information is entered into the radionuclide database in order to create the production document SDR 487 (Figure 7.9). The order in which the injections are prepared depends on the time of administration, the nature of the product, and pharmaceutical considerations, such as the boiling stage necessary for the production of ^{99m}Tc-MAG3.

Finally, the activity to be added to each of the patient doses, the method of reconstituting and subdividing the kit is calculated depending on the method of production – manufacturer's method or "wet" method (Table 7.3). In both methods the activity contained in each patient dose should give an overage which allows the required activity to be easily withdrawn from the vial whilst giving some flexibility as to the intended time of injection. The calculated activity is entered into SDR 487, which is prepared in duplicate – one copy for the operator in the cleanroom and one for the operator in the preparation room.

Production

In Aberdeen a minimum of two operators are required to carry out this production procedure, one operator in the cleanroom and the other in the preparation room that services it. Their duties are outlined below.

Operator 1:

1. enters the cleanroom following a written three-stage change procedure for entry into this controlled environment;
2. elutes the generator in the specific elution volume;
3. disinfects the workstation before switching on.

Operator 2:

1. enters the preparation room following a written change procedure for entry into this controlled environment;

2. performs and records the daily calibration checks on the radionuclide calibrator (see Section 5.5);
3. disinfects and then loads the double-ended hatchway with the trays containing the materials for manufacturing the radiopharmaceuticals. All materials transferred via the hatchway are disinfected, the hatchway being the link between the preparation and cleanrooms. Currently it is expected that this disinfection stage, or the one carried out by operator 1 on the workstation, should involve wiping of the materials with sterile alcohol wipes;
4. measures and records (SDR 486, Figure 7.10) the ^{99}Mo contamination level in the eluate (Section 7.4.3);
5. measures and records (SDR 486, Figure 7.10) the ^{99m}Tc activity of the eluate;
6. calculates the volumes of eluate to be used in each of the patient doses to complete and record in SDR 487 (Figure 7.9).

The operator in the cleanroom disinfects, either by spraying or wiping with sterile alcohol, and then transfers the contents of the tray into the workstation. The patient doses are manufactured in the workstation following the instructions given in SDR 487, employing aseptic technique throughout.

On completion these doses, contained within their lead pots, are passed out to the preparation room via the hatchway. Here "operator 2" treats the doses as follows:

1. The ^{99m}Tc activity is measured in the radionuclide calibrator and recorded in the production document SDR 487. This is performed automatically using the computerized database where the activity is directly read from the calibrator and is linked, via the internal clock in the computer, to the time of calibration.

2. With each activity measurement being entered into SDR 487 the database creates a label complying with the specifications given above.

3. The vial is returned to the lead pot and is sealed in a plastic securitainer to which the label is attached.

Aberdeen Royal Infirmary, Department of Pharmacy
Technical Services: Radiopharmacy

Study Type: Bone

Instructions:
Reconstitute kit with 10.5 ml of NaCl 0.9% for injection and subdivide into 1ml doses, add required volume of eluate made up to 1ml with NaCl 0.9% for injection.

Batch Number: MDP_14044

Additional Materials:	Batch Numbers:	Expiry Dates:	Radionuclide:	Letter:	Batch Number:
Sodium Chloride Inj. 0.9%	S03801	31/01/2005	99mTc	D	3994 Z01136566
Medronate	538	10/02/2004			

Patient	Ward	Admin (MBq)	Dispensed Activity (08:30)	Eluate/Stock (ml)		Final Vol (ml)	Measured Act (MBq)	Time Measured	Returned
A.N. Other	ARI 44 OP	600	850 MBq	0.35	(D)	2	866	08:52	√
A.N. Other	Albyn OP	600	1000 MBq	0.4	(D)	2	978	09:06	√
A.N. Other	ARI 44 OP	600	1000 MBq	0.4	(D)	2	941	09:04	√
A.N. Other	Roxburgh Ho OP	600	1000 MBq	0.4	(D)	2	965	09:05	√
A.N. Other	ARI 1	600	1000 MBq	0.4	(D)	2	954	09:04	√

SDR 487 (03/0404/D.Graham)   Supersedes SDR 62(05/95)   Approved By:

Figure 7.9. Radiopharmacy dispensing record (SDR 487).

99mTc Generator Report

Generator Details		Quality Control		QC Carried Out By
Supplier	Amersham Health	**Al Content**	<10mcg/ml mcg/ml	Janice Johnston
Delivered	05/06/2004	**Tc04 Content**	99.9 %	Janice Johnston
Reference	40 GBq on 11/06/2004	**Sterility 1**	Pass	Susan Denning
Batch	4058 Z01353847	**Sterility 2**	Pass	Susan Denning
Expiry	27/06/2004			

Elutions

Letter	Activity (MBq)	Reference Time	Reference Date	Volume (ml)	Activity (MBq/ml)	Vial Batch	99Mo (KBq)	Eluted By
A	99950	08:32	07/06/04	19.65	5087	10241060	Pass	J Johnston
B	4163	11:02	07/06/04	20	208	10241060	Sterility	J Johnston
C	70946	08:03	08/06/04	19.91	3563	10241060	Pass	M Christie
D	55265	08:33	09/06/04	19.94	2772	10241060	Pass	M Christie
E	42367	08:01	10/06/04	10.11	4191	10241060	Pass	M Christie
F	33141	08:29	11/06/04	9.95	3331	10241060	Pass	M Christie
G	18217	15:54	11/06/04	10.13	1798	10241060	Pass	M Christie
H	15527	08:37	14/06/04	9.6	1617	10241060	Pass	M Christie
I	12064	07:56	15/06/04	10.12	1192	10241060	Pass	M Christie
J	8524	08:08	16/06/04	10.07	846	10241060	Pass	D Graham
K	7120	08:09	17/06/04	10.08	706	10241060	Pass	M Christie
L	5443	08:08	18/06/04	9.99	545	10241060	Pass	M Christie
M	606	11:14	18/06/04	20	30	10241060	Sterility	M Christie

Final Check By: **Date:**

Figure 7.10. Elution record for sterile ^{99m}Tc generator (SDR 486).

4. The activity, time of calibration, and final volume are recorded on the nuclear medicine order form (Figure 7.8).

5. All doses are checked by a pharmacist against the following requirements:
   (a) nature of the study;
   (b) radioactive concentration;
   (c) labeling requirements.

This procedure is repeated for the remaining trays until the production schedule is completed. At the end of each working session the workstation, cleanroom, and changing rooms are systematically disinfected in accordance with a written procedure.

7.3.5 Non-^{99m}Tc Radiopharmaceuticals

These are supplied either as ready-to-use products or where dilution and subdivision are required. Where no further pharmaceutical manipulations are necessary prior to administration of the product, it is only necessary to check the manufacturer's label details for correctness. These products tend to be single use products where any remaining stock is discarded after administration.

Non-^{99m}Tc radiopharmaceuticals with long half-lives can also be supplied where it is necessary to dilute or subdivide the radiopharmaceutical. Subdivision may also be required on separate occasions a number of days apart. When diluting a radiopharmaceutical it is important to check the compatibility of the diluent with the manufacturer. Also, consideration should be given to radiopharmaceuticals containing preservatives, the concentration of which should be maintained when diluted to ensure its continued effectiveness. Dilution and/or subdivision must be carried out in the facilities as outlined in Table 7.1 (long-lived radiopharmaceuticals prepared by closed or open procedures).

7.3.6 Manufacture of Monoclonal Antibodies and Peptides

In recent years there has been a great interest shown in the use of monoclonal antibodies (MAB) and peptides as a means of targeting the radiopharmaceutical to the organ or tissue of interest. These have mainly, although not exclusively, been developed for the diagnosis and/or treatment of malignant disease. The manufacture of MAB is a lengthy, complex, and expensive business and it is rare for such a task to be undertaken in a hospital-based radiopharmacy. However, there have been a number of MABs and peptides that have become commercially available in a kit form, which allows the radiolabeling of the proteins to be carried out in the radiopharmacy.

Radiolabeling techniques vary depending on the radionuclide being used and the physical properties of the MAB or peptide itself. Generally many of these kits involve open procedures and the environmental conditions in which they are produced must comply with those given in Table 7.1. Currently there is much debate around the segregation of facilities used for the handling of these products and it is recommended that risk assessments are carried out on each product individually to determine what precautions are necessary for the safe handing of these agents.

Radiolabeling with any of the radionuclides of iodine may result in the accidental release of radioiodine gas and hence such techniques must be carried out in a total exhaust workstation. Radiolabeling with indium (^{111}In) involves working with ^{111}In-indium chloride, which is strongly acidic. Metal ion contamination can adversely affect the labeling efficiency of the radionuclide to the MAB and hence the use of disposable plastic containers rather than glass may be necessary. Also the use of needles to transfer the indium may have to be avoided by using automatic pipettes fitted with sterile tips. This technique would have to be carried out as an open procedure.

7.3.7 Blood Cell Labeling

The modern radiopharmacy is often involved in the radiolabeling of autologous erythrocytes, leukocytes, and platelets. Protocols for the cell separation and radiolabeling are beyond the scope of this chapter, but may be found in Chapters 6 and 7 of Sampson [17].

The facilities required for radiolabeling of blood cells are discussed in the DHSS circular of 1982 [3] and are also outlined in Table 7.1. Generally in radiopharmacy practice the problems of ensuring the sterility of the product as well as protecting the environment form ionizing radiation are to be considered. When handling blood components, however, there is the additional consideration of the risk of viral contamination (hepatitis B and HIV) of other products as well as the potential for the accidental infection of the operator. Personnel handling blood components may be offered hepatitis B vaccination as a precautionary measure.

It is preferable, especially when cell labeling is carried out frequently, to have a separate cleanroom facility for carrying out these procedures. A dedicated workstation (Table 7.1) should be operated, with no other manipulations being carried out in the cleanroom at the same time. This prevents cross-contamination with other products [3]. Additionally, it has now become accepted that changing facilities for entry into cell labeling facilities should be separate from changing facilities for other purposes.

Closed procedures are recommended to be used for cell labeling where possible [3], but we have found open procedures to be a preferable option since they avoid handling the blood components with syringe and needle thus eliminating the risk of needle-stick injury. It is good practice when handling radioactive substances to work over drip-trays as a method of containing any spillage. This is equally important in the handling of blood components, where the drip-tray used should be large enough to hold any spills.

In the cell separation processes, which are employed in cell labeling techniques, the use of a centrifuge is essential. Centrifuges with sealable buckets should be used for these methods.

The surfaces of the workstation, benches, and all apparatus used in a cell labeling procedure must be disinfected after use to prevent cross-contamination with subsequent samples as well as contamination of other areas of the radiopharmacy. The local disinfection policy of the hospital should be consulted for the choice of the disinfectant, but one that is active against hepatitis B and HIV is essential. Consideration must be given to the COSHH regulations [18] when handling such agents as many are toxic as well as being corrosive.

It is a requirement of the DHSS circular [3] that simultaneous labeling of blood from more than one person should not be carried out in the same workstation.

7.4 Quality Assurance of Radiopharmaceuticals

The quality assurance (QA) of a product involves a series of processes that are designed to guarantee the fitness of that product for a given purpose [19]. It includes not only analytical procedures, but also the monitoring of other production processes that will affect the quality of the final product.

In routine pharmaceutical production it is essential to quarantine final products until they are proven suitable for their intended use. Only after the products are shown to comply with all specifications, compendial or otherwise, may they be released for use.

The radiopharmaceuticals most commonly produced in the radiopharmacy are formulated as sterile, apyrogenic injections and are intended for administration to patients for a diagnostic or therapeutic purpose. These injections have to comply with the same standards of safety and efficacy as conventional parenteral pharmaceuticals. Due to the short useful shelf-life of the majority of radiopharmaceuticals, it is necessary to release products before some tests are completed. Analytical tests to check radionuclidic, radiochemical, and chemical purity must be carried out routinely, although some results are only obtained retrospectively. This especially applies to the routine sterility testing carried out on parenteral radiopharmaceuticals. As a result, these tests cannot guarantee the quality of these products alone and greater emphasis must be placed on process controls to ensure the continued quality of the radiopharmaceuticals produced. This is achieved by:

1. all operating procedures being documented and strictly observed;

2. the keeping of accurate and up-to-date records;

3. routine monitoring of the production environment with respect to microbiological, particulate, and radiological contamination;

4. planned preventative maintenance (PPM) on equipment and instruments routinely used within the department, including calibration checks.

It is a principle of GMP [4] that quality control (QC) and production procedures should be carried out by different personnel. The nature of radiopharmaceuticals make it necessary for many QC tests to be carried out by the production staff. Therefore the responsibility for the approval and release of final products may lie with the radiopharmacist and not the QC pharmacist. The role of both should be clearly defined at a local level.

There are a number of other official documents that give additional guidance on production procedures and to the level of QA deemed to be acceptable for the preparation of aseptically prepared pharmaceuticals in the UK [11, 20, 21].

7.4.1 Radioactivity Measurement

In the radiopharmacy three main types of radioactivity measuring devices or detectors may be found:

1. the radionuclide calibrator or ionization camber;
2. the Geiger-Muller (G-M) detector;
3. the scintillation counter.

For each of these detector/measurement devices it is essential that a quality assurance program is in place to check that these instruments are operating correctly for all the radionuclides being measured. Such a program is discussed in Section 5.5.

7.4.2 Radionuclidic Purity

The British Pharmacopoeia (BP) [22], the European Pharmacopoeia (EP) [23], and the United States Pharmacopoeia [24] all define radionuclidic purity as the ratio, expressed as a percentage, of the radioactivity of the radionuclide concerned to the total radioactivity of the source. Radionuclides used medicinally are of a high radionuclidic purity as laid down in the individual monographs of the Pharmacopoeias concerned.

There are three main sources of radionuclidic impurities in radionuclides:

1. the manufacturing process, giving rise, for example, to fission "by-products";
2. daughter radionuclides;
3. parent radionuclides.

It is very important to have a strict control of the levels of radionuclidic impurities in radiopharmaceuticals as their presence could potentially increase the radiation dose to the patient and/or affect the imaging processes.

The monograph for sodium pertechnetate (^{99m}Tc) injection (fission) BP [22] sets the limits for the radionuclidic impurities allowable in the injection. The test method described involves gamma scintillation spectroscopy, where the impurities are determined on a sample of eluate retained for a sufficient length of time to allow the impurities to be detected. This procedure, because of the instrumentation required, is beyond the scope of most radiopharmacies. The purchase of product licensed (EC) or Food and Drug Administration (FDA) approved (USA) ^{99m}Tc generators should guarantee that the quality of the sodium pertechnetate (^{99m}Tc) injection (fission) produced complies with the appropriate compendial standard and that these tests need not be carried out by the user. There is the possibility, however, of accidental elution of the parent ^{99}Mo from the column during elution of the generator and a limit test for the ^{99}Mo should be performed. It is recommended that at least the first eluate from each generator be assayed and this should be repeated if the generator is moved [21].

The ^{99}Mo level present in eluate can be quickly and easily tested prior to the use of the eluate in compounding injections. The method relies on the principle that the activity of the eluate due to ^{99m}Tc may be attenuated by a factor of 10^{-6} by 6 mm thickness of lead shielding. By placing the eluate-bearing vial in a lead pot of these dimensions and by placing the shielded vial in a radionuclide calibrator, the amount of ^{99}Mo may be assessed. The activity due to any ^{99}Mo present in the eluate is, however, partly attenuated by the lead shield and this must be taken into account when carrying out the assay. The actual ^{99}Mo content may then be determined by multiplying the ^{99}Mo measured by a calibration factor given by the manufacturer of the lead pot.

7.4.3 Radiochemical Purity

The radiochemical purity (RCP) is the ratio, expressed as a percentage, of the radioactivity of the radionuclide concerned that is present in the source in the chemical form declared to the total radioactivity of that radionuclide present in the source [23]. To determine RCP it is first necessary to separate the various radiochemical forms present in the radiopharmaceutical.

For ^{99m}Tc radiopharmaceuticals, RCP may be measured by chromatographic means, for example using planar chromatography, electrophoresis, and high performance liquid chromatography (HPLC). Planar chromatography is the method of choice as it provides a rapid, simple, and inexpensive method of determining the RCP. Also, the measurement of the radiochemical species present along the length of the developed chromatography paper may be easily determined and only requires inexpensive equipment. This technique's strength lies in the fact that it can be used both qualitatively (to identify the radiochemical species present) and quantitatively (to determine how much is present).

Before describing methods for the determination of RCP of ^{99m}Tc radiopharmaceuticals, it is necessary to consider briefly how ^{99m}Tc-labeled compounds are produced and how radiochemical impurities might be formed.

Labeling with ^{99m}Tc

Generator-produced ^{99m}Tc exists in its most stable oxidation state of $+7$ in the pertechnetate ion ^{99m}TcO$_4^-$, which is chemically unreactive. Reduction of the ^{99m}Tc (VII) to a lower oxidation state (most commonly the $+1, +3$, and $+5$) is necessary to form the ^{99m}Tc complex and is carried out using a reducing agent. The oxidation state of ^{99m}Tc to form the complex is dependent on:

1. the nature of ligand and reductant;
2. pH of the complexation reaction;
3. the temperature at which the complexation reaction takes place.

Stannous (Sn^{2+}) salts (usually the chloride or fluoride) are the most commonly used in commercial kits to reduce the ^{99m}Tc, which will then combine with a wide variety of chelating compounds or ligands. The amount of ^{99m}Tc present in the vial is very small (typically 10^{-9} M), when compared to the amount of Sn^{2+}, which is present in excess.

There are a number of competing reactions that result in impurities being produced within the kit vial:

1. Free ^{99m}TcO$_4^-$ may result from failure of the reducing agent to work. Also reduced ^{99m}TcO$_4^-$ can become reoxidized back to ^{99m}TcO$_4^-$ which may not relabel. Oxidation can occur due to the introduction of air during production procedures in the radiopharmacy. The potential for oxidation can be reduced by using N$_2$-filled vials for subdividing patient doses.

2. Sn^{2+} can reduce and label TcO$_4^-$ itself to form a stable dioxide, TcO$_2$, which is commonly known as hydrolyzed/reduced technetium (H/R-Tc). Formation of this impurity is dependent mainly on the rate of complex formation and complex stability.

These competing reactions make it important to routinely check the RCP of radiopharmaceuticals produced in the radiopharmacy. Manufacture of radiopharmaceuticals, even when using commercial kits, is not just a simple reconstitution of the contents but a complex chemical reaction which goes on within the vial and it is important to determine whether this reaction has taken place. Impurities will have a different biodistribution from the expected product, which could result in a distorted image in the nuclear medicine clinic. This will lead to organs being irradiated unnecessarily and, if not noticed, could lead to a misdiagnosis. For these reasons it has been recommended that RCP should be determined on all radiopharmaceuticals prepared from unlicensed kits or from 'in-house' formulations. Kits from commercial sources, on the other hand, can be tested less frequently and as a minimum the first vial from any new batch should have its RCP tested [21].

General Principles of Planar Chromatography

Planar chromatography is usually considered to include paper chromatography (PC), thin layer chromatography (TLC), and instant thin layer chromatography (ITLC). There are examples of all of these techniques being employed in the determination of RCP of most radiopharmaceuticals. The test procedure is similar for all and is outlined above.

Generally a few microliters of the product under test is applied near the bottom (origin) of the chromoplate (Figure 7.11). The chromoplate (stationary phase) is then placed in a solvent (mobile phase), ensuring that the origin is not immersed in the solvent. The solvent is allowed to migrate along the chromoplate (by absorption and capillary action) separating the chemical species present. The different species distribute themselves between the mobile and stationary phases, with the most soluble moving fastest.

When the solvent has moved the desired distance along the chromoplate (known as the solvent front, S$_f$), it is removed from the solvent and allowed to dry. The distribution of activity is then determined as described later.

The distance each of the radiochemical species has traveled along the chromoplate is expressed as a fraction of the distance that the solvent front has moved. This fraction is known as the relative front and is denoted as the R$_f$ value for the radiochemical species. The R$_f$ value is characteristic of the species and should be constant for the stationary and mobile phases used, as long as the operating conditions are carefully controlled.

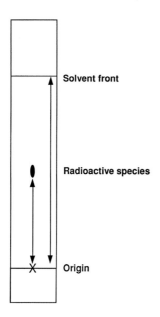

Figure 7.11. A chromatographic strip with the position of the origin and solvent front shown. The sample is placed at the point marked on the origin.

Paper Chromatography (PC)

Paper chromatography has some applications in RCP determination, but has three main disadvantages:

1. poor resolution compared with the other planar methods available;
2. long developing times required;
3. poor structural strength when wet resulting in the chromoplate collapsing into the solvent during development.

One paper used widely in radiochromatography is Whatman 31ET, which due to its open texture develops very rapidly and also remains strong when wet.

Thin Layer Chromatography (TLC)

TLC is a widely used technique, usually where the stationary phase is layered onto a glass plate for support. For radiopharmaceutical applications plastic or foil support mediums are more appropriate since they can be cut to a size to fit the application.

The ability to cut the chromoplate is an advantage, since the analysis of the distribution of radioactivity along the length of the chromoplate may involve cutting the chromoplate into seg-

ments and then counting the segments. Some TLC plates have surfaces that chip on cutting, leading to loss of counts, and care should be exercised when using these materials.

Instant Thin Layer Chromatography (ITLC)

Gelman Scientific Inc. have produced ITLC materials that have proved to be very useful particularly in the RCP determination of ^{99m}Tc radiopharmaceuticals. The material consists of a glass fiber web support medium onto which is impregnated the silica gel (ITLC-SG) and the silic acid (ITLC-SA) stationary phase. The rapid developing times of these chromoplates have made them popular and useful as long as resolution is not critical, it being similar to that of paper chromatography.

Sample Application

Sample application can influence chromatographic separation and operators should develop a technique that is accurate and reproducible. The BP [23] suggests the application of volumes of 5–10 μl, but both generally and specifically for ^{99m}Tc radiopharmaceuticals we have found it is better to apply samples by drawing up the radiopharmaceutical under test using a 1 ml syringe and expelling a partially formed drop of the material from a 25-G (orange) needle. (NB this method should be modified for the determination of the RCP of ^{99m}Tc-MAA by using a 21-G (green) needle since the particles are trapped in the 25-G needle.)

Drying spots prior to developing in the solvent should be avoided for ^{99m}Tc radiopharmaceuticals, unless specified in the manufacturer's instructions, as sample decomposition can occur due to oxidation, which would lead to an incorrect determination of RCP. The sample should be placed centrally on the chromoplate, not near the edge, since solvent evaporation at the edge can affect the movement of the test material.

Size of Chromoplate

Methods for the determination of RCP usually state the size of the chromoplate to be used and normally employ origin to solvent front distances of 10–20 cm. These can, depending on the stationary and mobile phases used, be quite time-consuming to perform and hence miniaturized methods described by Robbins [25] have been developed for most routine RCP determinations (Table 7.4). Here chromoplates are prepared, 1 × 8 cm, with an origin to solvent front distance of 6 cm. It is important to validate these miniaturized

THE RADIOPHARMACY

Table 7.4. Chromatography systems for the determination of the RCP of commonly used radiopharmaceuticals

Product	Medium	Solvent	R_f values		
			Complex	TcO^{4-}	H/R-Tc
Pertechnetate	ITLC.SG	Acetone 50% Aq	N/A	1.0	0.0
	ITLC.SG	Methanol 85% Aq	N/A	1.0	0.0
Tc-MAA	Whatman 31ET	Acetone	0.0	1.0	0.0
Tc-DTPA	ITLC.SG	H_2O or NaCl 0.9%	1.0	1.0	0.0
	Whatman 31ET	Acetone	0.0	1.0	0.0
Tc-MDP	ITLC.SG	H_2O or NaCl 0.9%	1.0	1.0	0.0
	Whatman 31ET	Acetone	0.0	1.0	0.0
Tc-Pyrophosphate	ITLC.SG	H_2O or NaCl 0.9%	1.0	1.0	0.0
	Whatman 31ET	Acetone	0.0	1.0	0.0
Tc-Mebrofenin	ITLC.SG	H_2O	1.0	1.0	0.0
	ITLC.SA	NaCl 20%	0.0	1.0	0.0
Tc-exametazime[a]	ITLC.SG	Butan-2-one	0.8–1.0	0.8–1.0	0.0[b]
	ITLC.SG	NaCl 0.9%	0.0[b]	0.8–1.0	0.0[b]
	Whatman No. 1	Acetonitrile 50% Aq	0.8–1.0[b]	0.8–1.0[b]	0.0
Tc-nanocolloid	Whatman 31ET	Acetone	0.0	1.0	0.0
Tc-tin colloid	ITLC.SG	NaCl 0.9%	0.0	1.0	0.0
Tc-sestamibi	"Baker-flex" Al_2O_3 IB-F	Ethanol 95%	0.5–1.0	0.0–0.5	0.0
Tc-tetrofosmin[c]	ITLC.SG	Acetone 35; dichloromethane 65	0.5[d]	1.0	0.0

[a] Not a miniaturized method but can be carried out with 10 cm origin to solvent front distance.
[b] Secondary Tc-exametazime complex migrates with this R_f in addition to the complex.
[c] Not a miniaturized method but a 15 cm origin to solvent front distance is recommended by the manufacturer.
[d] We have found that this value is very variable unless the assay conditions are tightly controlled.

methods to show that the likely radiochemical species which may be present can be resolved by the method.

These methods are useful when the radiochemical species either remains on the origin or moves to the solvent front and this is the case with the miniaturized methods described by Robbins. In these methods the RCP is determined by using two different stationary and mobile phases. One determines the level of H/R-Tc impurities, while the other determines the free TcO_4^-. By calculating the ratio of activity associated with the impurity to the total activity of the chromoplate, the amount of impurity present may be quantified and the RCP may be calculated by using Equation 7.1:

$$\%RCP = 100 - (\%free\ TcO_4^- + \%H/R - Tc).$$
$$(7.1)$$

Mobile Phases or Solvents

Solvents used as the mobile phase should be of a grade suitable for chromatography, HPLC grade usually being sufficient. Solvents are best if freshly prepared on the day of the RCP determination.

Chromatography Tanks

There are a number of chromatography tanks commercially available which can be used for the more traditional methods of performing PC and TLC. With miniaturized methods it has been found that beakers with Petri dishes for lids make practical and cheap chromatography tanks. Gas jars with ground glass lids can be used for chromatograms of a longer length.

Assessment of the Radioactive Distribution along the Length of the Chromoplate

There are a number of methods for the determination of the radioactive distribution along the length of the chromoplate. These include:

1. autoradiography;
2. chromatogram scanning;
3. cutting the chromoplate and counting the segments;
4. imaging the chromoplate using the gamma camera, determining regions of interest to carry out quantitative analysis.

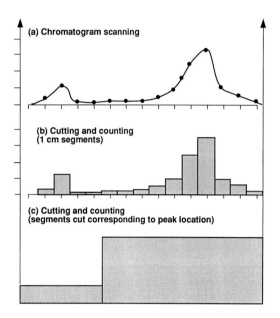

Figure 7.12. a Scan of an imaginary chromatographic strip used in the determination of the RCP of a ^{99m}Tc radiopharmaceutical. **b** Distribution of the radioactivity described as a bar chart if the same chromatogram were cut into 1 cm segments and counted in a well counter. **c** Distribution of the radioactivity described again as a bar chart if the same chromatogram were cut into two segments corresponding to known peak locations.

We will describe the method of chromatogram scanning and of cutting and counting since they use equipment that is readily available to most facilities.

The radiochromatogram scanner uses a scintillation detector to scan the chromoplate by allowing the chromoplate to pass under the detector. The radiation is detected as it passes through a narrow single-slit lead collimator which lies between the chromoplate and the detector. As the chromoplate passes underneath the detector, the count rate is recorded by a ratemeter and this signal is traced on a chart recorder, producing a scan (Figure 7.12a).

The R_f values for each of the peaks detected can be determined from the scan, allowing identification of the radiochemical species present and thus providing the qualitative analysis. If the scanner incorporates an integrator then it can be used to determine the area under the radioactive peaks, which is directly proportional to the concentration of the radiochemical species present on the corresponding part of the chromoplate. The percentage of a radiochemical species may be calculated using

Equation 7.2, where peak A is that corresponding to one of the components and peak B to all other species present.

$$\% \text{ Component A} = (100 \times \text{area peak A})/$$
$$(\text{area peak A} + \text{area peak B}). \quad (7.2)$$

Using the different mobile and stationary phases to quantify each of the components the RCP may be determined using Equation 7.1.

It is important when using radiochromatogram scanners to validate and periodically check the instrument. This should be carried out for the following parameters for each radionuclide where appropriate:

1. setting the upper and lower discriminator levels of the NaI detector;
2. setting the EHT voltage of the NaI detector;
3. determination of the resolution of the instrument;
4. determination of the scanner response linearity of the NaI detector;
5. determination of the band area stability.

Methods may be found for these procedures in Sampson [17].

When the distribution of radioactivity is not known, it is simplest to cut the chromatogram breadth-wise into 1 cm segments and count each in a scintillation well counter – the method of cutting and counting. From the counts in each segment the distribution of the activity along the length of the chromoplate can be determined (Figure 7.12b). The method of identifying which segment contains which radiochemical species is to assume that a new species is present in a segment that has a greater number of counts than the previous one. The percentage of a radiochemical species may be calculated using Equation 7.3.

$$\% \text{ Component A} = (100 \times (\text{sum of counts}$$
$$\text{assigned to component A}))/(\text{sum of}$$
$$\text{counts on whole plate}). \quad (7.3)$$

As described earlier, the RCP can then be calculated using Equation 7.1.

When the distribution of radioactivity is known, for example by scanning, then the chromoplate can be cut into two or three segments corresponding to a radiochemical species (Figure 7.12c). In the method advocated by Robbins [25], cutting in half is suggested since the assay methods employed result in either the product or impurity being present at either the origin or solvent front. The percentage of a radiochemical species may be calculated using Equation 7.4.

$$\% \text{ Component A} = (100 \times (\text{counts in segment A})/(\text{counts in segment A} + \text{counts in segment B}). \quad (7.4)$$

As previously described, RCP can then be calculated using Equation 7.1.

When counting, it is important to maintain the same counting geometry for all segments, large or small. All counts should be background corrected.

As with scanning, it is important to validate the instruments and the methods being employed for each radionuclide where appropriate by:

1. setting the upper and lower discriminator levels of the NaI detector;
2. setting the EHT voltage of the NaI detector;
3. determination of the linearity of the detector and ensuring all assays are carried out within the linear range.

Method for the Determination of the RCP of ^{99m}Tc Radiopharmaceuticals

Chromatographic systems suitable for determining the RCP are given in Table 7.4.

The kit under test should be reconstituted in the same manner as for patient use and assessed using the following procedure.

1. Place sufficient of the appropriate solvent into each of two developing tanks. The depth of the solvent should be sufficient to come in contact with the chromoplate without covering the origin. Allow volatile solvents to equilibrate to give a saturated atmosphere in the tank.
2. Place a drop, as described earlier, of the radiopharmaceutical under test on the origin of each of the chromoplates as indicated in Figure 7.11. It is good practice to mark the origin and the solvent front on the chromoplate with a sharp soft pencil prior to sample application. It might also be prudent to mark the chromoplate with the name of the solvent in which it is to be developed and the name of the product under test.

3. Immediately place the chromoplate in the tank, taking care to develop it in the correct solvent.
4. Allow the solvent to migrate to the solvent front line and then remove the chromoplate from the tank. It can be difficult to observe the progress of the mobile phase moving along the chromoplate. Back lighting can be of help since the wet chromoplate becomes translucent. Alternatively, an ink spot applied about 20 mm below the solvent front at the side of the chromoplate will be carried by the solvent, allowing the progress of the solvent to be followed. The exact position of the solvent front should be marked with a soft pencil and the chromoplate can then be allowed to dry.
5. Measure the distribution of the activity along the length of the chromoplate as described earlier, working out the RCP using the appropriate equations as detailed.

Once the tests have shown that a radiochemically pure product has been produced (usually an RCP of 95% is acceptable, but individual manufacturers' product data sheets should be consulted), the kits may be approved for patient use, released from quarantine, and transferred to approved stock.

7.4.4 Chemical Purity

The EP and BP monographs for sodium pertechnetate (^{99m}Tc) injection (fission) give a limit test for the aluminum (Al^{3+}) content of ^{99m}Tc eluates. Al^{3+} may originate from the generator column, being produced during the absorption process of the ^{99}Mo onto the alumina column. It is important to perform this test since Al^{3+} can affect the stability of some colloidal radiopharmaceuticals.

The limit test given in the EP is complicated and time-consuming to carry out and the use of a commercially available kit (Du Pont) is recommended. The kit consists of Al^{3+} indicator papers and a standard Al^{3+} solution of 10 μg/ml. A drop of this standard solution is placed on the indicator paper next to a sample drop from the eluate. If the intensity of the color produced by the eluate is less than that from the standard, then the eluate has passed the test and contains less that 10 μg/ml (equivalent to 10 ppm – USP monograph limit;

EP limit is 20 ppm). This test may be carried out from a test sample taken from the first elution of the generator and from any subsequent eluates to be used in compounding colloidal radiopharmaceuticals affected by the presence of Al^{3+} [21].

The pH of the generator eluate and of any other radiopharmaceutical may be tested by placing a drop of the radiopharmaceutical under test onto a piece of pH indicator paper, the color change indicating the pH. Narrow range pH papers should be used in conjunction with standard pH buffers. A drop of the buffer is placed onto the pH paper to give reference colors corresponding to the upper and lower limits of the radiopharmaceutical's pH. A drop from the radiopharmaceutical under test is then placed alongside for comparison.

7.4.5 Sterility Assurance

All preparations intended for parenteral administration must be tested to ensure that they comply with the EP test for sterility [23]. There are problems, however, in applying this test to ^{99m}Tc radiopharmaceuticals. Because of their short shelf-life, preparations have to be released prior to the results of the sterility test being known. This is recognized by the Pharmacopoeias, which require that the test still be carried out, constituting a control on the quality of production procedures. Also if the test sample is to be tested outside the radiopharmacy, then they must be stored to allow the radioactivity to decay before they are handled for testing.

Radioactive injections have been shown to support microbial growth [26], but are far from ideal growth media for long-term microbiological survival. Even in the absence of radioactivity, generator eluates and reconstituted kits have been shown not to support long-term microbiological growth [27]. This has brought the value of the test into doubt, for although it might indicate that the product is sterile at the time of testing, it cannot show whether the product was sterile at the time of production, or, more importantly, at the time of administration.

We have devised a test protocol that is in general compliance with the current recommendations [21]. The second elution (taken as early as possible after the first), and the final elution from each generator are used as sterility test samples. Also each week a different prepared dose is sent as a sterility test sample so that over a period of time the range of injections commonly manufactured in the department have all been tested. The test method used is a closed filtration system using a Millipore two-unit sterility testing system.

Broth transfer trials (validation of operator's aseptic technique) and process simulation tests (validation of the aseptic process) should be performed on a regular basis by each member of staff preparing aseptically prepared radiopharmaceuticals. Operators new to the unit should have their aseptic technique validated using an authorized broth transfer trial and should pass a number of consecutive validations prior to receiving trained confirmation that they are authorized to prepare radiopharmaceuticals. In addition to this, the aseptic processes carried out within the department should also be mimicked using broth simulations.

The broth transfer trial tests the ability of the operator to aseptically prepare products free from microbial growth. The process simulation test should be designed to demonstrate that the procedures in the facilities being used during aseptic preparation as well as the staff undertaking aseptic processes are capable of maintaining the sterility of the product [21].

Guidance is given in "Quality Assurance of Aseptic Preparation Services" [11] on how broth transfer trials and process simulations should be carried out. Both rely on pre-sterilized stock solutions of broth being aseptically subdivided in a manner that should mimic those used in production procedures. Those procedures at highest risk of becoming contaminated should be targeted in particular (e.g. open procedures). The resulting samples of broth from the mimicked process may then be incubated at 20–25°C and 30–35°C for 14 days to check for absence of growth of microorganisms.

We feel that the broth transfer trials and process simulations are additional process controls, offering further evidence as to the assurance of the sterility of the final product. These should be carried out in conjunction with sterility testing and not as a substitute procedure.

7.4.6 Pyrogen Testing

Pyrogens are non-volatile, water-soluble substances that, when injected into the body, cause a rise in temperature. Commonly this reaction is caused by substances derived from the cell walls of bacteria, mainly lipopolysaccharides known as endotoxins. The presence of pyrogens is particularly undesirable in large-volume parenterals where patients receive large volumes of the infusion. As a result, all single dose parenterals of 15 ml or more must be pyrogen free.

It will not normally be necessary to carry out pyrogen testing on ^{99m}Tc radiopharmaceuticals due to their small volumes. If pyrogen testing is thought desirable, then the Limulus amoebocyte lysate (LAL) test may be more appropriate than the rabbit test [21]. The latter involves measuring the temperature invoked in rabbits following the parenteral administration of the preparation under test.

The LAL test is a laboratory in vitro test which provides a very sensitive limit test for the presence of endotoxin in parenteral pharmaceuticals. It should be noted that, while the LAL test is more sensitive than the rabbit test in terms of its detection limit, it can only detect the presence of endotoxins. Pyrogens may be present that are not of endotoxin origin.

The adoption of the LAL test by the EP follows that of the USP (XX) in 1963. At this time the USP also included the LAL test in the official monographs for several radiopharmaceuticals, including some ^{99m}Tc radiopharmaceuticals.

7.4.7 Gross Particulate Contamination

All solutions intended for parenteral administration should be free from any gross particulate contamination. This may be readily and easily checked by viewing the injection through a polarizing filter with back-lighting.

Applying this method to radiopharmaceuticals results in exposing the operator to ionizing radiation. The operator must be given protection while viewing the injections, and this may be carried out by the means of a lead glass screen. In addition to this, the operator should be continuously monitored, by wearing, for example, a suitably positioned thermoluminescent dosimeter.

7.4.8 Environmental Monitoring

In the UK, the quality of the environment in which parenteral radiopharmaceuticals are manufactured must comply with BS EN/ISO 144146-2 as well as the additional specifications for microbiological cleanliness given in the GMP [4]. The maintenance of this environment is of the utmost importance in assuring the sterility of the injections being produced in such units.

To ensure that the working environment meets with these specifications, an environmental monitoring program must be carried out:

- on the commissioning of new cleanrooms,
- following any maintenance of the facilities,
- routinely following a written program at an agreed frequency.

A proposed program is given in Table 7.5 and should be used as an illustration of an approach. Any program of environmental monitoring should drawn up as an operational procedure to meet the needs of the individual unit [21].

Environmental monitoring procedures are common to all pharmaceutical production areas manufacturing sterile products. However, in the radiopharmacy there is the additional aspect of monitoring for radiation contamination, the performance of which should be recorded in a written log.

7.4.9 Planned Preventive Maintenance

In order to ensure medicinal products of a consistently high quality can be prepared, documented evidence is required to show that all equipment involved in production procedures continues to function properly within the manufacturer's specification. This is a necessary control requirement of GMP [4] and an essential component of quality assurance.

Those items of equipment that require planned preventive maintenance (PPM) should be included on a program, allowing such equipment to be maintained at a predetermined frequency, agreed between maintenance and the user.

7.4.10 Audit

Chapter 9 of the GMP [4] requires that a system of self-inspection or audit be conducted on all areas where aseptic preparation takes place. Also since the publication of Executive Letter (97) 52: Aseptic Dispensing in NHS Hospitals in 1997, a program of external audits of NHS unlicensed aseptic production premises has been undertaken by regional quality controllers in collaboration with regional officers. A written procedure should be followed on a regular basis which monitors implementation and compliance with all aspects of

Table 7.5. Environmental monitoring program

(a) Physical tests				
Parameter monitored	**Area monitored**	**Monitoring equipment**	**Standard requirements**	**Test interval**
Record pressure differential across HEPA filters	(1) Cleanrooms	Manometers	Manufacturer's specification	(1) Monitor continuously – record daily
	(2) LFW and isolators	Manometers	Manufacturer's specification	(2) Monitor continuously – record daily
Record pressure differential between cleanroom and adjacent areas	(1) Cleanrooms	Manometers	(1) ISO 14644	(1) Monitor continuously – record daily
	(2) Isolators[a]	Manometers	(2) BS EN 12469	(2) Daily
Air change rate	(1) Cleanrooms	Vane anemometer or balometer	(1) ISO 14644	(1) Monthly
	(2) Isolators	Vane anemometer	(2) Usually > 60 air changes per hour	(2) Monthly
Air velocity – downflow and inflow	LFW (class II)	Vane anemometer	BS EN 12469	Quarterly
Airborne particulate matter	Cleanrooms, LFW, and isolators	Electronic airborne particle counter	ISO 14644 and GMP	Monthly
HEPA filter integrity	Cleanrooms, LFW, and isolators	Dioctyl-phthalate (DOP) test	ISO 14644	Annual
Operator protection	LFW	Potassium iodide disk test	BS EN 12469	Annual

[a] Isolators should also have (1) gauntlet integrity checked sessionally, (2) pressure alarms checked weekly, and (3) leak test checked weekly.

(b) Microbiological tests				
Parameter monitored	**Area monitored**	**Monitoring equipment**	**Standard requirements**	**Test interval**
Airborne microbial contamination	LFW and isolator	Settle plates (90 mm)	<1 cfu/4 hour (GMP grade A)	Each aseptic work session
		Centrifugal air sampler	<1 cfu/m^3 (GMP grade A)	Monthly
	Cleanroom	Settle plates (90 mm)	5 cfu/4 hour (GMP grade B) 100 cfu/4 hour (GMP grade D)	Weekly
		Centrifugal air sampler	10 cfu/m^3 (GMP grade A) 200 cfu/m^3 (GMP grade D)	Monthly
Surface microbial contamination	LFW and isolator	Contact plates (55 mm) or surface swabs	<1 cfu (GMP grade A)	Weekly
	Cleanroom	Contact plates (55 mm) or surface swabs	5 cfu (GMP grade B) 50 cfu (GMP grade D)	Weekly Monthly
	Materials entering cleanroom or isolator through hatch	Surface swabs	[a]	
	Gloved fingers of operator	Finger dabs onto settle plate	<1 cfu (GMP grade A)	Each aseptic work session

[a] No specification exists but action limits should be set locally with trend analysis applied. Any microbes should be identified.

GMP. The audit should result in a written report of the observations made and propose, if necessary, any corrective action. These should be reviewed at the next audit. It has been proposed that self-audit may be conducted by senior staff at a local level, with an annual inspection by a suitably qualified independent person conducted annually [21]. An example of an audit document to assess a radiopharmacy service has been published on the U.K. Radiopharmacists' Group website (www.ukrg.org.uk) and can be used for guidance. It is expected that these audits will be conducted in addition to inspection by Medicines Healthcare products Regulatory Agency (MHRA) inspectors as part of the licensing requirements of some departments.

7.5 Radiation Protection in the Radiopharmacy

The legislative controls, regulations, and dose limits that govern radiation protection requirements for radiopharmacies are the same as for other premises dealing with ionizing radiation. Since these are dealt with in detail in Chapter 6, only the specialist areas of pharmaceutical work and safety requirements will be discussed here.

7.5.1 Shielding Techniques and Materials

Radiopharmaceutical production manipulations are basically the same, regardless of the design of the premises and the nature of the work being undertaken. From the radiopharmacist's point of view it is important to achieve maximum safety for the operator and the product at all times. Appropriate shielding may be obtained by using a variety of materials such as lead, tungsten, aluminum, plastic, or lead glass. Lead should be encased or painted so as to give a safe, cleanable surface and one that will prevent accidental absorption.

Other important factors to be considered when dealing with radiation are manipulative time, distance from the source, the radioactivity and type of radiation from the source. Any practice that affords the operator a favorable balance with respect to these four factors must be employed wherever practicable.

7.5.2 Shielding Equipment

Workstations

All parenteral radiopharmaceutical manipulations should be carried out in workstations which offer both operator and product protection, conforming to the standards for LFWs and isolators given in Table 7.1. While such workstations can be provided with lead glass windows the addition of an appropriate thickness of lead sheeting in the base and the back of the workstations gives useful additional protection.

All aseptic transfers for parenteral radiopharmaceuticals should be carried out with syringes shielded with either lead, lead-tungsten or lead glass syringe shields. All manipulations in these workstations should be carried out over drip trays, allowing easier containment in event of accidental spillage.

Secondary Lead Shielding

Different systems are employed to shield ^{99m}Tc generators depending on the generator type and its activity rating. Secondary shielding systems may be obtained commercially either from the generator supplier or constructed locally.

Lead Pots

Lead pots 3 mm thick provide sufficient shielding during the preparation, storage, and handling of ^{99m}Tc radiopharmaceuticals. They should also be painted to give a safe, cleanable surface and one that is safe to handle.

7.5.3 Monitoring Equipment

A Geiger monitor placed in the preparation rooms and cleanrooms can be used to continuously monitor the radiation levels. By providing an audible response to radiation, it alerts staff to any increase in the background count rate.

Film badges are the most widely used method of personnel monitoring and are very effective. One problem we have encountered is the presence of a fog on the film due to disinfection of the badge as part of the procedure for entering the cleanrooms. The problem may be avoided by covering the badge with a plastic film. Electronic dosimeters are also now available which display real time measurement of radiation dose and may be a useful addition to staff monitoring systems.

Finger doses are a particular problem for the radiopharmacy staff, hence the use of long-handled forceps and tongs. Finger doses may be monitored by the wearing of thermoluminescent dosimeters on the fingers of the hand receiving the most radiation dose. Electronic extremity dose monitors (e.g. Advanced Extremity Gamma Instrumentation System or AEGIS) are also now available which can be used to investigate doses received for individual manipulations near to the fingertip. We feel that these AEGIS type systems are more useful for risk assessment of new procedures or investigating problems rather than routine dose monitoring.

7.6 Glossary of Terms

Aseptic procedure: a method of handling sterile materials by employing techniques that minimize the chance of microbial contamination.

Antioxidant: a chemical agent used to retard the oxidation of ingredients in a medicinal product.

Bactericide: a chemical agent which under defined conditions is capable of killing bacteria but not necessarily bacterial spores.

Buffers: chemical compounds or mixtures of compounds which when in solution resist changes in the pH of the solution, upon the addition of acids or bases, dilution of the solvent or when there is a temperature change.

Closed procedure: a procedure whereby a sterile pharmaceutical is prepared by the addition of sterile ingredients into a pre-sterilized container via a system closed to the atmosphere (e.g. by injection with a syringe and needle through the rubber bung).

Contact plate: a plate containing sterile nutrient agar designed so as to allow the agar to come into contact with any surface (floor, wall, and benching). This allows the microbiological contamination of the surface to be assessed.

Open procedure: a method of preparation whereby at some stage the radiopharmaceutical or other ingredients are exposed to the controlled environment with the consequent risk of the ingression of microorganisms or other contaminants.

Parenteral: administration of a medicinal product not through the alimentary tract but rather by injection by some other route (e.g. intramuscular and intravenous).

Settle plates: a sterile Petri dish containing sterile nutrient agar. This when open to the environment acts like a container and allows the assessment of airborne microbiological contamination.

Sterile: a state in which there is complete absence of living organisms (the state of sterility is absolute: there are no degrees of sterility).

References

1. Medicines Act 1968. London: HMSO.
2. The National Health Service and Community Care Act 1990. London: HMSO.
3. Department of Health and Social Security. Premises and Environment for the Preparation of Radiopharmaceuticals. London: DHSS; 1982.
4. Department of Health. Rules and Guidance for Pharmaceutical Manufacturers and Distributors, 6th edn. London: HMSO; 2002.
5. Commission of the European Communities. The Rules Governing Medicinal Products in the European Communities Vol. IV: Good Manufacturing Practice for Medicinal Products. Luxembourg: European Commission; 1992.
6. Ionising Radiation Regulations 1999. (SI 1999 No. 3232). London: HMSO.
7. Radioactive Substances Act 1993. London: HMSO.
8. Institute of Physics and Engineering in Medicine (IPEM). Medical and Dental Guidance Notes: A good practice guide on all aspects of ionising radiation protection in the clinical environment. York: IPEM; 2002.
9. Health and Safety Commission. Work with Ionising Radiation. Approved Code of Practice and practical guidance on the Ionising Radiation Regulations 1999. London: HSE; 2000.
10. Commission of the European Communities. EC Guide to Good Manufacturing Practice Revision to Annex 1. Brussels: European Commission; 2003.
11. Beanes AM, ed. Quality Assurance of Aseptic Preparation Services, 3rd edn. London: Pharmaceutical Press; 2001.
12. BS EN ISO 14644. Cleanrooms and Associated Controlled Environments. London: BSI; 1999.
13. BS EN ISO 12469. Biotechnology, Performance Criteria for Microbiological Safety Cabinets. London: BSI; 2000.
14. Midcalf B, Phillips WM, Neiger JS, Coles TP. Pharmaceutical Isolators A Guide to their Application, Design and Controls. London: Pharmapress; 2004.
15. Millar AM, Best JJK, Merrick MV, Muir AL. An alternative method for the preparation of ^{99m}Tc radiopharmaceuticals from freeze dried kits. Nucl Med Commun 1981; 3:147–151.
16. Millar AM, Brydon J, Williamson D, Forsyth IF. A radiopharmacy label processor. Br J Radiol 1984; 57:741–743.
17. Sampson CB. Textbook of Radiopharmacy: Theory and Practice, 2nd edn. Yverdon, Switzerland: Gordon and Breach Science Publishers; 1994.

18. Control of Substances Hazardous to Health (COSHH) Regulations. Sheffield: HSE; 1999.

19. Couper I, Driver N. Quality Assurance. In: Allwood AC, Fell JT, eds. Textbook of Hospital Pharmacy. Oxford: Blackwell Scientific Publications; 1980.

20. Department of Health. Aseptic Dispensing for NHS patients – A Guidance Document for Pharmacists in the UK. London: DoH; 1995.

21. Quality Assurance of Radiopharmaceuticals. Report of a Joint Working Party: The UK Radiopharmacists Group and the NHS Pharmaceutical QC Committee. Nucl Med Commun 2001; 22:909–916.

22. The Pharmacopoeial Commission. British Pharmacopoeia (XVII). London: HMSO; 2003.

23. The Council of Europe. European Pharmacopoeia, 4th edn. France: Maisonneuve SA; 2002.

24. US Pharmacopoeial Convention. United States Pharmacopoeia and National Formulary, 27th Revision. Rockville: USPC; 2004.

25. Robbins PJ. Chromatography of ^{99m}Tc-radiopharmaceuticals – a practical guide. New York: The US Society of Nuclear Medicine Inc; 1984.

26. Abra RM, Bell NDS, Horton PW. The growth of microorganisms in some parenteral radiopharmaceuticals. Int J Pharm 1980; 5:187–193.

27. Brown S, Baker MM. The sterility testing of dispensed radiopharmaceuticals. Nucl Med Commun 1976; 7:327–336.

8

The Skeletal System

Margaret E. Brooks

8.1 Introduction

Imaging of the skeleton using radioactive substances has been possible for over 40 years. Improvements in radiopharmaceuticals and instrumentation have taken place over this time, most notably the introduction of technetium-labeled phosphates in the 1970s and the development of the dual-headed gamma camera in the 1990s. However, the basic technique of the radionuclide bone scan has changed very little. Despite advances in other forms of imaging, the bone scan remains an extremely valuable diagnostic tool and is still one of the most common procedures performed in nuclear medicine departments. It has sustained its position because of several noteworthy qualities.

It is exquisitely sensitive and demonstrates abnormality early in the disease process, often at a stage where no lesion is evident on plain radiographs. The whole skeleton can be imaged in a single examination which most patients can tolerate. It is widely available and comparatively inexpensive, with relatively low radiation dose compared to computed tomography (CT). There are no known contraindications.

The bone scan has an oft-quoted lack of specificity, but this is less of a problem if scan interpretation takes account of the clinical context, including the patient's age, and other available imaging. Indeed, part of its utility stems from this non-specificity, making its application appropriate and helpful in a wide variety of clinical settings.

8.2 Anatomy and Physiology

The skeleton consists of over 200 individual bones which can be classified as belonging to either the axial or the appendicular skeleton. The axial skeleton includes the bones of the spine, ribs and sternum, skull and facial bones, while the pelvis, scapulae and limb bones comprise the appendicular skeleton.

Microscopically bone consists of a fibrous matrix, composed mainly of collagen, and mineral matrix of inorganic salts, including calcium, phosphate, and carbonate, with the principal component being crystals of hydroxyapatite. Bone is a highly vascular, living tissue with remarkable resilience and capacity for regeneration and remodeling.

Two cell types in bone perform this remodeling process: the osteoclasts, which are large phagocytes responsible for bone resorption and removal, and the osteoblasts, which form new bone. It is the synthesis of bone by osteoblasts that accounts for the accumulation of radiolabeled phosphate on a bone scan, with the radiopharmaceutical being incorporated into newly formed crystals of hydroxyapatite.

This system of bone resorption and synthesis is finely balanced and continues throughout life, with complete skeletal turnover approximately every 20 years. In normality the process occurs diffusely in the skeleton and uptake of radionuclide is uniform and of low intensity. In disease states causing increased bone turnover there is a greater accumulation of radionuclide with respect to normal [1].

8.3 The Bone Scan

8.3.1 Indications

Many pathologies cause increased bone turnover, and the most frequent indications for a radionuclide bone scan are listed in Table 8.1. This extensive but not exhaustive list reflects changing referral patterns in recent years. While previously the majority of examinations were performed for the assessment of malignant disease, there are now increasing numbers of referrals for benign conditions.

8.3.2 Technique

The main agent in current clinical use for bone scanning is ^{99m}Tc methylene diphosphonate (MDP), a phosphate analogue. Following intravenous injection MDP circulates in the vascular system for a short time then equilibrates to the extravascular space. Its subsequent accumulation in bone is rapid, with excretion of the residual MDP via the urine. Approximately half of the administered dose is eliminated within 4 hours, producing a high bone-to-background ratio of activity, except in situations where renal function is poor.

Table 8.1. Indications for radionuclide bone scan (not in order of frequency)

Tumors	Primary: benign malignant Secondary
Infection	Osteomyelitis Diskitis Septic arthritis
Trauma	
Surgery	Joint prostheses Bone viability
Metabolic bone disease	
Pediatrics	Suspected non-accidental injury Tumors: primary secondary
Unexplained musculoskeletal pain	
Abnormal bone biochemistry	

Table 8.2. Bone imaging

Radiopharmaceutical	^{99m}Tc methylene diphosphonate (MDP)
Activity administered	600 MBq (15 mCi) 800 MBq (20 mCi) for SPECT; scaled dose based on weight for pediatric patients
Effective dose equivalent	3 mSv (300 mrem)
Patient preparation	Good hydration; empty bladder prior to imaging
Collimator	Low-energy, high-resolution
Imaging	Dual-head camera—scan speed 8–10 cm/min Spot views—minimum 500 kcounts per view

The protocol for a radionuclide bone scan is outlined in Table 8.2. The patient is advised to maintain good hydration with oral fluids and to empty their bladder regularly to reduce unnecessary radiation dose to the pelvic organs. No other patient preparation is required.

Two to four hours after injection whole body imaging takes place. This is performed either on a dual-head gamma camera, acquiring anterior and posterior views simultaneously, or on a single-head facility, performing spot views. Additional views are obtained as necessary, depending on the clinical problem being investigated and the findings on the initial images. These may include, for example, oblique views of the sternum and ribs, lateral views of the lower legs or squat views of the pelvis. The latter is designed to separate bladder activity from the pubic bones, as these structures are superimposed on the anterior view. Although the patient should empty his bladder prior to commencement of imaging, refilling inevitably takes place during the examination, promoted by the good hydration.

Magnification views may be useful for improving visualization of the hands and wrists in the adult, and for the hip joints in pediatric patients.

The degree of uptake of MDP is not governed by osteoblastic activity alone, but also by blood flow. By imaging an area of interest immediately after MDP administration it is possible to visualize indirectly the vascularity of a lesion (flow phase) and assess any hyperemia of adjacent soft tissues (blood pool phase). Delayed phase images are then acquired as normal, completing a triple-phase bone scan. It is the combination of increased vascularity and increased vascular permeability that accounts for the early accumulation of MDP in bone tumors, healing trauma, inflammatory and infected conditions of bone, and the triple-phase scan may be usefully employed when these pathologies are suspected. An alternative protocol is to combine the flow and blood pool images which, with the delayed images, produces a dual-phase study.

Single photon emission computed tomography (SPECT) of the skeleton is performed as an addition to planar imaging and provides extra information about complex areas such as the lumbar spine, knees, base of skull, and facial bones. It improves the detection and anatomical localization of lesions and is more readily compared with other tomographic imaging such as CT and magnetic resonance imaging (MRI).

8.3.3 Normal Appearances and Interpretation

In the normal adult skeleton individual bones are visualized, and uptake is symmetrical about the midline (Figure 8.1). There may be some background soft tissue uptake, particularly in an obese patient. Both kidneys and the urinary bladder should be readily identifiable. Knowledge of skeletal and urinary tract normal variants is necessary to avoid misinterpretation (Figure 8.2).

In the normal immature skeleton the greatest uptake of MDP occurs at the epiphyseal plates, the sites of active bone growth. Uptake fades when the epiphyses fuse and growth ceases. This phenomenon can be useful when early or delayed epiphyseal closure is suspected.

Interpretation needs to take account of the age of the patient and findings which may be considered incidental at that age. Full and accurate clinical information is vital, including any history of trauma or surgery. Current medication may also be relevant. With this knowledge the bone scan appearances can be placed in clinical context. Previous bone scans should be available for comparison at the time of reporting as their contribution can be pivotal. If there is any doubt about the significance of an abnormality, the availability of other imaging can be invaluable, and these studies should be viewed alongside the bone scan to gain most benefit from the exercise.

If further imaging of an area is deemed necessary, plain films are still the best first-line investigation. These may demonstrate and even

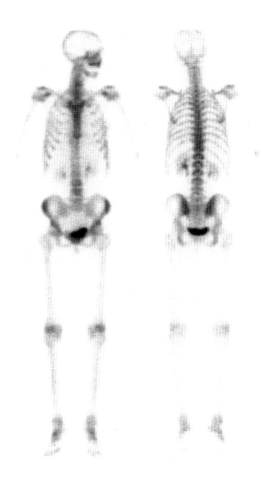

Figure 8.1. Normal adult ^{99m}Tc-MDP bone scan, anterior and posterior views.

characterize a lesion to account for the bone scan uptake. In view of the increased sensitivity of the bone scan over plain film, if the radiographs are normal, CT or MRI should be considered. The choice of modality will depend on the area of the body in question, and the suspected pathology.

8.3.4 Tumors

Metastases

The bone scan remains an efficient means of detecting skeletal metastatic disease because of its high sensitivity and whole body coverage, despite competition from other modalities such as MRI. Secondary tumor deposits usually spread to bone by the hematogenous route, although direct

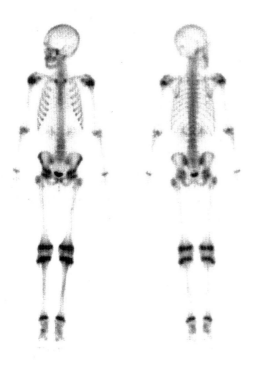

Figure 8.2. Normal immature skeleton, anterior and posterior views, with horseshoe kidney.

invasion also occurs. The usual sites of distribution throughout the skeleton are explained by the predilection of metastases for red marrow [2]. Thus in adults the axial skeleton is preferentially involved, though some tumors (e.g. bronchial carcinoma) notably produce distal appendicular lesions.

Tumor deposits stimulate local osteoclastic activity, producing bone resorption, followed by increased osteoblastic activity in an attempt at bone repair. The balance of this process determines whether the outcome is a purely osteolytic or osteosclerotic lesion, or a combination of both. Obviously a mainly osteoblastic response increases the lesion's chances of detection on a bone scan. Predominantly osteolytic lesions, which produce a photopenic defect, are more difficult to appreciate. However, they may incite osteoblastic activity at their leading edge, which improves visualization (Figure 8.3).

The cardinal features of skeletal metastatic disease are multiple focal areas of increased MDP uptake, randomly distributed but favoring the axial skeleton, with asymmetric involvement (Figure 8.4a and b). Over a series of examinations, without therapeutic intervention, these increase in size, number, and intensity of uptake. Solitary metastases can be more problematic, but consideration of the type of primary tumor and the site of the single abnormality can inform interpretation. A solitary asymmetric sternal lesion in a patient with breast cancer has a very high chance of malignancy. Single rib lesions, even with a known primary tumor, are much more likely to be due to simple trauma than metastatic disease [3]. If in doubt, complementary imaging should be arranged.

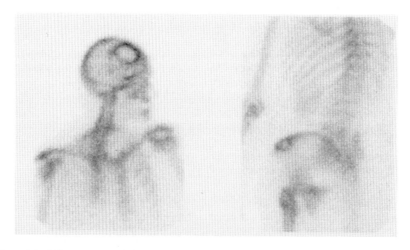

Figure 8.3. Oblique spot views of the skull and pelvis with osteolytic metastases from primary renal carcinoma.

THE SKELETAL SYSTEM

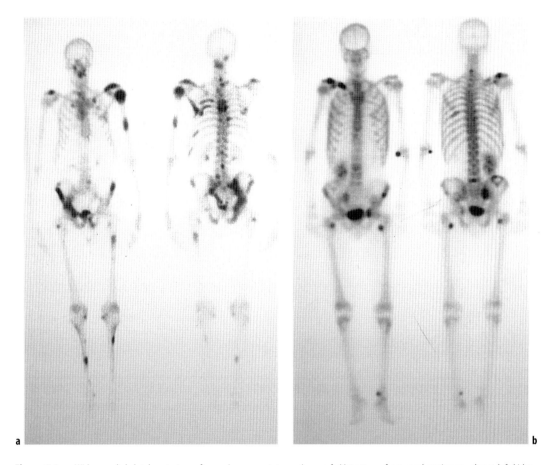

Figure 8.4. a Widespread skeletal metastases from primary prostate carcinoma. **b** Metastases from renal carcinoma, absent left kidney (nephrectomy).

Difficulties in the appreciation of photopenic lesions, such as in myeloma where the tumor process is purely osteoclastic, are in part technical, because they are obscured by surrounding normal activity, and in part perceptual. Unless large in size or number, defects are naturally more of a challenge to detect than areas of excess uptake. However, the bone scan can be useful in myeloma, as lesions may present themselves by virtue of associated pathological fracture and subsequent healing (Figure 8.5).

Diffuse intense skeletal uptake with reduced renal visualization (the "superscan" appearance) occurs when there is high bone tumor load, most commonly in carcinoma of the prostate or breast (Figure 8.6). In this situation MDP accumulates in the numerous bone lesions to such an extent that there is little available for renal excretion. Although this may give the illusion of normal skeletal uptake, recognition that the uptake comprises multiple separate foci, together with reduced renal activity, should prevent misinterpretation.

Diffuse increased uptake along the margins of the long bones may be seen with malignancies of the lung and pleura, benign pleural tumors, and other diseases of the chest and gastrointestinal system. This is hypertrophic pulmonary osteoarthropathy (HPOA), which is a non-metastatic manifestation of the primary tumor, with a classic appearance on scintigraphy (Figure 8.7).

In children, metastases adjacent to the epiphyseal growth plate can be masked by the normal intense uptake at that site. Close comparison with the contralateral limb is recommended, and where there is doubt, alternative imaging strategies should be employed.

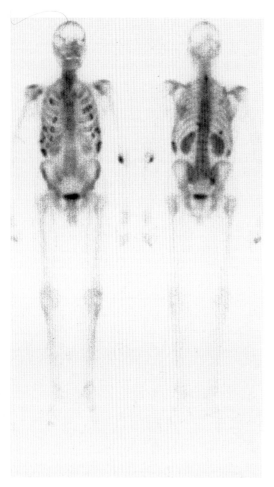

Figure 8.5. Myeloma with multiple rib and vertebral pathological fractures.

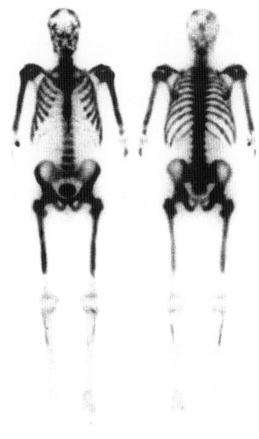

Figure 8.6. "Superscan" appearance of prostatic metastases, kidneys not visualized.

Another situation most commonly encountered with breast and prostate cancer is the "flare phenomenon". This refers to an apparent deterioration in appearances after commencement of therapy, with increased activity in existing metastases and the apparent development of new lesions, despite improvement in the patient's clinical condition. Follow-up studies show resolution, and this flare of uptake is likely to reflect increased osteoblastic activity in healing lesions and unmasking of previously undetected disease.

Currently the bone scan is established as the best technique for the assessment of suspected bone metastases, whatever the primary tumor, but indications change regarding which category of patients should be investigated. At present the use of the bone scan in patients with early clinical stage of certain cancers is controversial as the yield of abnormalities is low. However, some authors advocate a bone scan at presentation to act as a baseline against which later studies can be compared.

New musculoskeletal symptoms or biochemical abnormalities, rising tumor markers, and abnormal radiographic findings are all suitable reasons for referral.

Primary Bone Malignancy

In osteosarcoma and Ewing's sarcoma the bone scan is not performed to assess the primary lesion but to evaluate the remainder of the skeleton for metastatic disease. The pulmonary and other soft tissue secondaries of osteogenic sarcoma may also be avid for MDP and detectable on the bone scan, but CT is the method of choice for their demonstration.

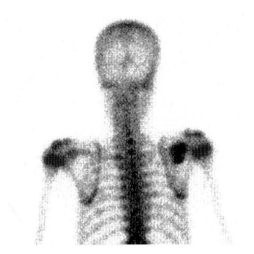

Figure 8.8. Posterior view of osteochondroma, right scapula.

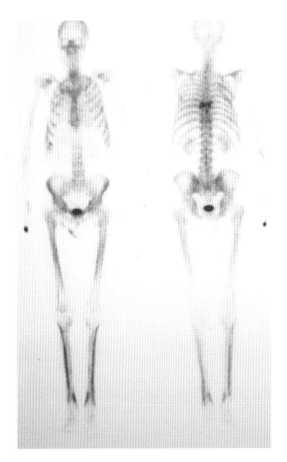

Figure 8.7. Hypertrophic pulmonary osteoarthropathy (affecting femora and tibiae), with spinal and rib metastases and left pleural effusion, secondary to bronchial carcinoma.

Benign Bone Tumors

There are no typical features on a bone scan which reliably differentiate benign and malignant neoplasms. In osteoid osteoma there is typically increased uptake in the early phases and intense MDP accumulation on the delayed images, but a similar pattern is visualized in other benign tumors (Figure 8.8), and in malignant lesions [4]. However, the bone scan can be valuable when plain radiographs have been unhelpful in localizing an abnormality.

8.3.5 Trauma

The bone scan is useful in both acute and subacute trauma [5]. There is focal MDP accumulation at fracture sites reflecting the increased vascularity and bone formation of the healing process. This is detectable as early as 24 hours following fracture. As an injury heals, the accumulation of activity becomes less intense, and uptake in 90% of fracture sites will have returned to normal by 2 years.

Occult Fractures

The most common clinical scenario is an elderly patient with suspected femoral neck fracture. Plain radiography will have failed to demonstrate an abnormality to account for the patient's clinical presentation. The strengths of the bone scan are its sensitivity for fracture detection (Figure 8.9), and its potential to expose associated but unsuspected injuries, or other diagnoses to explain the symptoms.

Carpal bone fractures are notorious for remaining radiographically occult for some weeks after injury. While MRI is superior for anatomical resolution of the fracture site, the bone scan has similar high sensitivity and may be more readily available.

Stress Fractures

This term refers to fractures occurring in normal bone that has been subjected to repetitive stress [6]. Produced by unaccustomed or over-strenuous activity, such as running, these injuries are common in athletes. Stress fractures can occur at many sites in the skeleton but are most common in the lower limb, particularly the tibia, and may be bilateral.

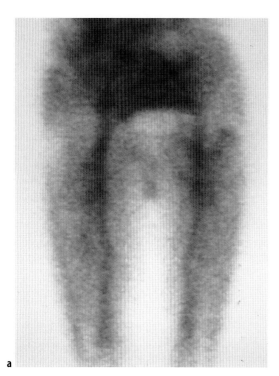
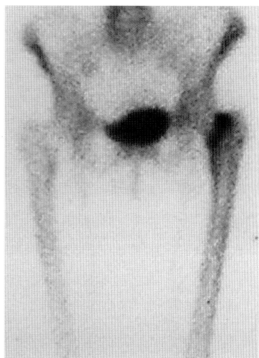

Figure 8.9. (a and b). Anterior views of intertrochanteric fracture, left femoral neck. **a** Blood pool and **b** delayed phase.

The bone scan has high sensitivity for these lesions and is typically abnormal one to two weeks in advance of radiographic changes. Dual- or triple-phase imaging is recommended, including several views of the symptomatic area on the delayed study to improve lesion localization and characterization. For tibial lesions this should include medial views and for metatarsal injuries plantar views. Acute fractures demonstrate local increased MDP uptake on all phases, while injury involving only the soft tissues will be normal on the delayed phase. The spectrum of tibial stress injury includes the condition of shin splints, which is a soft tissue disorder. On the bone scan there is abnormality along the posteromedial tibial cortex, usually confined to the delayed phase images, thereby allowing differentiation from tibial stress fracture.

8.3.6 Metabolic Bone Disease

Osteoporosis

Osteoporosis is characterized by reduced bone density and increased risk of fracture, and is found most commonly in elderly females. Vertebral compression fractures are the hallmark of this disease (Figure 8.10). When presented with a patient who has multiple collapsed vertebrae, the bone scan can assist in identification of the symptomatic level, which can guide therapeutic intervention such as vertebroplasty. Demonstration of the entire skeleton has the added advantage of detecting other fractures which may coexist in this vulnerable patient group, or may suggest an alternative diagnosis to account for the patient's pain.

The classic appearance of osteoporotic collapse is a vertebral body that is reduced in height with intense linear MDP uptake across its width, but these findings are not specific, and vertebral collapse secondary to metastases can be indistinguishable. This is most problematic when only a single vertebral body is involved, in which case plain radiography of the area can be helpful. However, progression to MRI or even biopsy may be necessary.

Another typical fracture in the osteoporotic patient is the sacral insufficiency fracture, which produces a classic appearance on the bone scan (Figure 8.11). There is vertical linear increased

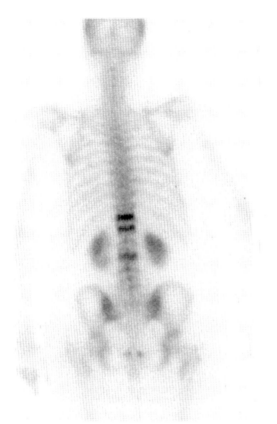

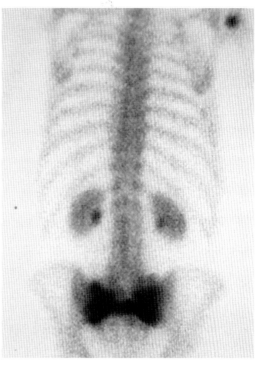

Figure 8.11. Posterior view of sacral insufficiency fracture.

Figure 8.10. Posterior view of multiple vertebral fractures due to osteoporosis.

uptake through each sacral ala, bridged by horizontal uptake across the sacral body, forming the pathognomonic "H" sign. The bone scan is particularly important in the diagnosis of this condition, as the fracture is usually not evident on a plain film.

The radionuclide bone scan is not used in the assessment of bone density. This is the province of bone densitometry.

Osteomalacia

In this metabolic disease bone is poorly mineralized and liable to specific lesions known as pseudofractures. These occur typically in the ribs, scapulae, pelvis, and proximal femora (Figure 8.12). The bone scan has a limited role in osteomalacia but is highly sensitive for the demonstration of pseudofractures and is often the first investigation to identify and characterize them by virtue of their situation [7].

Paget's Disease

This is a relatively common disorder of bone metabolism which is of unknown etiology. It shows geographical variation in prevalence, being most common in northern Europe. Often asymptomatic, it may be discovered incidentally on radiographs or a bone scan, but can also present with pain or with secondary complications, which include fracture and sarcomatous change.

Paget's disease can occur in any bone, but the pelvis, femora, tibiae, spine, and skull are most frequently involved. The bone scan is more sensitive than plain films for its demonstration, with intense MDP uptake in the affected part of the bone. In the long bones the process extends from the articular surface into the shaft and has a typical flame-shaped leading edge. This has a similar characteristic appearance on the bone scan, which may also demonstrate bone expansion and bowing deformity (Figure 8.13a and b). In 20% of cases only a single bone is involved (monostotic Paget's) but often the pattern of uptake can still allow a confident diagnosis to be made.

cumstances, if there is doubt about the specificity of the bone scan appearance, additional imaging with another modality should be performed.

The bone scan can be difficult to evaluate when Paget's disease and skeletal metastases coexist. This is a particular problem if the Paget's disease has been treated, as this can result in atypical appearances with multifocal lesions. Again, correlative imaging is recommended in situations of uncertainty.

8.3.7 Infection

Infection in the musculoskeletal system can be classified as involving bone (osteomyelitis), joints (septic arthritis), intervertebral disks (diskitis), or soft tissues (cellulitis).

Osteomyelitis

Organisms reach bone by three mechanisms: hematogenous spread, contiguous spread from adjacent soft tissues, and direct inoculation. The hematogenous route is the most common cause of childhood osteomyelitis, which will be discussed in the Pediatrics section (8.3.9). Contiguous spread and direct inoculation are the more frequent routes in the adult. Typical patients at risk of bone involvement from soft tissue infection are diabetics with neuropathic ulceration of the feet and bedridden patients with dependent ulceration. Direct inoculation may be caused by penetrating injury, but is more often seen as a complication of surgery.

Plain radiographs can remain normal for up to 3 weeks from the time of infection, but should still be the initial investigation.

On a triple-phase bone scan the classical findings of osteomyelitis are localized increased uptake on all phases, which becomes more focal and intense on the delayed images. This type of study is sensitive for infection, particularly in the absence of a preexisting bony abnormality. Unfortunately, many patients referred for the investigation of suspected osteomyelitis have underlying conditions which reduce the specificity of the bone scan.

In the diabetic population neuropathic joints are common and can mimic osteomyelitis both clinically and radiologically. Labeled white cell scintigraphy can be very useful in this scenario, but often requires to be combined with a bone scan

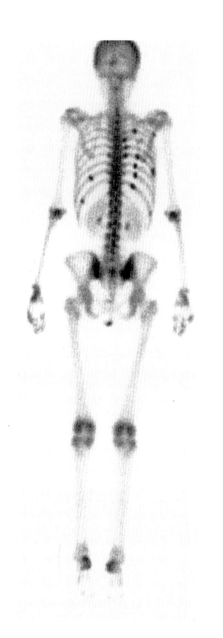

Figure 8.12. Posterior view of osteomalacia with multiple rib fractures and pseudofracture, lateral border right scapula.

Complications of the disease can also be visualized by the bone scan, for example pathological fracture or degenerative joint disease. However, activity in the primary lesion can obscure these secondary findings. Sarcoma development is rare and normally associated with relatively reduced MDP uptake. As in other cir-

THE SKELETAL SYSTEM

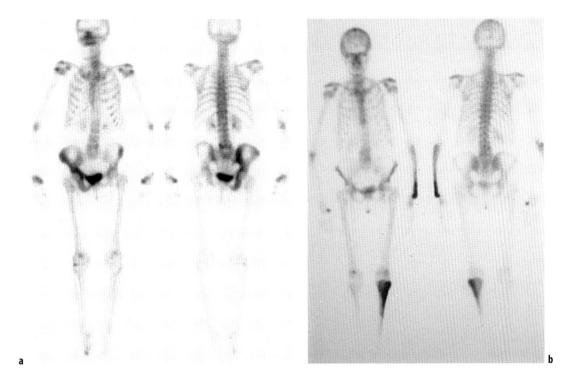

Figure 8.13. **a** Paget's disease of right hemipelvis. **b** Paget's disease of left ulna and tibia.

for accurate anatomical localization of abnormalities. However, labeled white cells also accumulate in normal marrow, the distribution of which is highly variable, particularly in the presence of systemic disease. This can lead to false positive interpretation. The addition of marrow imaging, with technetium-labeled colloid, can identify the location of marrow. Thus white cell accumulation in the absence of marrow activity on the colloid study can be assumed to represent infection. This combined technique has a reported accuracy of over 90% [8].

Similar problems exist in the investigation of potentially infected joint prostheses. This is a rare but extremely important complication which requires reliable differentiation from aseptic loosening. Unfortunately, following a hip replacement there is normally increased MDP uptake around the prosthetic components for many months. Knee replacements also demonstrate this prolonged periprosthetic activity, particularly around the tibial component. The phenomenon is even more pronounced with more recent cementless prostheses, which also cause increased white cell

accumulation [9]. Interpretation can therefore be difficult, but knowledge of the timing and type of surgical procedure is helpful.

While a normal bone scan is therefore very useful, positive findings require to be taken in context with other features. Diffuse periprosthetic uptake has been described as suggestive of infection (Figure 8.14a and b), while local uptake at the tip of the femoral prosthesis is more in keeping with loosening, but there is some overlap in these appearances. A combined approach to this problem using other agents can improve specificity. This can be achieved by performing both bone and gallium scans, with accepted criteria for interpretation relying on the congruity or otherwise of the site and intensity of uptake. Incongruous distribution of uptake, which is more intense on the gallium study, is reported to be accurate for the presence of infection. Other appearances may be less helpful, and increased gallium uptake can occur in aseptic loosening and heterotopic new bone formation.

An alternative approach involves combined white cell and marrow scintigraphy, with reported

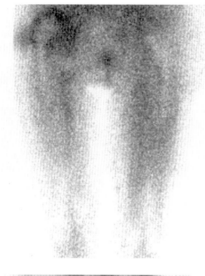

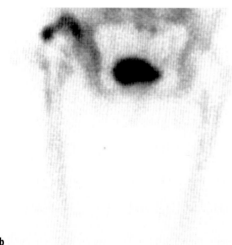

Figure 8.14. (a and b). Posterior views of left total hip replacement, with infected acetabular component. **a** Blood pool and **b** delayed phase.

accuracy of over 90%, similar to its results in investigation of the diabetic foot.

Diskitis

This term applies to infection centered on the intervertebral disk, which spreads to involve the adjacent vertebrae. It is most common in the lumbar spine, and recognized risk factors include recent surgery of the spine or genitourinary tract. The clinical features are often non-specific but the classical presentation is of back pain and

fever. *Staphylococcus aureus* is the most common causative organism but the possibility of other infections, particularly tuberculosis, should be considered.

On the bone scan there is increased uptake on all phases in the endplates of adjacent vertebrae. This may be present before any discernible radiographic changes and allow earlier identification of the level for diagnostic aspiration. MRI will also show specific appearances and is the investigation of choice if diskitis is suspected on a bone scan.

Vertebral Osteomyelitis

Infection may arise in the vertebra rather than the disk, though the risk factors, common sites, pathogens, and clinical features are similar. There is increased MDP accumulation in the affected vertebra, which is usually confined to a single level.

Labeled white cell scintigraphy is not recommended in this condition as the affected site appears more commonly as a photopenic defect than an area of increased accumulation. This defect is a non-specific finding and may result from other processes including tumor or Paget's disease (Figure 8.15a and b).

The addition of a gallium study may increase specificity of the bone scan and has the advantage of demonstrating adjacent soft tissue infection such as a paravertebral abscess.

Other Sites

Septic arthritis is rare and usually affects only a single joint. It may occur secondary to instrumentation or penetrating trauma, while underlying conditions such as rheumatoid disease or diabetes are predisposing factors.

MDP bone scan, gallium and white cell imaging may all demonstrate increased activity in relation to the joint, usually on both sides of the joint space, but are non-specific. Similar findings will be found in acute sterile inflammatory monoarthropathy such as gout. The diagnosis is made by joint aspiration.

In cellulitis the early phases of the bone scan will demonstrate diffuse increased activity in the soft tissues, which becomes less intense on the delayed phase.

8.3.8 Joint Disease

The bone scan is not usually employed for the diagnosis of an arthropathy, although the pattern of

THE SKELETAL SYSTEM

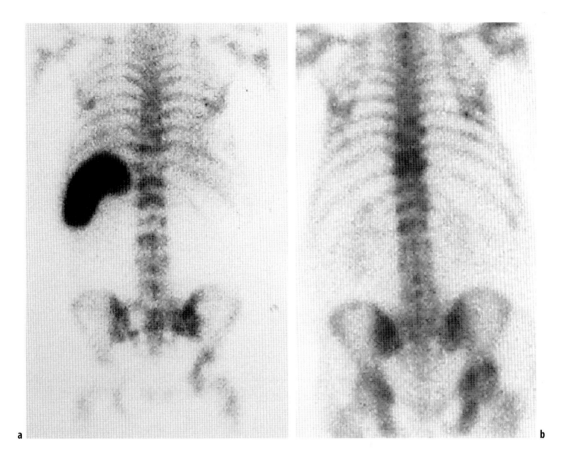

a   b

Figure 8.15. **a** Metastases producing photopenic defects in lower thoracic and lumbar spine, and left side of sacrum, on a labeled white cell scan. **b** MDP bone scan in the same patient, with increased uptake at corresponding sites.

uptake can help to characterize a disorder if the distribution is typical. However, increased uptake occurs before radiographic changes are evident, which allows a more accurate estimate of disease extent and may indicate involvement in joints that are as yet asymptomatic. In rheumatoid arthropathy the degree of uptake mirrors disease activity and can therefore guide therapy.

In the investigation of the seronegative arthropathies, for example ankylosing spondylitis or Reiter's syndrome, which cause sacroiliitis, often early in the disease, it can be useful to evaluate the sacroiliac joint activity against a reference region. The ratio is elevated in sacroiliitis, though this condition is not specific for these arthropathies. The ratio is also raised following strenuous physical activity. Enthesopathy, another complication, can be recognized by focal MDP uptake at the site of tendon insertion (Figure 8.16).

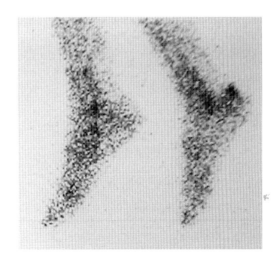

Figure 8.16. Left Achilles tendinitis with increased uptake at the site of tendon insertion to the calcaneum.

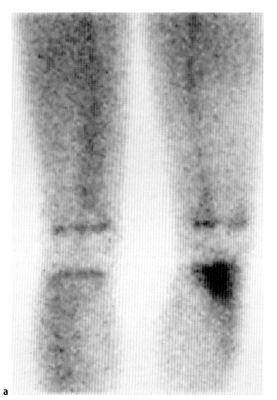
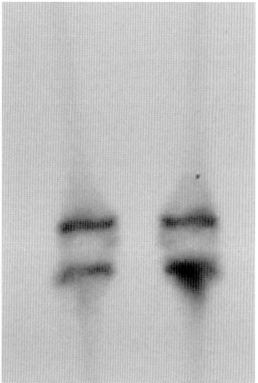

Figure 8.17. a and b. Anterior views of osteomyelitis left proximal tibial metaphysis in a child. **a** Blood pool and **b** delayed phase.

Crystal deposition diseases, such as gout, may present as an acute inflammatory arthritis, and the clinical and radiological findings are often confused with infection. Bone, gallium, and white cell scintigraphy can all be positive and the diagnosis is made biochemically or by joint aspiration.

8.3.9 Pediatrics

On a bone scan the epiphyseal growth plates are recognizable as thin linear accumulations of intense activity with sharp margins. Loss of clarity of the plate can be indicative of adjacent pathology in the epiphysis or metaphysis, common sites of osteomyelitis in children. Comparison with the contralateral limb is useful when abnormality is suspected.

Hematogenous spread is the most frequent route of infection. In infants, infection may reach the epiphysis via vessels which cross the growth plate from the metaphysis. In the growing period from approximately 1 to 16 years the epiphysis and

metaphysis each have a separate blood supply and hematogenous infection has a predilection for the metaphysis, without epiphyseal involvement.

Infection in either the epiphysis or metaphysis produces similar bone scan appearances with increased uptake on all phases (Figure 8.17). This is a non-specific pattern which may also be seen in some bone tumors, such as osteoid osteoma or Ewing's sarcoma. Clinical history and radiographic correlation are essential for differentiation. The bone scan's strength lies in its ability to demonstrate the presence of multifocal infection (Figure 8.18).

Septic arthritis in childhood must be diagnosed promptly. It occurs most often in the lower limb, particularly the hip joint, and may be a primary site of infection or secondary to adjacent osteomyelitis, the possibility of which should be considered when interpreting the bone scan. In this condition the femoral head can appear photopenic, secondary to raised intra-articular pressure, and urgent joint aspiration is the required treatment.

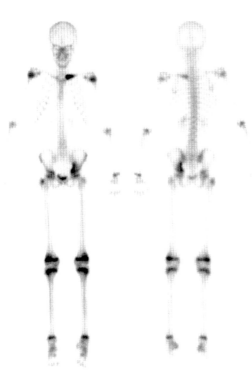

Figure 8.18. Multifocal osteomyelitis in a child involving medial left clavicle and pelvis.

Another condition that affects the hip is transient synovitis [10]. This is the most common cause of hip pain in children and does not usually require scintigraphy for diagnosis. If performed, the bone scan can be normal or can demonstrate mild increased activity in early and delayed phases. However, the bone scan is not reliable for the differentiation of these two entities, and the clinical context and results of joint aspiration are more important in establishing a diagnosis.

Diskitis and vertebral osteomyelitis in children can present with non-specific symptoms, and radiographs can remain normal for several weeks into the illness. The bone scan becomes abnormal at an earlier stage and the appearances in each condition are similar to the findings in adults.

The type of skeletal trauma sustained in childhood varies with age. Use of bone scintigraphy tends to be restricted to the younger child, where the clinical symptoms and their localization can be unreliable, and reluctance to walk may be the only clinical sign [11].

The characteristic "toddler's fracture", a spiral fracture of the tibia, may produce only subtle radiographic changes, but a bone scan will demonstrate increased uptake along the tibial shaft, though the spiral configuration may not be appreciable. In this age-group isolated tarsal bone fractures also occur and can similarly be demonstrated by scintigraphy.

Skeletal trauma may be a manifestation of child abuse. The high sensitivity and total body inclusion of the bone scan are useful in such cases, particularly in areas such as the ribs or scapulae where conventional radiography may fail to demonstrate the injuries.

Perthes' disease is a condition that occurs in the early school years where the capital femoral epiphysis undergoes osteonecrosis. It may be the result of repeated trauma or infarction, but the precise etiology is unknown. It is more common in males and can be bilateral, though it is not necessarily synchronous. The bone scan will reliably demonstrate the disease earlier than radiography. Initially there is relative photopenia in the affected epiphysis which progresses to increased uptake in the healing stages.

8.3.10 Reflex Sympathetic Dystrophy

There are many pseudonyms for this entity, including algodystrophy, Sudck's atrophy, and complex regional pain syndrome. Reflex sympathetic dystrophy occurs typically in a limb that has been subjected to trauma, but sometimes no cause can be identified. It is characterized by a combination of intense pain, vasomotor disturbance, soft tissue swelling, and skin changes, but its definition is imprecise and varies from specialty to specialty, with no gold standard for its diagnosis [12].

The bone scan appearances are dependent on the stage of the disease process and are variable, reflecting the complex physiological changes inherent in this condition. The most suggestive pattern of uptake is increased activity on all phases of a triple-phase study, with diffuse uptake and periarticular accumulation on the delayed phase. However, in late stages of the disease decreased uptake may be the case in the early phases of the scan. Comparison with the normal side is obviously crucial.

8.3.11 Avascular Necrosis

This disorder occurs most commonly in the femoral head and has many causes, including trauma, certain drugs, and systemic diseases. The bone scan appearances change with the age of the process. Initial photopenia of the femoral head, reflecting reduced vascularity, is gradually replaced by increased uptake secondary to new bone formation.

The sensitivity of the bone scan for the demonstration of avascular necrosis varies with the etiology, and while it is greater than plain radiography, it is surpassed by MRI, which is also more specific and is therefore the technique of choice. Scintigraphy may still have a role to play if MRI is not possible.

8.3.12 Non-skeletal Uptake

While a radionuclide bone scan is performed primarily to assess the skeleton, there can be findings in other systems. These may be incidental or relevant to the bone pathology. It is important therefore not to overlook the urinary tract and the soft tissues when evaluating the examination.

By virtue of the renal excretion of MDP, normal variants in the urinary tract are exposed. They should be recognized as such and documented, as this may be their first demonstration. Uptake in only a single kidney implies absence or impaired function of the other. Ectopia, malrotation, ptosis, and fusion abnormalities (e.g. horseshoe kidney) are all well visualized if renal function is adequate (Figure 8.19).

In bladder or prostatic malignancy the bone scan, executed primarily for identification of skeletal metastases, can also highlight urinary obstruction, though this is likely to have been detailed on a prior ultrasound examination. In other clinical circumstances the referrer may not be aware of, or expecting, this finding and its detection may prompt further investigation. Urine leaking from a ruptured collecting system can have a bizarre appearance (Figure 8.20).

In renal malignancy the primary mass lesion, if large enough, can be appreciated as a photopenic defect. Occasionally this will be noted unexpectedly, and while it is not specific for a neoplasm, further investigation is mandatory to exclude renal carcinoma.

Some soft tissue MDP uptake is normal and the amount varies with body mass and renal function. Once again, demonstration of abnormal soft tissue uptake may be incidental or of significance, depending on the clinical setting. This uptake occurs when there is soft tissue calcification or os-

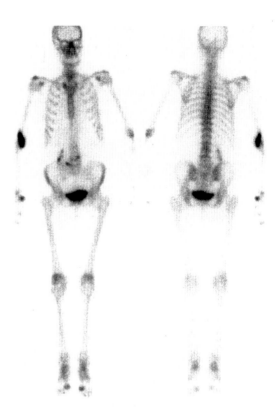

Figure 8.19. Normal renal variant (crossed fused ectopia).

Table 8.3. Some causes of extra-osseous MDP uptake

Normal breast tissue
Breast carcinoma
Liver metastases
Osteosarcoma metastases
Soft tissue sarcomas
Tumoral calcinosis
Pleural effusion
Ascites
Calcified uterine fibroids
Injection sites
Surgical scars
Old hematomas

sification (Figures 8.21 and 8.22), or when MDP accumulates for other reasons, such as in a pleural effusion. This latter example can have a subtle appearance, particularly if bilateral, and is best appreciated on the posterior view (Figure 8.23). The more common causes of extra-osseous uptake are listed in Table 8.3.

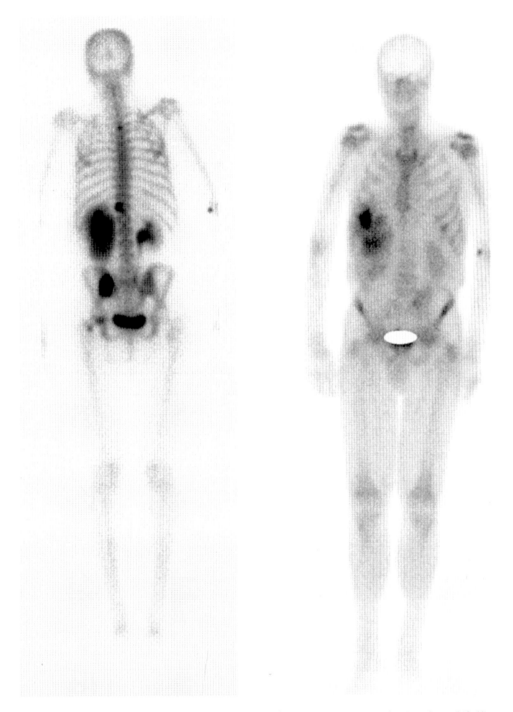

Figure 8.20. Posterior view of leakage of urine and MDP from left kidney obstructed by bladder carcinoma, with bone metastases.

Figure 8.21. Anterior view of MDP uptake in calcified liver metastases.

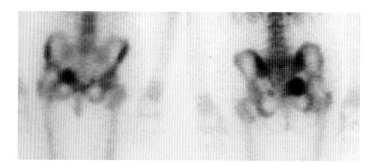

Figure 8.22. MDP uptake in calcified uterine fibroid.

8.3.13 Artifacts and Pitfalls

Artifactual abnormalities on the bone scan are areas of increased or decreased activity that are non-pathological and are recognized by their typical position or configuration.

Metal, either inside or outside the patient, attenuates gamma rays and produces a photopenic defect on the image. Pacemakers and orthopedic hardware are usually easily recognized (Figure 8.24), as are belt buckles, but smaller defects due to coins in a pocket or jewelry may be missed, or, of more concern, misinterpreted.

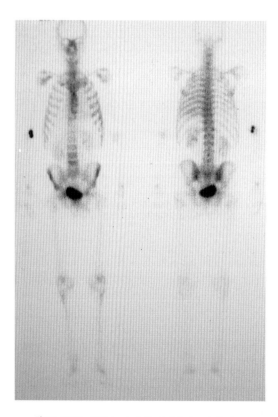

Figure 8.23. MDP accumulation in left pleural effusion.

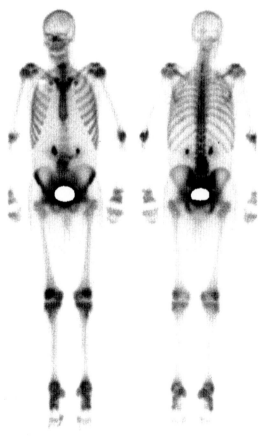

Figure 8.24. Photopenic defect due to pacemaker; normal renal variant (horseshoe kidney).

Focal increased activity at the injection site is unlikely to be mistaken for pathology. If the site is unusual this should be documented at the time of MDP administration. Contamination by direct spillage or by urine is usually self-evident by its pattern. It can occur on the patient's clothing or the camera face and can cause confusion until its true nature is appreciated.

Slight alterations in patient positioning can lead to apparent disparity in the activity between right and left sides. This is particularly true in the pelvis. Here the degree of rotation can be assessed by comparing the obturator foramina, which should be symmetrical.

In the situation where overlying soft tissue is reduced, most often by surgery (e.g. mastectomy), the underlying bone will appear to have increased activity relative to the normal side. The diffuse nature of this apparent discrepancy and the altered soft tissue outline of the affected side should allow appropriate interpretation.

8.4 Summary

The radionuclide bone scan is a sensitive technique which is applicable in a wide variety of pathologies. Advances in technology during the last four decades have allowed the bone scan to maintain its important role in the management of musculoskeletal disorders, alongside the other imaging options now available. Its lack of specificity can be countered by interpreting scan findings in the context of the clinical setting and in the light of other imaging.

References

1. McCarthy EF. Histopathologic correlates of a positive bone scan. Semin Nucl Med 1997; 27:309–320.
2. Krasnow AZ, Hellman RS, Timins ME, et al. Diagnostic bone scanning in oncology. Semin Nucl Med 1997; 27:107–141.
3. Tumeh SS, Beadle G, Kaplan WD. Clinical significance of solitary rib lesions in patients with extraskeletal malignancy. J Nucl Med 1985; 26:1140–1143.
4. Brown ML. Bone scintigraphy in benign and malignant tumours. Radiol Clin North Am 1993; 31:731–738.
5. Holder LE. Bone scintigraphy in skeletal trauma. Radiol Clin North Am 1993; 31:739–781.
6. Spitz DJ, Newberg AH. Imaging of stress fractures in the athlete. Radiol Clin North Am 2002; 40:313–331.
7. Ryan PJ, Fogelman I. Bone scintigraphy in metabolic bone disease. Semin Nucl Med 1997; 27:291–305.
8. Palestro CJ, Torres MA. Radionuclide imaging in orthopaedic infections. Semin Nucl Med 1997; 27:334–345.
9. Turpin S, Lambert R. Role of scintigraphy in musculoskeletal and spinal infections. Radiol Clin North Am 2001; 39:169–189.
10. Mandell GA. Nuclear medicine in paediatric orthopaedics. Semin Nucl Med 1998; 28:95–115.
11. Connolly LP, Treves ST. Assessing the limping child with skeletal scintigraphy. J Nucl Med 1998; 39:1056–1061.
12. Fournier RS, Holder LE. Reflex sympathetic dystrophy: diagnostic controversies. Semin Nucl Med 1998; 28:116–123.

9

The Cardiovascular System

Malcolm J. Metcalfe

9.1 Introduction

In a healthy individual both during exercise as well as at rest all four heart chambers contract in a co-ordinated fashion, the valves function normally and the heart muscle is perfused uniformly by the coronary arteries. Disease states can result in abnormalities of valves, ventricular contraction, and reduced perfusion of the heart muscle. Nuclear cardiology is a very useful clinical tool which can help to assess and treat these problems.

9.2 Anatomy and Physiology

The heart is a four-chambered structure lying behind the lower sternum and centered slightly to the left. Its orientation leads to the right atrium and ventricle being anterior whilst the left atrium and ventricle are posterior. The long axis through the complete heart is roughly along a line from upper mid-right sternum to the edge of the ribcage at 14:30 o'clock as viewed from head to foot. Thus simple cross-sectional (transaxial) and longitudinal views do not lead to anatomically correct short and long axis images of the heart and image reconstruction has to take this into account.

The right atrium (RA) receives blood back from the great veins and passes it into the right ventricle (RV). This pumps the blood through the lungs (for oxygenation) to return to the left atrium (LA). This structure then passes blood into the left ventricle (LV), which in turn pumps it around the body to satisfy the body's needs. Both atria and ventricles are dynamic structures with their own individual contraction patterns. For example, the left ventricle has radial, longitudinal, and torsional contraction components.

Blood is prevented from going backwards by the heart valves. The tricuspid valve is between RA and RV. Between RV and lungs is the pulmonary valve, between LA and RV is the mitral valve (which has only two rather than three leaflets) and between LV and the aorta is the aortic valve.

As the blood pressure on the right side is only approximately 20% of that on the left, the RV has a much thinner muscular wall than the LV. Heart muscle is unique in that it has the ability to contract spontaneously; this is called automaticity. However, there is also a hierarchical system which ensures that certain parts of the heart "overdrive" others so ensuring a coordinated contraction pattern. Normally, electrical depolarization starts at the sinoatrial node (SAN) situated at the free margin of the right atrium. The SAN's rate of depolarization is controlled by both the sympathetic system (increasing heart rate) and the vagal system (decreasing heart rate). The wave of depolarization spreads to both atria leading to contraction. The electrical wave then meets an inert insulating layer between atria and ventricles, the atrioventricular ring. The only way though this is via the atrioventricular node (AVN) which delays passage of the depolarization wave into the ventricular conducting system by 120–200 ms. This allows the ventricles to be optimally filled before they, in turn, contract. Loss of atrial contraction, as in atrial fibrillation, leads to a significant reduction in cardiac output for equivalent heart rates.

Passage of the electrical wave of depolarization in the ventricles is via two left-sided pathways (anterior and posterior left fascicles) and one on the right. Abnormalities of conduction via these pathways lead to characteristic patterns on the surface electrocardiogram (ECG) of left and right bundle branch block (LBBB and RBBB), respectively.

The sympathetic system innervates not only the SAN but also the ventricular muscle. The parasympathetic system only innervates the SAN. The sympathetic nervous system is responsible for a "fight or flight" effect in the body. Thus stimulation leads to an increase in heart rate and contraction. The heart is capable of increasing its output when required by up to approximately eightfold, for example during exercise. It does this by increasing both the heart rate and increasing the amount of blood ejected per heart beat (ejection fraction).

Imaging of the heart is rendered more complex than usual by factors such as the heart's motion, respiratory motion and also its position in the lower thorax. It is surrounded by tissues of varying density with different abilities to both absorb and scatter radiation. It also overlies the diaphragm and activity can be sometimes difficult to separate from sub-diaphragmatic activity. In females there can also be problems with increased attenuation from overlying breast tissue whilst in males there may be problems related to diaphragmatic attenuation.

Conventional radionuclide tracers can be used to assess myocardial perfusion, myocardial infarction, blood pool distribution, sympathetic nervous system activity, and free fatty acid utilization. Using positron emission tomography (PET) imaging, special tracers can be synthesized to investigate virtually any biochemical/physiological pathway.

9.3 Cardiac Imaging

Although tomographic imaging has rendered planar imaging obsolete for general myocardial perfusion imaging (MPI) [1], planar imaging is still important in certain circumstances particularly, for example, radionuclide ventriculography. Planar imaging is usually performed by angling the gamma camera to the desired position; for example, in radionuclide ventriculography the gamma camera is usually positioned in the 45 degree left anterior oblique (LAO) projection with 15–30 degrees of caudal tilt. The LAO angle is then adjusted to obtain clear separation of the ventricles (known as the "best septal view") and the caudal tilt can also be adjusted to obtain separation of the atria from the ventricles [2]. In sympathetic innervation studies and myocardial perfusion imaging an anteroposterior (AP) planar image is an important part of the examination, as will be expanded upon later.

Cardiac tomographic imaging usually employs 32 or 64 steps ("step and shoot") over a 180 degree arc from the right anterior oblique (RAO) projection to the left posterior oblique (LPO) projection. This 180 degree arc has the advantage of avoiding the variable and significant attenuation effects from the spine. Even with attenuation correction it is generally found to be superior to 360 degree acquisitions and is much quicker – particularly if a twin-headed (or triple-headed) camera is used [3, 4]. Even when ECG gated images are required (which need more counts) a complete examination can usually be completed within 20–25 minutes.

Tomographic imaging has significant advantages over planar imaging of much improved contrast, enhanced sensitivity/specificity, and reduced artifact. For MPI it has conclusively been shown to be superior to planar imaging.

Attenuation can be a particular problem in MPI. Although methods of correcting for attenuation are available (see Section 2.2.4) they all suffer from a variety of problems and hence their clinical value is uncertain [5]. Breast binding, using a broad strap, around the chest can be useful in both sexes as it prevents movement and may help to reduce breast attenuation artifact. However, it is essential that consistency in application is achieved, especially in myocardial perfusion imaging.

Care must also be taken over image display. It is important when undertaking image reconstruction that true short and long axis segments are obtained. Error in this regard may make images difficult to interpret and compare in MPI. Although many computer systems conveniently display MPI stress and rest images adjacent to each other, they frequently scale to the maximum activity within a set (e.g. stress or rest images). Although this is generally an advantage, occasionally high adjacent cardiac activity (e.g. from bowel) can lead to a suboptimal display of the cardiac myocardium. It is useful in these circumstances to be able to modify the image display. Examples of this are the ability to be able to "mask" extraneous myocardial activity at the reconstruction phase and to be able to independently set background subtraction and scale maximum. These maneuvers often lead to the image sets being interpretable.

Differing color scales can have quite a dramatic effect upon interpretation of images. When using a gray or thermal scale it can sometimes be difficult to distinguish areas of mildly differing activity. Use of a coarse graduated scale can lead to overinterpretation of minor differences. As a consequence it is suggested that a continuously variable scale be used where the colors graduate progressively from one to another across the whole scale. Some centers nevertheless prefer to use either a gray or thermal scale. However, whatever scale is chosen it is imperative that experience is built up using the same scale.

9.4 Radionuclide Ventriculography

Radionuclide ventriculography is known by a number of synonyms and acronyms such as radionuclide ventriculography (RNVG), equilibrium radionuclide ventriculography (ERNVG), or multigated acquisition (MUGA). Although echocardiography is the usual method of choice for assessing left ventricular function, RNVG studies remain very useful for a number of reasons. This modality is able to assess left ventricular performance, even when it is not possible to obtain adequate echocardiographic images, it provides more accurate/reproducible information with respect to left ventricular ejection fraction (LVEF), and it can provide important information with respect to the timing of ventricular contraction (phase imaging) [6]. LVEF is the amount of blood ejected per heart beat as a ratio of end-diastolic volume (EDV).

An RNVG study is simple to perform and involves the intravenous administration of 800 MBq (20 mCi) of ^{99m}Tc pertechnetate after priming with 5 mg of stannous chloride (Table 9.1). The latter binds the radionuclide to the patient's own red blood cells so that "blood pool" imaging can

Table 9.1. Gated blood pool imaging

Radiopharmaceutical	^{99m}Tc pertechnetate in vivo labeled red blood cells
Activity administered	800 MBq (20 mCi)
Effective dose equivalent	7 mSv (700 mrem)
Patient preparation	Injection of stannous agent 15–20 minutes prior to ^{99m}Tc pertechnetate. ECG electrodes applied to allow gating to cardiac cycle
Collimator	Low-energy, general purpose
Images acquired	45° LAO (best septal) + 15–30° of caudal tilt
	List mode: 5 million counts within region if interest
	Formatted to 16–24 frames
	Frame mode can be used if list mode unavailable

be undertaken (in vivo labeling). This is almost always successful but occasionally a patient is found in whom this procedure is unsuccessful. In this case in vitro labeling of the patient's red blood cells can be undertaken in the radiopharmacy and the labeled blood subsequently returned to the patient (see Section 14.14).

The gamma camera is positioned in the "best septal" projection (with suitable caudal tilt) and imaging performed. An acquisition of approximately 5 million counts within the cardiac field is usually sufficient for satisfactory statistical analysis for 16 frames (divisions of the cardiac cycle). It is usual to employ a "zoom mode" to maximize data collection within the cardiac field of view. The cardiac cycle is gated by simultaneously recording the ECG and allocating appropriate counts to the appropriate part (frame) of the heart beat. The computer therefore builds up images of the heart over the desired number of frames. There are two main ways of doing this either in real time, known as "frame mode", or retrospectively, known as "list mode" (see Section 1.4.2). List mode is generally preferred as it allows rejection of "bad beats", for example caused by ventricular ectopics. When this sequence is played in cine mode the activity within the cardiac chambers (blood pool) can be observed over the cardiac cycle. By drawing a region of interest around, say, the left ventricle a time–activity curve can be obtained as shown in Figure 9.1. After correcting for background activity, the LVEF can be obtained by measuring the total counts in a region of interest drawn around the left ventricle

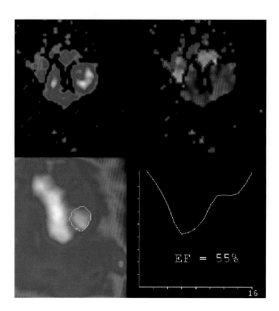

Figure 9.1. Normal RNVG in a patient pre-chemotherapy. Bottom left is the summed image showing the regions of interest. Bottom right is the time–activity curve, which gives a normal LVEF of 55%. Above these are the parametric images, amplitude on the left and phase on the right, both showing the four cardiac chambers.

and using the formula [6]:

$$\text{LVEF} = (\text{counts at end diastole} \\ - \text{counts at end systole})/ \\ \text{counts at end diastole}.$$

LVEF values can vary considerably depending upon the method used for their derivation. For example, if a simple end-diastolic background area is used values will be less than if a dynamic region (which moves with the cardiac cycle) is used. The smaller the background area the higher the value obtained but at the expense of reproducibility. As a result of this it is important that a normal range and reproducibility coefficients are established in each center. Furthermore, it should be realized that values obtained may not be directly comparable between centers or to values obtained using other imaging modalities [6, 7]. This problem is not confined to RNVG [7].

With further mathematical processing of the counts within each frame, parametric images of extent of contraction (amplitude) and timing of contraction (phase) can be obtained (see Section 1.4.2) [6] (Figure 9.1). In a patient with a septal myocardial infarction it would be expected to find a reduced LVEF, abnormal wall motion indicated

by delayed (phase) and reduced (amplitude) septal motion.

It should be appreciated, however, that one disadvantage of planar RNVG is that the derived ejection fraction is depth dependent. This effect leads to an over- and under-assessment of true LVEF values in the presence of inferior and anterior wall motion abnormalities, respectively, when imaging is performed in the usual LAO projection. For example, with an inferior wall motion abnormality the counts arising from this wall are further from the collimator than the anterior activity. Due to scatter, fewer counts will be able to pass through the collimator from the inferior wall than from the anterior wall and consequently the time–activity curve will be biased towards the anterior activity. Hence the LVEF will be overestimated from its true value. In an anterior wall motion abnormality the converse will occur. This is, however, not usually of clinical significance [2].

The number of frames acquired can also influence accuracy. More frames leads to improved accuracy of the time–activity curve but requires increased counts. There are two ways of increasing the number of counts obtained, either by increasing the duration of acquisition or by giving more activity. The latter is undesirable as it will increase the radiation dose so there has to be a "trade-off" between accuracy and length of acquisition and generally 16–24 frames per cardiac cycle are employed.

It can also be useful to obtain planar images of the blood pool in projections other than the LAO, such as anteroposterior (AP), right anterior oblique (RAO), and left lateral (LL). These views when observed dynamically can help to assess both right and left ventricular wall motion. It is also quite possible to perform tomographic imaging with advantage but in practice this is rarely done at present.

One of the most common applications of the RNVG is for measurement of LVEF, particularly in oncology patients receiving chemotherapy. This technique is of especial benefit due to the inherent excellent reproducibility ($\pm$4%) [8]. Thus sequential measurement can detect early impairment to LV performance with a greater degree of certainty than echocardiography, allowing treatment to be modified accordingly at an earlier stage. Figure 9.1 shows a normal RNVG in a pre-chemotherapy patient.

RNVG studies can also be used to subjectively assess the degree of valvular regurgitation, objectively measure diastolic relaxation, and assess intraventricular phase dispersion. The latter may be a useful and robust method of assessing suitability for resynchronization pacing therapy (RPT) in patients with severe symptomatic heart failure [9].

9.5 First-pass Imaging

This is another method of assessing right and left ventricular function [6]. It involves injecting a bolus of radionuclide into the venous circulation and following its passage through the right and then left heart. Time–activity curves can be constructed for each chamber and, with background correction, ejection fractions obtained. It is also possible to measure "recirculation" through an interatrial or interventricular defect and calculate the size of the shunt. However, despite this method's attractions, it needs either a gamma camera with very high count rate capability or a multicrystal camera to be successful. As echocardiography and cardiac magnetic resonance (CMR) are now without question the modalities of choice for investigation of these problems, first-pass imaging has consequently become a technique carried out in only a few centers worldwide and hence will not be considered further.

9.6 Myocardial Perfusion Imaging

9.6.1 Introduction

Myocardial perfusion imaging (MPI) is the foremost nuclear cardiology procedure, being responsible for more than 75% of cardiac imaging in most centers. It is of consummate benefit to the cardiologist as it has a number of advantages that are difficult to emulate using other imaging modalities. It also has the advantage of being robust and reproducible, although occasionally there can be difficulties as with any imaging technique [1].

It is performed using a tomographic imaging protocol, following the injection of either ^{99m}Tc-labeled tetrofosmin or MIBI (Table 9.2), or ^{201}Tl thallous chloride (Table 9.3). It is carried out in two parts either on the same day (single day protocol) or on separate days (two day protocol). One part of the examination is performed with stress

Table 9.2. Myocardial perfusion imaging (^{99m}Tc agents)

Radiopharmaceutical	^{99m}Tc tetrofosmin
Activity administered	2 day protocol:
	400 MBq for stress (10 mCi)
	400 MBq for rest (10 mCi)
	1 day protocol:
	200 MBq for stress (5 mCi)
	800 MBq for rest (20 mCi)
Effective dose equivalent	2 day: 8 mSv (800 mrem)
	1 day: 10 mSv (1 rem)
Radiopharmaceutical	^{99m}Tc-MIBI
Activity administered	As per tetrofosmin
Effective dose equivalent	2 day: 10 mSv (1 rem)
	1 day: 12.5 mSv (1.25 rem)
Patient preparation	No caffeine for minimum of 12 hours if dipyridamole/ adenosine stress being used
	Consider fasting, withdrawing anti-anginal and vasodilator therapy
	Consider fatty meal/water load after radionuclide
	Chest binding
Collimator	Low-energy, general purpose
Images acquired	2 day protocol superior but may be impractical
	Follow chosen stress protocol (Table 9.4)
	Tomographic acquisition
	Image 30–60 min after administration
	Gate images if at all possible (8 frames minimum)

Table 9.3. Myocardial perfusion imaging – ^{201}Tl chloride

Radiopharmaceutical	^{201}Tl chloride
Activity administered	80 MBq (+ 40 MBq for reinjection protocol)
Effective dose equivalent	18 mSv (1.8 rem)
Patient preparation	No caffeine for minimum of 12 hours if dipyridamole/adenosine stress being used
	Consider fasting, withdrawing anti-anginal and vasodilator therapy
	Chest binding
Collimator	Low-energy, general purpose
Images acquired	Follow chosen stress protocol
	Tomographic acquisition
	Should not be gated
	Stress imaging should start immediately after stress ends
	Reinject and reimage as appropriate

and the other at rest, allowing a comparison of myocardial perfusion to be made. If the amount of tracer in a particular segment is observed to be relatively low on the stress image and then increases at rest, known as a reversible defect, this is taken as showing ischemia. If there is a fixed defect, this indicates myocardial infarction. There may also be a mixed pattern as a mixture of infarction and ischemia.

The commonly used terminology is unfortunate as defects are not "reversible" but what is being imaged is a difference in perfusion between areas of the myocardium. During stress, that myocardium supplied by unobstructed coronary arteries experiences an increase in perfusion and hence delivery of the radiopharmaceutical. Areas of myocardium supplied by obstructed coronary arteries cannot increase perfusion with exercise to the same degree and hence the supplied area of myocardium gets proportionately less tracer delivered.

9.6.2 Radiopharmaceuticals

Thallium-201 Imaging

Thallium acts as a potassium analogue in the body and is taken up into the myocardial tissue both actively by sodium/potassium cellular pump and also passively along an electrochemical gradient. Its 90% first-pass extraction is better than other current radiopharmaceuticals and uptake is linearly proportional to flow except at high blood flow rates. Once inside the myocyte it then redistributes along an electrochemical gradient back to the bloodstream. Thus whilst thallium is an excellent marker of myocardial perfusion it also fairly rapidly redistributes, reaching an equilibrium at 3–4 hours. The latter is taken as the rest or redistribution images. Thus it is important that stress imaging is started as soon as possible after injection.

Thallium has the disadvantages, however, of not only delivering a relatively high radiation dose, so the administered activity is limited to 80 MBq (2 mCi), but also of emitting low-energy gamma rays which are subject to more attenuation than those of higher energy. Its use is also associated with a particular artifact known as "upward creep". Since stress imaging starts immediately after exercise then as the patient relaxes and breathing is restored to normal, the heart's position moves towards the head. Thus during acquisition there can be upwards movement of the myocardium. It

can be usually compensated for by adjustment at the stage of image reconstruction.

This tracer does, however, have the advantage of being taken up in the lungs in patients with high left ventricular end-diastolic pressures (EDP). This is a very useful prognostic marker, a high uptake denoting a high risk assessment.

Technetium-99m Tracers

Two ^{99m}Tc tracers are currently commercially available; 2-methoxy-isobutyl-isonitrile (sestamibi or MIBI) and tetrofosmin [1]. There is little clinical difference between them and choice will depend upon local circumstances.

These tracers have the advantages over thallium of fewer attenuation artifacts owing to the higher energy gammas, and better dosimetry allowing greater activity to be given. The usual allowable dose is 1000 MBq (25 mCi) for a single day protocol (usually divided as 200 MBq (5 mCi) for "stress" and 800 MBq (20 mCi) for rest) or 400 MBq (10 mCi) for each part of a two day protocol. It is allowable to increase the dose in certain circumstances, for example obesity.

These tracers rely on a functioning myocyte, as extraction is an active process, and first-pass extraction is less than with thallium. However, both tracers have the advantage of becoming "locked" in the myocardium, in proportion to delivery, which is useful as it means that imaging can be delayed. This allows the tracers to be administered to patients presenting with chest pain in the emergency room, a normal scan facilitating early discharge.

The ability to be able to defer imaging is also important as the tracers are also avidly taken up in the sub-diaphragmatic organs, particularly the gallbladder. Thus a delay of 30–60 minutes (sometimes longer) can improve the target to background ratio and optimize imaging conditions. To try and improve clearance of the radiopharmaceutical from the abdominal organs, a fatty meal and/or water is often given. However, there is no conclusive evidence that this is beneficial and indeed it may increase retrogressive passage of the radiopharmaceutical from duodenum to stomach.

Although the radiopharmaceutical is rarely taken up in the lung in response to a high EDP, the higher dose that can be administered allows imaging to be performed with ECG gating thus permitting simultaneous examination of both myocardial perfusion and left ventricular contraction patterns. This not only allows an

Table 9.4. Stress protocols

Method	Protocol	Radionuclide injection
Exercise	Bruce protocol (or equivalent)	Inject tracer at peak stress and continue exercise for 2 minutes. Start imaging as soon as possible after administration of thallium. With ^{99}Tc radionuclides delay for 30–60 minutes to clear splanchnic uptake
Dipyridamole (vasodilator)	140 µg/kg/min for 4 minutes Aminophylline "antidote"	4 minutes after completion of injection Effects may last 25–30 min
Adenosine (vasodilator)	140 µg/kg/min for 6 minutes Short-acting	At 4 min
Dobutamine (inotrope – safe for asthmatics)	Start at 5 µg/kg/min Increase by 5–10 µg/kg/min every 4 minutes up to 40 µg/kg/min If target heart rate (200 – age of patient) not reached consider atropine Relatively short-acting	At peak stress. Either precipitation of characteristic symptoms or target heart rate

assessment of LV contraction but helps to distinguish real from apparent myocardial infarction, for example the anterior wall in females (see Figure 9.5).

9.6.3 Major Indications for Myocardial Perfusion Imaging

It is important to recognize the patient groups in whom MPI will be useful. In patients without a robust diagnosis of ischemic heart disease (IHD), MPI is used:

1. to exclude or diagnose IHD in patients with inadequate ETT (exercise treadmill testing), preexisting ECG changes e.g. LBBB (left bundle branch block), or in females;
2. as a screening test for those felt to be at high risk when unsuitable for, or with inadequate, ETT;
3. in high-risk surgical patients (e.g. after major vascular surgery).

In patients with a diagnosis of IHD, MPI is used for:

1. risk stratification in patients with inadequate ETT, those unable to exercise, preexisting ECG changes, or females;
2. risk stratification in intermediate risk patients as assessed by ETT;
3. assistance in directing revascularization after determining coronary anatomy;

4. post-myocardial infarct (MI) risk stratification;
5. detection of restenosis following PCI (percutaneous coronary intervention) or angioplasty;
6. detection of ischemic burden after CABG;
7. assessment of patients with severe LV impairment for detection of "hibernating myocardium".

9.6.4 Imaging Technique

Patient Preparation

Patients should be prepared for MPI as follows:

1. Withdraw drugs that may interfere with either physiological exercise response or reduce apparent "ischemic response", e.g. anti-anginal therapy and vasodilators unless medically contraindicated.
2. Avoid caffeine for 12 to 24 hours prior to the stress examination.
3. Consider fasting.
4. Give appropriate information about nature of test, side effects of therapy, etc.

Stress Procedures

There are several methods for stressing the patient and these are outlined in Table 9.4. It is important that these guidelines are followed when stressing patients for MPI.

Table 9.5. Major side effects of pharmaceutical stress (%)

Side effect	Dipyridamole (3911 patients)	Adenosine (9256 patients)	Dobutamine (144 patients)
Chest pain	20	35	31
Dyspnea	3	35	14
Flushing	3	37	14
Headache	12	14	14
Palpitation	3	1	29
Dizziness	12	9	–
Hypotension	5	2	15
Serious heart block	2	5	0
Dysrhythmias	5	3	4

1. The patient should give full informed consent to the technique and have been apprised of the associated risks (Tables 9.5 and 9.6).

2. Must be undertaken by appropriately trained individual with ready access to emergency cardiac care.

3. ECG monitoring, either single- (or preferably) multi-lead, is mandatory.

4. All patients should have venous access readily available.

5. The patient demographics, clinical history, current medication, and caffeine status should be rechecked and advice sought before proceeding if potential problems are identified.

6. Justification and authorization for the test should be confirmed in accordance with current legislation.

7. Exercise, alternative stress or both are then undertaken.

8. Hemodynamic variables are measured at rest and at each stage during the test.

9. The radionuclide is administered at peak stress and in the case of exercise this is continued at a lower level for one to two minutes further.

10. Exercise duration, symptoms, reason for stopping, and ECG changes should be noted.

11. When the patient is deemed clinically stable transfer to the nuclear medicine department can be made (if appropriate).

Imaging

In order to achieve good quality MPI the following should be observed:

1. The patient is placed upon the imaging couch in a supine position with both arms above the head; the majority of tables have hand-grips to facilitate this. Knee support can be helpful.

2. A breast band is then applied as appropriate.

3. Imaging is then performed usually over a 180 degree arc from 45° RAO to 45° LPO. Dual-headed cameras should ideally have the heads at 90° to each other.

4. For ^{201}Tl and ^{99m}Tc radionuclides a low-energy, general purpose collimator should be employed.

5. For thallium imaging 20% dual energy windows set at 72 and 167 keV are used while for technetium a 20% window at 140 keV is utilized.

6. A zoom mode can be used with care taken to ensure the heart is contained within the field of view.

7. Imaging is then undertaken either by "step and shoot" with 32 or 64 steps or in a continuous mode. The rotation can be circular, elliptical or body contouring depending upon the equipment and expertise available. A good quality AP image should be obtained prior to camera rotation. ECG gating can be used with technetium tracers to produce gated images. If this is done it is usually necessary to increase the acquisition time and, thereby, the counts acquired. The planar projection set should be immediately reviewed at the end of the acquisition to ensure that they are of sufficient quality, for example with no significant movement.

Table 9.6. Summary of reported serious adverse effects for various forms of stress (%)

	Exercise	Dobutamine	Dipyridamole	Adenosine
Number of patients Event:	170 000	3011	3911	9256
Cardiac death	0.01	0	0.05	0
Major non-fatal cardiac event	0.02	0.3	0.05	0.01

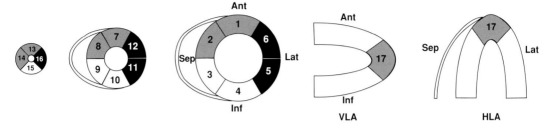

Figure 9.2. A schematic diagram showing three SA sections together with the VLA and HLA sections, which are approximately equivalent to those in the clinical images shown in Figures 9.3 to 9.9. Also shown are the 17 segments referred to in Table 9.7. The assignment of these segments to coronary territories is demonstrated by the shading (*gray*, LAD; *black*, LCX; *white*, RCA). The septum, lateral wall, anterior wall, and inferior wall of the left ventricle are indicated by "Sep", "Lat", "Ant", and "Inf" respectively. LAD, left anterior descending; LCX, left circumflex; RCA, right coronary artery.

Image Processing

From the three-dimensional data the long axis of the LV is defined either manually or automatically. It is defined as the line between the apex of the LV and mid-mitral valve and, if performed automatically, the processing should be checked for accuracy. It is obviously essential that this axis is the same between stress and resting images. Three sets of images are then constructed: horizontal long axis (HLA), vertical long axis (VLA), and short axis (SA) (Figure 9.2). The horizontal long axis is a plane through the LV to incorporate the septum, lateral wall, and apex in the shape of a horseshoe. The vertical long axis is the plane through the LV incorporating free anterior wall, inferior wall, and apex. The short axis views are perpendicular to the long axis views and show the LV as a ring except towards the base, when the myocardium becomes crescent shaped.

The images are then inspected for quality and problems such as poor orientation and artifacts. If deemed to be of sufficiently good quality they are then stored for interpretation.

Image Reporting

The ideal report should include the following:

1. Patient details.
2. Type of study (e.g. gated MPI) and stress method used.
3. Clinical reasons for study.
4. Quality of study.
5. Findings, e.g. severity, extent, and location of any defects. Often reported in decreasing order of importance. If the study is normal this should be explicitly stated.

6. Gated data.
7. Special findings (e.g. suggestion of neoplasm, hibernation status etc.).
8. Conclusions including prognostic assessment.

9.6.5 Image Interpretation

The best quality and most meaningful reports are produced when clinical details, stress details, and images are interpreted together by a suitably qualified clinician and physicist [1]. Of particular importance are the clinical question being asked, the adequacy of stress, symptoms precipitated by stress, and the quality of the images.

The planar images should be first examined in cine display mode with regard to the following:

1. The heart is always within the field of view.
2. To look for sources of artifact such as patient movement, breast tissue, subdiaphragmatic activity, injection site extravasation etc.
3. To check on the presence of external objects influencing the images.
4. To note heart–lung uptake ratio (thallium only).

The image sets should then ideally be displayed adjacent to one another and adjusted to optimize matching slices. The displays should be viewed on a high-resolution computer screen avoiding paper or film interpretation as the latter reduces sensitivity. All three tomographic axis sets of images should be displayed using an appropriate color scale and examined either together or sequentially.

In gated imaging the moving images should be examined with particular regard to ensuring that any automatic contours used for derivation of volumetric data (e.g. LVEF) are accurate. It is usually helpful to examine the moving display using both a gray and a continuous color scale. The former is better for wall motion whilst the latter helps to aid interpretation of wall thickening. Reference to a "heart beat length histogram" can also be a useful method of assuring good quality.

First a qualitative assessment as to the size of both left and right ventricles should be made. If the cavity of the LV appears larger in the stress images than the rest images then this should be noted. It is an important prognostic sign and results from either sub-endocardial ischemia or genuine left ventricular enlargement. It was previously called pseudo-cavity dilation but this is both confusing and inaccurate so has been replaced with the term "transient luminal dilation" (TLD).

The images are then assessed visually in a semi-quantitative fashion to assess the extent, severity, and location of any defects. The extent to which any defects improve at rest is also noted. It is usual to do this using either a 9 or 17 segment model, the latter being recommended by the American Society of Nuclear Cardiology [10] (Figure 9.2). The extent of both fixed and "reversible" defects provides important prognostic information; the greater the evidence of ischemia or infarction the worse the outlook. A suggested scale is given in Table 9.7.

Occasionally what is termed reverse redistribution is noted, with the rest images appearing to develop a "defect". The reasons for this are uncertain but it is usually of no clinical consequence. It can, however, occur if imaging is undertaken shortly after MI and in the presence of an open infarct-related artery [1].

A useful display format is the polar map or "bulls-eye" image. This is a circular representation of the left ventricular perfusion. It is displayed as if the cone-shaped LV is flattened into a pancake. Thus conventionally the apex is in the center, the anterior wall to the top, the lateral wall to the left, the septum to the right, and the inferior wall to the bottom. The periphery is also the base of the heart. Images can also be quantitatively analyzed by comparison with pooled "normals", although even when available this may not be necessary for the majority of studies. The usual method of comparison is via the polar map [11].

Table 9.7. A suggested "scoring system" for assigning extent of myocardial perfusion per segment and hence risk of myocardial event (using the American Society of Nuclear Cardiology 17-segment model, see Figure 9.2).

Degree of perfusion identified per segment	Assigned score
Normal[a]	3
Mildly reduced	2
Moderately reduced	1
Severely reduced or absent	0

[a] In males inferior activity up to 70% maximum can be normal. Similarly in females mild "fixed" anterior defects may be due to breast attenuation and can be regarded as "normal" too.

Total perfusion score for all segments	Risk
51 (17 × 3 = maximum possible)	Very low
	↓
45	Low
	↓
40	Intermediate
	↓
30	High
	↓
20	Very high

Subtract 5 (i.e. increase risk) for:
• anatomically different areas of abnormality;
• LV transient luminal dilation (TLD);
• high lung uptake (thallium images).

Normal

When interpreting the images only the left ventricular muscle is readily identified, due to its thickness compared to that of the right ventricle and atria. The right ventricle can, however, frequently be seen in good quality studies but is usually disregarded unless obviously enlarged. As the short-axis sections approach the base (atria) of the heart the intraventricular septum becomes membranous and the valve plane becomes included in the slices. As neither of these structures contains muscle, the short axis section becomes a crescent shape rather than a circle with the "gap" at the high part of the septum. MPI images from a normal male are shown in Figure 9.3.

Figure 9.4 shows MPI images from a male subject that demonstrate a slight reduction in inferior activity compared to other areas. This is a normal variant for a male and is due to diaphragmatic attenuation.

MPI images from a female subject in Figure 9.5 show a reduction in counts anteriorly in both stress and rest images. The lack of history of MI and

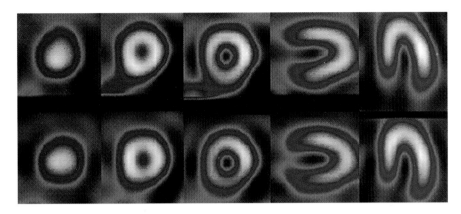

Figure 9.3. Stress (top) and rest (bottom) MPI images from normal male subject.

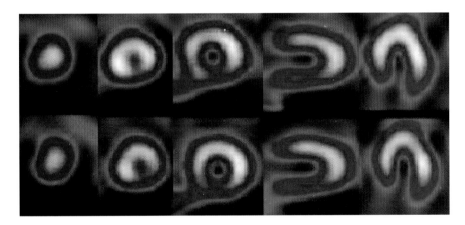

Figure 9.4. Stress (top) and rest (bottom) MPI images from a male subject, showing a slight reduction in inferior activity compared to other areas.

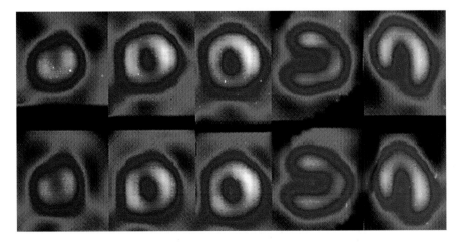

Figure 9.5. Stress (top) and rest (bottom) MPI images from a female subject showing a reduction in counts anteriorly in both stress and rest images.

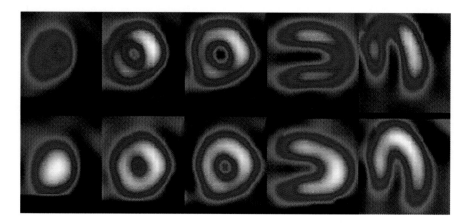

Figure 9.6. Stress (top) and rest (bottom) MPI images from a subject with apical ischemia.

normal wall motion on the gated images strongly suggest breast attenuation artifact, which is common in females.

Patterns of Abnormal Perfusion

MPI images from a subject with apical ischemia are shown in Figure 9.6. One can clearly see the reduction in apical perfusion with stress compared to normal perfusion at rest.

Figure 9.7 displays MPI images from a patient with prior extensive antero-apical MI and no residual ischemia. The large fixed antero-apical defect is easily distinguished.

In the presence of left bundle branch block one can see the reduction in septal activity in both stress and rest images characteristic of this electrical abnormality, although the defect can be variable in position (Figure 9.8).

Hibernating Myocardium

Many patients with heart failure have left ventricular dysfunction which may improve following revascularization [12]. This can be due to a variety of physiological states such as chronic ischemia, recurrent stunning, or hibernation. Damaged myocardium may consist of a complex mixture of scar tissue, stunned and hibernating myocardium. Careful evaluation is therefore needed before considering a patient for revascularization as attempts to do this in a patient with only scar tissue may result in an adverse outcome.

Hibernating myocardium is thought to occur when the blood supply to a region of myocardium becomes chronically reduced with the result that

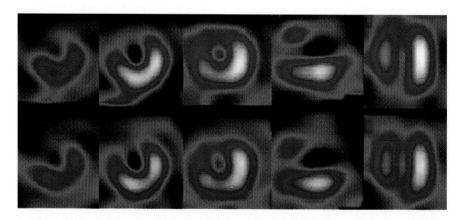

Figure 9.7. Stress (top) and rest (bottom) MPI images from a patient with prior extensive antero-apical MI and no residual ischemia.

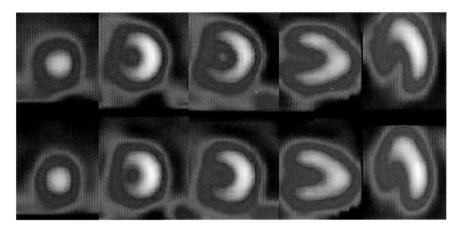

Figure 9.8. Stress (top) and rest (bottom) MPI images from a patient with LBBB.

the myocardium regresses into a physiologically alive, but functionally inert, state. Strictly, this state is associated with specific cellular changes but there is controversy whether or not pure hibernating myocardium can be made to contract again following revascularization. The term "hibernating myocardium" is therefore generally used more loosely. However, tissue identified as being viable (alive) and either hypocontractile (reduced contraction) or akinetic (no contraction) appears to have a good chance of functional improvement following revascularization [12].

Although thallium, being essentially a flow tracer, has advantages over the technetium tracers, in practice there is evidence that all three tracers can be used. It is important, however, to give the myocardium the best chance of taking up the tracer, for example when using thallium, by employing either delayed 24-hour imaging or a reinjection protocol. The latter involves giving oral or sublingual nitrates after the redistribution images have been acquired, then injecting a further 40 MBq (1 mCi) of ^{201}Tl and repeating the imaging. It is not uncommon to find that an area of myocardium felt to be a fixed defect then takes up tracer following the "reinjection". Both akinetic and viable myocardium, together with these areas, is felt to represent hibernating myocardium [12]. PET imaging, however, has probably the highest sensitivity and specificity for the detection of hibernating myocardium [12], as is discussed later in Section 9.10.

It is important to realize that due to the complex mixture of myocardial tissue, merely finding viable myocardium in the presence of ischemic damage does not guarantee that revascularization will successfully restore contraction. Stress echocardiography can be helpful and complementary here as it has the opposite characteristics to perfusion imaging, namely a relatively high specificity but modest sensitivity. If the identified region of hibernating myocardium can be seen to contract during stress echo then there is an increased chance it will improve following revascularization.

MPI images from a thallium study performed to find hibernating myocardium are shown in Figure 9.9. The stress images show a large inferolatero-apical perfusion defect. The redistribution images show improved perfusion of the anterior, inferior, and lateral walls. Following reinjection/nitrates a further substantial improvement in perfusion is seen in these areas, restoring the distribution to virtually normal for a male (Figure 9.9), although the heart remains considerably enlarged. This patient would be likely to benefit from coronary artery bypass grafting.

9.7 Acute Infarction Imaging

Two tracers have been historically used to identify myocardial necrosis, ^{99m}Tc stannous pyrophosphate and ^{111}In-labeled antimyosin antibodies. However, with the advent of very reliable and sensitive markers of myocardial damage, such as troponin, they have little, if any, place in modern practice and hence will not be considered further.

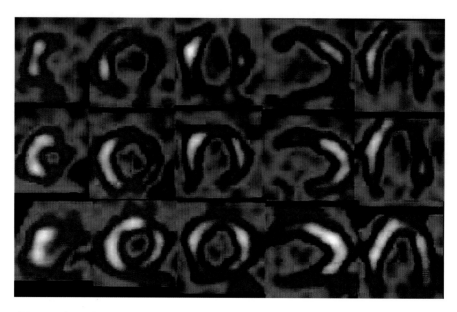

Figure 9.9. MPI images from a thallium scan carried out to look for hibernating myocardium showing stress (top), redistribution (middle), and reinjection (bottom) images.

9.8 Sympathetic Nervous System Imaging

Meta-iodo-benzylguanidine (MIBG) is a nore-pinephrine (noradrenaline) analogue and is taken up into vesicles within the presympathetic sympathetic nerve endings. It can be labeled with a variety of radionuclides, but for diagnostic purposes ^{123}I is usually used. Its main use is in diagnosing pheochromocytomas. However, it is also taken up by the left ventricle in proportion to the sympathetic nervous supply [13]. Although an experimental tool from the cardiac point of view, it has provided some important information, such as the extent of the penumbra of denudation outside an MI scar being proportionate to ventricular dysrhythmias. It has also provided an insight into how beta-adrenergic blockers and heart failure affect the heart [13, 14].

9.9 Fatty Acid Labeling

Although not yet incorporated into clinical practice, metabolic imaging using conventional radionuclides is possible and may become clinically useful. Iodine-123 labeled B-methyl-iodo-

pentadecanoic acid (BMIPP) is one of the most promising tracers being able to image fatty acid metabolism [12]. It may have a particular use in acute chest pain imaging as it seems to retain a "memory" for an ischemic event when conventional perfusion tracers may be normal. Hence an ischemic event precipitated by coronary artery spasm will have an abnormal BMIPP image but a normal perfusion image both following stress and at rest.

9.10 Positron Emission Tomography

PET imaging is an exciting method of imaging, in theory, any biochemical metabolic process and is discussed in detail in Chapters 3 and 17. It relies on the incorporation of a PET emitting radionuclide into either the study molecule itself or an analogous compound. Images can be attenuation corrected and provide quantitative measurements.

This technology has led to a much greater understanding of blood flow characteristics within the myocardium and is still the "gold standard" for the detection of hibernating myocardium [12]. Hibernating myocardium classically changes from free fatty acid to glucose metabolism. Thus ^{18}fluoro-2-deoxyglucose (FDG) is more avidly taken into an area of hibernating than normally perfusing myocardium. It becomes "trapped" as it cannot be utilized further in the metabolic pathway. Simultaneous perfusion assessment using either $H_2^{15}O$, $^{13}NH_3$ or ^{82}Rb demonstrates either reduced or near-normal perfusion in the hibernating zone. Thus the characteristic appearance of hibernating myocardium is a "mismatch" of FDG versus perfusion.

FDG has a relatively long half-life and can be imaged remotely from the producing cyclotron and by gamma cameras adapted for PET imaging. Perfusion imaging is more of a problem and only generator-produced ^{82}Rb is feasible. Because of these problems, together with the only small perceived advantage over conventional perfusion imaging, it has very limited use in cardiology.

References

1. Anagnostopoulos C, Harbinson M, Kelion A, et al. Procedure guidelines for radionuclide myocardial perfusion imaging. Heart 2004; 90 (Suppl):i1–i10.

2. Metcalfe MJ, Norton MY, Jennings K, Walton S. Improved detection of abnormal left ventricular wall motion using tomographic radionuclide ventriculography compared to planar radionuclide and single plane contrast ventriculography. Br J Radiol 1993; 66:986–993.

3. Germano G. Technical aspects of myocardial SPECT imaging. J Nucl Med 2001; 42:1499–1507.

4. Eisner RL, Nowak DJ, Pettigrew R, et al. Fundamentals of 180-degree acquisition and reconstruction in SPECT imaging. J Nucl Med 1986; 27:1717–1728.

5. O'Connor MK, Kemp B, Anstett F, et al. A multicenter evaluation of commercial attenuation compensation techniques in cardiac SPECT using phantom models. J Nucl Cardiol 2002; 9:361–376.

6. Radionuclide angiography. In: Iskandrian AS, Philadelphia VMS, eds. Nuclear Cardiac Imaging: Principles and Application. Philadelphia: FA Davis; 1996: 144–218.

7. Bellenger NG, Burgess MI, Ray SG, et al. Comparison of left ventricular ejection fraction and volumes in heart failure by echocardiography, radionuclide ventriculography and cardiovascular magnetic resonance: are they interchangeable? Eur Heart J 2000; 21:1387–1396.

8. Van Royen N, Jaffe CC, Krumholz HM, et al. Comparison and reproducibility of visual echocardiographic and quantitative radionuclide left ventricular ejection fractions. Am J Cardiol 1996; 77:843–850.

9. Botvinick EH. Scintigraphic blood pool and phase image analysis: The optimal tool for the evaluation of resynchronization therapy. J Nucl Cardiol 2003; 10:424–428.

10. Cerqueira M, Weissman N, Dilsizian V, et al. Standardized myocardial segmentation and nomenclature for tomographic imaging of the heart. Circulation 2002; 105:539–542.

11. Mahmarian JJ, Boyce TM, Goldberg RK, et al. Quantitative exercise thallium-201 single photon emission computed tomography for the enhanced diagnosis of ischemic heart disease. J Am Coll Cardiol 1990; 15:318–329.

12. Underwood SR. Bax JJ, vom Dahl J, et al. Imaging techniques for the assessment of myocardial hibernation. Report of a Study Group of the European Society of Cardiology. Eur Heart J 2004; 25:815–836.

13. Hattori N, Schwaiger M. Metaiodobenzylguanidine scintigraphy of the heart: what have we learnt clinically? Eur J Nucl Med 2000; 27:611–612.

14. Baliga RR, Narula J, Dec GW. The MIBG tarot: is it possible to predict the efficacy of beta-blockers in congestive heart failure? J Nucl Cardiol 2001; 8:107–109.

10

The Lung

Henry W. Gray

10.1 Introduction

Lungs are the principal organs of the respiratory system. They function in concert with the heart to provide a gas exchange unit that facilitates uptake of oxygen and elimination of carbon dioxide from the blood as it traverses the pulmonary capillaries. Oxygen from the lungs is required for the production of energy for all biological processes and carbon dioxide is a by-product of energy release and metabolism. The techniques of nuclear medicine can provide a window through which the normal functioning of lung (physiology) and the abnormal function resulting from disease processes (pathology) can be studied. This unique view of lung function has assisted the diagnosis of venous thromboembolism (VTE), otherwise known as pulmonary embolism (PE), from chronic obstructive or parenchymal lung disease for more than thirty years. The recent introduction of computed tomographic pulmonary angiography (CTPA) has been a most welcome addition to the diagnosis of VTE. It is an elegant technique for direct imaging of thrombus within segmental and larger pulmonary arteries and is complementary with the nuclear medicine tests.

10.2 Anatomy and Physiology

10.2.1 Lung Structure

The lungs can be likened to two thin-walled elastic sponges within the chest. Communication with the atmosphere is via the mouth, nose, pharynx, trachea, and bronchi. A series of branching airways from segmental bronchi down to small bronchioles (about 25 divisions in all) conduct air in and out of alveoli (Figure 10.1). The further down the branches one goes, the smaller the diameter of the airways and the greater their number. The cross-sectional area of airway increases as the total number of airways increases. Airflow is maximum in the trachea (200 cm s^{-1}) and slows toward the periphery such that gas flow occurs solely by diffusion in the terminal bronchioles and beyond.

The alveoli are grouped into acini that are each supplied by a terminal bronchiole and acinar arteriole. Alveoli are minute sacs (200 μm diameter) that bud from an alveolar duct and respiratory bronchiole (Figure 10.2). Their walls are made up of a thin layer of alveolar cells surrounded by a confluent mesh of fine-walled capillaries supported by interstitial tissue. There are approximately 300 million alveoli in each lung. The total surface area of alveolar wall for gas exchange is around 80 m^2 in the adult lung.

The lungs are organized into lobes with an upper, lower, and middle lobe on the right and an upper and lower on the left. The lobes are further subdivided into segments, each supplied by a specific segmental bronchus and pulmonary artery and drained by a pulmonary vein. The branching structure of the pulmonary vessels is similar to that of the bronchi and bronchioles (Figure 10.3). The main pulmonary artery carries venous blood pumped by the right ventricle. The lung arterioles (<100 μm diameter) supply groups of acini and

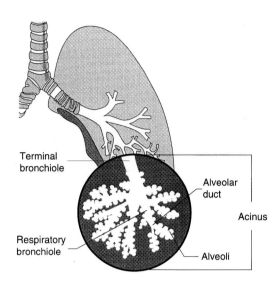

Figure 10.1. The air passages of the lung.

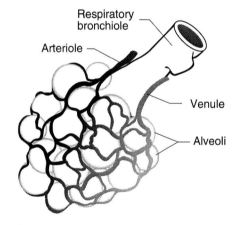

Figure 10.2. Clusters of alveoli budding from a respiratory bronchiole and alveolar duct (concealed) with surrounding capillary network.

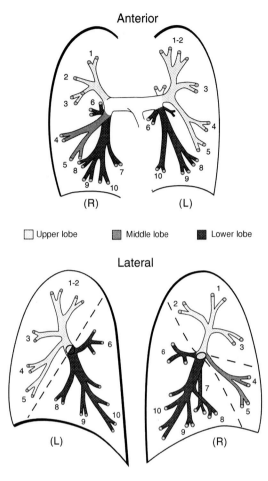

Figure 10.3. Branching structure of the larger pulmonary arteries. Segmental arteries include: 1, apical; 2, posterior; 1,2, apicoposterior; 3, anterior; 4, lateral (R) or superior lingular (L); 5, medial (R) or inferior lingular (L); 6, apical; 7, medial basal; 8, anterior basal; 9, lateral basal; 10, posterior basal.

10.2.2 Lung Function

Breathing is essentially a mechanical process controlled by nervous and chemical feedback mechanisms. Inspiration, which sucks air into the lungs, occurs by muscular effort of the diaphragmatic and intercostal muscles. The diaphragm expands the volume of both lungs downwards while intercostal muscles expand the lungs outwards as the ribs move upward and outward increasing both the anteroposterior and transverse diameter of the chest. Normal expiration, which pushes air out from lungs, occurs passively when those muscles relax.

their alveolar capillaries (7–10 μm diameter) with this blood for oxygenation. The acinar venules drain oxygenated blood into segmental, lobar then main pulmonary veins. These large veins transport the oxygenated blood from the lung to the left atrium and left ventricle. Thereafter, it is pumped to the aorta under pressure for distribution to body organs.

A separate bronchial circulation supplies arterial blood to lung tissues down to the level of the smallest bronchiole.

The respiratory center in the brainstem which controls the rate of breathing receives neurogenic and chemical feedback information by which it maintains the normal pressure of O_2 in arterial blood (P_aO_2) between 11 and 13 kPa (83–98 mmHg) and CO_2 (P_aCO_2) at 4.8–6 kPa (36–45 mmHg). A resting blood flow through the lungs of 5 liters min^{-1} carries 11 mmol min^{-1} (250 ml min^{-1}) of O_2 from lungs to body tissues. A resting ventilation of 6 liters min^{-1} carries 9 mmol min^{-1} (200 ml min^{-1}) of CO_2 out of the body. The normal lung has a great reserve capacity for increasing both the lung blood flow and the ventilation during exercise.

10.2.3 Ventilation Perfusion Matching

In an efficient gas-exchange unit, there should be a match between ventilation of alveoli and their perfusion. This match may not always be present in disease conditions. Indeed, in extreme circumstances, ventilation or perfusion can be considerably reduced relative to the other. If a sector of lung is ventilated but not perfused, then the ventilation of that sector takes no part in gas exchange and is called "physiological dead-space". Conversely, if a sector of lung is perfused but not ventilated, venous blood traverses the lung without an opportunity for gas exchange and passes through into the arterial system unoxygenated. This "physiological shunting" causes a reduction in the oxygen content of the arterial blood, sometimes called desaturation.

Regional under-ventilation leading to alveolar hypoxia can result from the partial airways obstruction of chronic bronchitis, asthma, or other parenchymal lung diseases. This local hypoxia usually stimulates an efficient reflex vasoconstriction of pulmonary arterioles supplying the under-ventilated region. This reflex diverts pulmonary blood flow away from hypoxic lung regions and serves to preserve the balance (matching) of ventilation and perfusion as close to normal as possible.

In an erect person, there is a tendency in normal lung for perfusion to be inadequate at the lung apices, and therefore mismatched to ventilation, while the reverse occurs at the bases. This is a result of gravitational forces acting on a low-pressure pulmonary circulation (2 kPa or 15 mmHg) and will therefore change when the person lies down. In that position, perfusion will be greatest posteriorly and least anteriorly.

Ventilation is often abbreviated to "V" in pulmonary physiology while "Q" represents perfusion from "quellen" in German meaning to spring or to gush forth.

10.3 Ventilation Perfusion Imaging

10.3.1 Perfusion Imaging

When a thoroughly mixed tracer in arterial blood is completely removed in a single passage through an organ, the final distribution of that tracer within the organ is proportional to the relative blood flow in different areas of that organ. The intravenous (IV) injection of ^{99m}Tc-labeled human albumin macro-aggregates (MAA) measuring 10–40 μm in diameter (Figure 10.4), results in impaction of the particles in the terminal arterioles

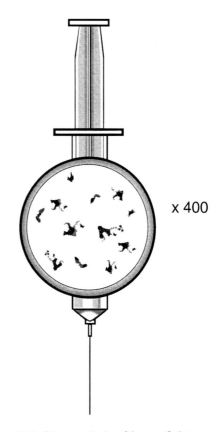

Figure 10.4. Diagrammatic view of the magnified structure of the protein clumps in macro-aggregates of albumin (MAA).

and other precapillary vessels. All commercial MAA has been manufactured from plasma known to be virus free. Subsequent gamma camera images of the chest show the relative pulmonary arterial blood flow. If 200 000 particles are given to a normal subject, fewer than 0.1% of the total number of arterioles are blocked, giving a safety margin of around 1000:1.

Prior to the withdrawal of a patient's dose into a syringe, the vial containing the MAA should be shaken to disaggregate the particles. The MAA is then injected slowly IV with the subject breathing normally. Blood should not be drawn into the syringe since clumping of MAA may result and manifest as large or small hotspots on the perfusion image. Injection of MAA is usually made with the subject supine to provide a more even apex-to-base distribution of perfusion. If the subject is breathless, injection in the erect position may be required. The effect of gravity in reducing apical pulmonary blood flow is then usually apparent on the images. This change from the normal procedure should be communicated to the person interpreting the images.

Imaging can be performed immediately after injection. Most centers acquire six views which include posterior, anterior, both posterior obliques, and either both anterior obliques or lateral views. These multiple views permit defects of perfusion to be visualized "in tangent" and "en-face" in at least one projection, thereby increasing the likelihood of detection. Imaging for 3 minutes will normally provide views containing more than 250 kcounts. The imaging protocol is described in Table 10.1. A normal perfusion study along with the Technegas ventilation images is seen in Figure 10.5.

After impaction, most particles will break up within hours due to macrophage activity and then pass through the lungs to be removed from the circulation by the liver and spleen. Full perfusion of the lung is then restored.

Perfusion scintigraphy is safe even in the most severely ill patients. Early after the technique was introduced, several deaths occurred following injection of MAA in patients of all age groups with pulmonary hypertension. In pulmonary hypertension, the number of lung arterioles and precapillaries is greatly reduced. It was recognized that a number of the cases had been injected with an excess of particles that presumably had blocked sufficient numbers of scarce pulmonary vessels to cause terminal heart failure. The number of particles

Table 10.1. Perfusion imaging

Radiopharmaceutical	^{99m}Tc MAA (macro-aggregated albumin)
Patient preparation	Patient flat or semi-recumbent
Injection technique	Slow IV injection. No withdrawal of blood into syringe
Activity administered	80 MBq (2 mCi)
Particles administered	$\leq$ 200 000 particles
Collimator	Low-energy, general purpose
Image acquisition	6 views
	Anterior, posterior, right and left posterior obliques, right and left anterior obliques or both laterals
	At least 200 kcounts per view
Effective dose equivalent	1 mSv (100 mrem)
Staff dose	1.5 μSv (150 μrem)

necessary for an artifact-free scan in normal individuals is >60 000 but injecting more than 200 000 particles will not improve the scan quality. Accordingly, most centers prefer to use around 200 000 particles per routine dose for perfusion scintigraphy and cut the number of particles by at least 50% for patients suspected of having pulmonary hypertension. No deaths have been reported in patients with pulmonary hypertension since this practice was instituted.

The dose of MAA should be reduced by 50% in pregnant women and children by a factor that relates to body weight. This lowers the radiation burden to acceptable levels. The number of particles will obviously be reduced pro rata but image quality is unaffected. Most departments will also cut the number of particles for injection in patients with right-to-left shunting to reduce the systemic embolism of brain and kidney (Figure 10.6).

10.3.2 Ventilation Imaging

Imaging of ventilation is undertaken with either gases or aerosols. This permits detection of areas of lung with matched (ventilation and perfusion both abnormal) or mismatched (ventilation normal but perfusion abnormal) perfusion abnormalities. The most commonly used gases are ^{81m}Kr and ^{133}Xe but aerosol imaging is by far the most usual technique for ventilation imaging.

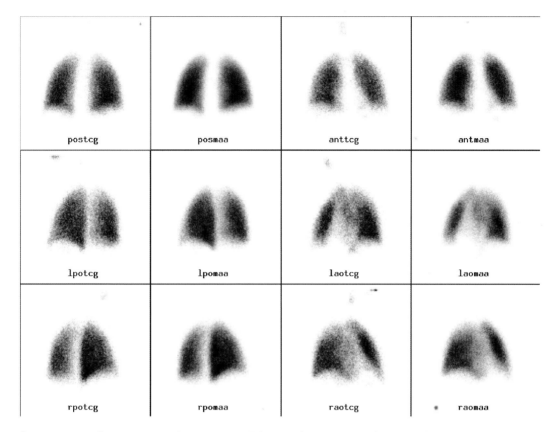

Figure 10.5. Normal category 6-view Technegas ventilation (left) and perfusion (right) scan of each pair performed sequentially. Count rate of perfusion was >5 times that of ventilation images.

Krypton-81m Imaging

^{81m}Kr, produced from a rubidium-81 generator, is the ideal gas for ventilation studies. The patient is first injected with MAA and the first perfusion image acquired. Next, the patient breathes a mixture of ^{81m}Kr in air or oxygen produced by passing a stream of water-humidified air or oxygen through the generator. This permits the ventilation image to be acquired in the same position after altering the energy window of the gamma camera. The procedure is then repeated after the acquisition of all subsequent perfusion images. The imaging protocol is given in Table 10.2.

The half-life of 13 seconds means that ^{81m}Kr decays very quickly within the lungs with none of the xenon tendency to build up in under-ventilated areas. The image signal is therefore equivalent to a "single breath" with xenon. It also results in a tiny radiation dose (effective dose equivalent 0.1 mSv). The photon energy of 190 keV is ideal

Table 10.2. Krypton ventilation

Radiopharmaceutical	^{81m}Kr gas in humidified air/oxygen
Patient preparation	Familiarization with face mask; good seal on mask
Activity administered	6000 MBq (150 mCi) is ARSAC limit
Collimator	Low-energy, general purpose
Images acquired	200–300 kcounts to match perfusion image
Effective dose equivalent	0.05–0.1 mSv (5–10 mrem)
Staff dose	0.1 μSv (10 μrem)

ARSAC, Administration of Radioactive Substances Advisory Committee.

for dual imaging with ^{99m}Tc and permits acquisition of separate perfusion and ventilation signals with excellent positional match and comparability (Figure 10.7).

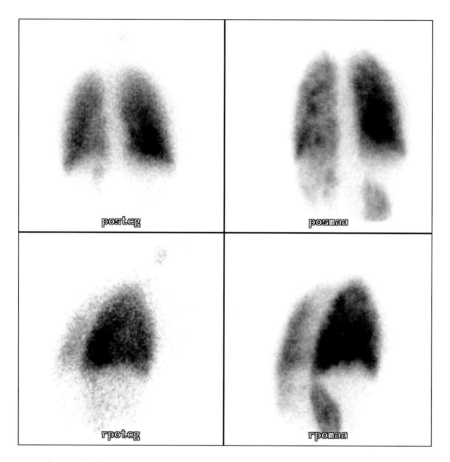

Figure 10.6. Ventilation and perfusion lung scan showing renal activity from right to left shunt. Brain images and activity not shown.

The short half-life of the generator (4.5 h), the twice-weekly cyclotron production of [81]Rb, and the considerable expense, however, limit its availability and application.

Xenon-133 Imaging

After 40 years of use in ventilation imaging, ^{133}Xe remains inexpensive and readily available. While its half-life of 5.3 days provides a conveniently long shelf life, the low gamma photon energy (81 keV) is a major disadvantage as it results in inferior image quality and resolution. Posterior view examination is usually best and must be performed before the MAA dose is injected. If the perfusion scan reveals a more anterior abnormality that cannot be visualized on the posterior ventilation view, a repeat ^{133}Xe study in the appropriate anterior projection is necessary. This must be deferred for 24 hours until the ^{99m}Tc has decayed as the pres-

ence of residual ^{99m}Tc will spill over into the lower energy ^{133}Xe window and fog the image. The imaging protocol is described in Table 10.3.

Table 10.3. Xenon-133 ventilation

Radiopharmaceutical	[133]Xe gas
Patient preparation	Familiarization with breathing circuit including mouthpiece and nose clip
Activity administered	37 MBq (1 mCi) per liter
Collimator	Low-energy, general purpose
Images acquired	Single view, usually posterior initially. Total study time 600 s, washout starting 300 s into study
	Dynamic acquisition of 100×6 s frames
Effective dose equivalent	0.3 mSv (30 mrem)
Staff dose	0.1 µSv (10 µrem)

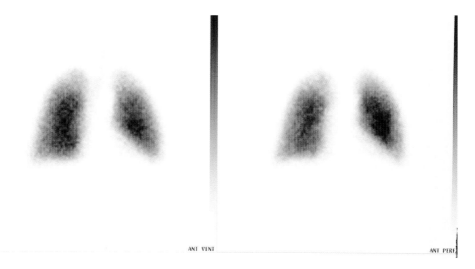

Figure 10.7. An anterior ^{81m}Kr ventilation image (left) and matched perfusion image with ^{99m}Tc-MAA (right) showing normal ventilation and perfusion (kindly provided by Dr Andrew Hilson).

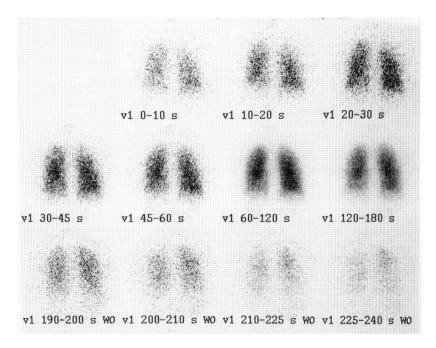

Figure 10.8. ^{133}Xe ventilation in the posterior projection. The wash-in until 120 s shows a decrease at right apex. The equilibration view between 120 and 180 s shows the right apex to be a functional part of the lung volume. Wash-out from 190 s onwards confirms ^{133}Xe trapping at the right apex, indicating parenchymal lung disease at that site.

First of all, the patient takes a single full inspiration from the ^{133}Xe mixed in 5 liters of air or oxygen in a closed ventilation circuit. Breath holding of that first deep breath for at least 15 seconds provides a "single-breath" image that reflects the ventilation rate of different lung regions. The "single breath" is the image most comparable with the ventilation signal from ^{81}Kr. The patient then continually breathes the ^{133}Xe/O$_2$/air mixture for 3–5 min until the gas reaches equilibrium within the different regions of lung. Images at this phase of the study demonstrate lung volume. The final phase occurs when the patient is switched to breathing air alone. During this "washout phase", the ^{133}Xe is exhaled into a bag for disposal and images show the regional rate of ^{133}Xe ventilation (clearance). Trapping of ^{133}Xe in areas of airways obstruction is revealed during this final phase. This trapping is probably the most sensitive imaging signal of parenchymal lung disease (Figure 10.8).

Aerosol Ventilation

When ^{81m}Kr is unavailable, ^{99m}Tc-aerosols provide a ventilation signal which has an ideal energy and which is provided in six views to position match with perfusion. An aerosol is a mixture of liquid droplets or solid particles that are stable as a suspension in air. Aerosols are usually defined by the size of their particles.

1. Aerosol droplet particles: These are produced by either a jet or ultrasonic device primed with ^{99m}Tc-DTPA that should produce a majority of particles less than 1 μm in size. The high activity required in the nebulizer bowl necessitates adequate shielding to protect patient and technologist. Most devices rely on the patient rebreathing through a mouthpiece so that the undeposited or unretained aerosol is collected on an exhalation circuit filter. Contamination of the atmosphere is possible. Ventilation studies performed under a ceiling extraction hood are much the safest method of preventing contamination of staff.

2. Technegas: Technegas is an ultra fine dispersion of small solid ^{99m}Tc-labeled carbon particles in argon gas produced by a commercial machine and a special patented heating technique. These particles are the smallest available at 5 nm maximum diameter. Since there is no O$_2$ in Technegas, patients with significant oxygen desaturation should inhale supplemental oxygen for 1 min prior to the procedure.

The imaging protocol for aerosol studies is described in Table 10.4.

Table 10.4. Aerosol ventilation

Radiopharmaceutical	^{99m}Tc-DTPA or ^{99m}Tc-dry particles
Patient preparation	Familiarization with breathing circuit including mouthpiece and nose clip Supplemental O$_2$ may be required
Activity administered to patient	20–40 MBq (1 mCi)
Activity in reservoir	1.5 GBq (40 mCi)
Activity in crucible	240 MBq (6 mCi)
Collimator	Low-energy, general purpose
Images acquired	Views to match perfusion images 200 kcounts per view
Effective dose equivalent	0.6 mSv (60 mrem)
Staff dose	0.3–0.5 μSv (30–50 μrem)

Importance of Particle Size

Particle size is of relevance for efficient aerosol imaging. Large particles of 5 μm are respirable with comfort but only those of 2 μm and less will reach peripheral respiratory bronchioles and alveoli. The very large and large particles suffer inertial impaction on large central air passages and also tend to sediment under gravity in the larger bronchi. Smaller particles will diffuse further downstream into alveoli and impact by that means. While 0.5 μm particles are most likely to reach the periphery, alveolar deposition is best between 0.05 and 0.2 μm. Even at that particle size, deposition mechanisms are very inefficient so most of the inhaled particles are exhaled to be safely collected for disposal.

Deposition of an aerosol increases with time and is inversely proportional to the airway diameter. Unfortunately, chronic obstructive airways disease with airway narrowing and distortion leads to marked localized central deposition and poor peripheral penetration of the particles. This results in central hotspots and will occur even with the smallest of particles (Figure 10.9). The larger particles deposit because of inertial impaction while the small particles are affected by turbulent diffusion. High inhalation flow rates in any situation will increase central airways deposition so patient training and encouragement to inhale in a calm and unhurried manner is most important.

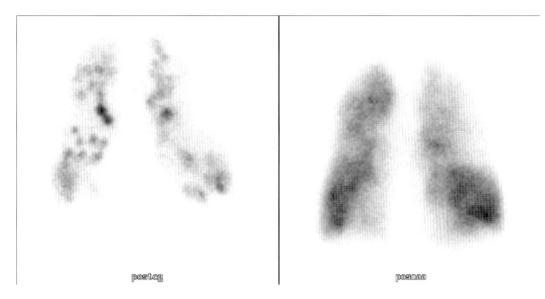

posteg   posmaa

Figure 10.9. Technegas ventilation image with a central deposition of tracer and poor peripheral penetration with focal deposition peripherally. Patchy perfusion (right) confirms chronic parenchymal lung disease.

Combination of Aerosol Ventilation and Perfusion Study

^{99m}Tc is the radionuclide for both aerosol ventilation and MAA perfusion studies and therefore simultaneous studies are not possible. Since aerosol droplet particles are cleared quite rapidly from the lung, a delay between ventilation and perfusion of 1 hour usually suffices to reduce the ^{99m}Tc lung background to acceptable levels. The alternative that allows better time management is to use a lower activity of ^{99m}Tc for the ventilation study and image longer to compensate. The perfusion dose should be increased to swamp the residual ventilation activity by least four-fold. This ideal four-fold preponderance of perfusion activity over ventilation should be checked for during each study. Too low a ratio could result in the ventilation signal filling-in mismatched perfusion defects, thereby obscuring the diagnosis of PE.

A normal Technegas ventilation and MAA perfusion scan is seen in Figure 10.5.

Pregnancy

Until recently, VQ imaging was the automatic investigation of choice for a pregnancy complicated by possible VTE. The widespread availability of multi-detector CT (MDCT) has led to a reassessment of this policy and this continues to-date. There is little doubt that the theoretical risk of inducing a cancer is double for the mother after CTPA given the effective dose of 1.7 mSv compared with 0.8 mSv for half-dose VQ imaging. However, the fetus is exposed to much more radiation dose from half-dose VQ scanning compared to MDCT because of the systemic administration of the tracers against the tight collimation of the CT beam on the upper torso. Against this of course must be weighed the risk to the fetus of maternal death from PE, and the use of contrast media which could lead to idiosyncratic reactions or fetal hypothyroidism due to the iodine load.

One other worry is that MDCT deposits significantly more radiation dose to the female breast tissue. This can be up to 8 mGy with modern machines but even higher with older equipment and compares with half-dose VQ imaging which gives a breast dose of approximately 0.3 mGy. CT doses in the UK and Europe tend to be lower than in the USA because of tighter acceptance criteria, annual dose checks, and strict scanning protocols optimized for dose reduction. A complication factor is that the theoretical lifetime risk of breast cancer after CT or VQ is highest in the young and reduces with age. The lifetime risks of radiation-induced breast cancer are seen in Table 10.5 [1].

Table 10.5. Lifetime risk of radiation-induced breast cancer

Age at exposure (years)	Lifetime risk (per million per mGy)	Risk from CT (For breast dose of 7.9 mGy)	Risk from VQ (for breast dose of 0.56 mGy)
20	18	1 in 7000	1 in 99 000
40	16	1 in 8000	1 in 110 000
60	10	1 in 12 5000	1 in 180 000
80	2.5	1 in 51 000	1 in 710 000

While a concern, this risk must be put in perspective. It would appear that the risk of breast cancer after the contraceptive pill equates to about 38 CTPAs so the risk from one CTPA is unlikely to concern the general population.

A compromise is usually arrived at locally to determine which patients receive which test and usually, the technique, VQ or MDCT, is chosen because of Ionizing Radiation (Medical Exposure) Regulations (IRMER) justification, clinical risk management, and the chest X-ray appearances. VQ imaging should be chosen and is of most value if the chest X-ray is normal, the patient is young and the PE risk is low to moderate (i.e. PE requires to be excluded).

10.4 Diagnosis of Venous Thromboembolism

10.4.1 Origin of Venous Thrombi

A deep vein thrombosis (DVT) often originates in the veins of the calf muscles or the venous valves of the ileofemoral veins in the thigh. The thrombus may be seeded de novo or start as a platelet cluster on damaged endothelium (vein lining). It grows when the strands of insoluble fibrin formed from soluble fibrinogen enmesh more and more red cells to form an expanding thrombus (clot) (Figure 10.10). As the thrombus grows in size, it can not only occlude the vein locally but also propagate and enlarge along the vein proximally to a larger vein. It is at this point that dislodgement from the endothelial tether can occur and, like a guided missile, the thrombus can drift passively with the venous return toward the right heart, eventually resulting in pulmonary embolism (PE). DVT and PE are separate but related aspects of the same dynamic disease process called venous thromboembolism (VTE). They not only share risk factors and treatment but also require a coordinated approach to diagnosis.

10.4.2 Risk Factors for VTE

Risk factors are conditions associated with an increased incidence of the disease [2]. Thrombus formation, its propagation and subsequent embolism increase in likelihood and frequency when two or more risk factors for VTE are present. These risk factors produce thrombosis by one or more of three mechanisms, namely stasis of venous blood, changes to the vessel wall, and changes to the composition of the blood. Vascular injury and damage to the endothelial lining of the vessel wall which increase the risk of a platelet thrombus can occur with the use of chronic indwelling central venous catheters, permanent pacemakers, internal cardiac defibrillators, or intravenous substance abuse but none are common. More commonly found is a genetic or acquired predisposition to thrombus formation (thrombophilia) caused by changes in the composition of the blood. A genetic predisposition often leads to recurrent VTE in members of the same family. Common causes include the presence of the factor 5 Leiden or prothrombin gene mutation or deficiencies in protein C, protein S and antithrombin 3. Normal factor 5 accelerates blood coagulation and the factor 5 Leiden variety is more resistant than normal to inactivation while protein C, S and antithrombin are normally inhibitors of coagulation.

The acquired risk factors that increase the coagulability of blood and hence predispose to thrombus formation include pregnancy, the oral contraceptive pill including progesterone only and specially the third generation pills, hormone replacement therapy, malignant tumors, and the presence of special antibodies that are associated with arterial and venous thrombosis (lupus anticoagulant and the anticardiolipin antibody).

Finally, environmental risk factors are usually associated with sluggish blood flow or venous stasis. These multiple risk factors for VTE include immobilization, paralysis, surgery, trauma, and the wearing of a leg plaster cast. Simply being an

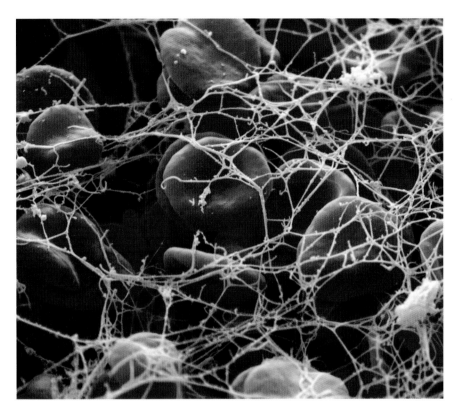

Figure 10.10. Thrombus with red cells enmeshed by fibrin strands. (Reproduced from Eye of Science. Medizin: Mensch: Blut. BMA News, 1 February 2004, page 1.)

inpatient in hospital and being over 65–70 years old is known to increase the risk. The economy-class syndrome of post-flight VTE is probably better called "traveler's thrombosis".

Medical illness too results in an increased risk of VTE. Cancer, congestive cardiac failure, chronic obstructive airways disease, diabetes mellitus, and inflammatory bowel disease are all recognized factors. Previous PE or DVT, however, are the most important factors of all.

All these various risk factors are additive so while the general population have a four-fold increase in the risk of VTE during prolonged travel, cases with factor 5 Leiden have a 12-fold increased risk.

10.4.3 Natural History of Venous Thromboembolism

It has recently become clear from studies originating in Brittany, France and the Mayo Clinic, USA that the annual incidence of VTE varies between 1 and 1.8 per 1000 while the incidence of DVT alone is between 0.6 and 1.2 per 1000. The studies have also shown that VTE is a condition of older age, particularly after 70 years. While the average incidence of VTE around the globe has probably remained constant around 1 event per 1000 person years since 1979, it reaches 1 event per 100 person years for those over 85 years. VTE continued to recur in cases recruited into the studies. At 1 year the recurrence was 13% while at 10 years, it had risen to 30%.

Survival after the first episode of DVT was found to be 96% but after PE it fell to 76%. It is thought that there are at least 200 000 cases of VTE in the USA each year comprising 105 000 with DVT alone and 95 000 with PE of whom 25% die within 7 days. For the majority who die quickly, no treatment or intervention is possible. Those who survive as far as the hospital may undergo treatment with thrombectomy, or thrombolysis is possible if the diagnosis is made quickly.

This most recent information has confirmed firstly that VTE remains a major ongoing health issue and, secondly, that as our populations age, the prevalence of VTE is likely to increase even further.

10.4.4 Clinical Presentation of Venous Thromboembolism

Thrombosis of the calf veins or more proximal deep veins of the thigh often presents with leg swelling and pain (DVT) but significant numbers of patients who develop DVT have no symptoms whatever (silent thrombosis). But PE can be even more difficult for clinical staff to detect, particularly in young, previously healthy individuals where the symptoms and findings can be subtle. The usual symptoms of chest pain and breathlessness are so prevalent in medical practice that they can often be justifiably ascribed to other common conditions but particularly primary heart or lung disease. The potential consequences of unrecognized PE are serious. Because of this, and because PE is difficult to diagnose clinically, particularly in the presence of other diseases, most physicians have a low threshold for investigating possible PE and this can pose logistical problems for imaging departments.

Symptoms and signs vary with the volume of thrombus passing through the right heart. Small volumes of thrombus may present with variable, intermittent, and usually unexplained breathlessness. Often, these minor symptoms can be completely unrecognized by patient and doctor and may presage a major embolus in the future. Moderate volumes of thrombus typically present with chest pain of a myocardial (not worsened by breathing) or pleuritic type (worsened by breathing) and breathlessness at rest. If the blood supply to a portion of lung becomes inadequate, death of pulmonary tissue occurs (infarction) which may cause intense pleuritic chest pain, blood in the sputum (hemoptysis), and an abnormality on the chest X-ray. In about 25% of cases the volume of thrombus passing through the right heart is such that the patient collapses immediately with chest pain and shock due to cardiac obstruction and cannot usually be resuscitated.

10.4.5 Clinical Diagnosis of Venous Thromboembolism

It requires perspicacity and a low threshold of suspicion to pick up the less clamant cases of VTE and experienced physicians who have been caught out by the condition in the past to the detriment of their patients are the most efficient in this regard. It cannot be stressed too often that nuclear medicine physicians and radiologists need an accurate assessment of this clinical risk of VTE for their VQ report to ensure an accurate diagnosis. This clinical information permits the VQ reporter to change the **relative** PE risk from the VQ lung scan category alone to the **absolute** risk obtained when the VQ category analysis is combined with an accurate clinical assessment. If a clinical opinion is not immediately available the alternative for the nuclear medicine service is the use of inhouse diagnostic tools or checklists that can stratify cases into the likely clinical prevalence of PE. Specifically, 10% prevalence is a low pre-test probability/risk, 30% is a medium pre-test and 70% prevalence is a high pre-test clinical risk. Wells et al [3] and Wicki et al [4] have developed sophisticated clinical algorithms and these appear to work well in the emergency room.

Simplified criteria focusing on the genetic, acquired, and environmental risk factors for VTE have been found useful in the author's practice (Table 10.6). Firstly, patients with a proven DVT by duplex ultrasound (including color flow and Doppler assessments) have a high clinical pre-test probability/risk of PE automatically because they are the group who succumb most often. Also included in this high-risk group are those who have three or more risk factors (see Section 10.4.2). Clearly, patients over 65 (one of the risk factors) need only two other risk factors to be in the high-risk group. Secondly, patients with one or two

Table 10.6. Clinical risk of PE

High (70–80%)	Medium (20–70%)	Low (5–20%)	Very unlikely (<5%)
≥3 Risk factors Documented DVT	1 or 2 risk factors	No risk factors Other symptoms/signs	D-dimer <500 ng/ml (Vidas)

Important risk factors include: past history of PE/DVT, immobilization, surgery in last 3 months, age >65 years, cancer ± chemotherapy, thrombophilia.

risk factors are given a medium clinical pre-test probability/risk of PE. Important risk factors in this algorithm include a history of previous DVT or PE, immobility for whatever reason (plaster cast, stroke, long journey etc.), surgery within the previous 3 months, age older than 65 years, cancer (particularly if prescribed chemotherapy) and thrombophilia indicated by other family members suffering from VTE. Thirdly, those younger than 65 years without risk factors but symptoms in relation to the cardiorespiratory system such as sudden breathlessness or pleuritic chest pain with a clear chest radiograph have a low clinical pre-test probability/risk of PE. PE is not excluded but it is much less likely.

10.4.6 Investigation for Venous Thromboembolism

Up until recently, a suspicion of pulmonary embolism would arise when a patient presented with chest pain and breathlessness with either an area of consolidation on chest X-ray, a change in the ECG trace, or the development of hypoxia. In general, however, such tests were too insensitive and unreliable to be of value as accurate screening tests for PE.

Today, the first screening test for VTE in the emergency department is often the rapid quantitative ELISA (Vidas) D-dimer measurement for cross-linked fibrin derivatives that are breakdown products of formed thrombus in the circulation. A negative test with D-dimer levels below 500 ng/ml can accurately exclude VTE with a specificity of 95% and usually eliminates the need for further investigation in those with low or medium pre-test clinical probabilities of PE. Regrettably, raised levels of D-dimer do not necessarily indicate VTE and are of no value in the diagnostic algorithm. However, raised levels without VTE are commonly found in hospitalized patients with myocardial infarction, pneumonia, sepsis, during the second and third trimester of pregnancy, peripheral vascular disease, cancer, many inflammatory diseases, and increasing age so unfortunately, this test may only be a valuable screening test in 10% of hospital patients. Conversely, it is sensible if patients with a high pre-test clinical risk of PE (three or more risk factors) and a negative D-dimer are investigated further. Such individuals are more likely to fall into the false negative D-dimer group and so conceal ongoing VTE [5].

Duplex ultrasound of the lower limb veins has replaced conventional contrast venography. It has been used for cases where a DVT was suspected clinically and where VQ imaging has been inconclusive. Clearly, identification of DVT in these clinical scenarios would render further investigation for VTE unnecessary and treatment mandatory. Ultrasound, however, has limited sensitivity for asymptomatic DVT and may be positive in as few as one-third of cases where PE has been definitely confirmed. This dismal performance may partially reflect the technical difficulties inherent in the technique or simply the likelihood of previously formed thrombus breaking from its tether in the vein wall and migrating to lung prior to lower limb ultrasound. It is acceptable clinical practice to withhold anticoagulant treatment in patients suspected of a DVT but with a negative ultrasound as long as arrangements are made to repeat the scan. However, it is unacceptable to withhold treatment in cases with suspected PE and an unhelpful VQ scan with a single negative ultrasound since VTE can be regularly missed under these circumstances. Unless a clinical decision had been made to anticoagulate, further investigation for PE would be advisable in this scenario.

In the past, echography was used non-invasively to screen suitable cases for PE. Both transthoracic and transesophageal echography have limited accuracy for detecting PE and with the advent of CT pulmonary angiography they are no longer indicated.

Pulmonary angiography used to be the gold standard for diagnosis of PE but it was never widely available. It involved passing a catheter from an arm or leg vein into the right side of the heart followed by an injection of contrast material into the pulmonary arteries. Opacification of the pulmonary arterial tree permitted visualization of thrombus in the larger vessels. Today, CT pulmonary angiography (CTPA) is available in most hospitals and has evolved in the last 10 years into an excellent test for PE [6, 7]. The advent of multi-detector (multislice) CT (MDCT) increasingly permits coverage of the whole chest with 1–2 mm resolution within a single breath-hold after injection of contrast. CTPA can detect thrombus in the main pulmonary arteries in at least 95% of cases although the sensitivity may fall to 75–80% for the smaller emboli in sub-segmental arteries. CTPA has rapidly become the gold standard for diagnosis of PE and has been revolutionary for clinicians. There was concern about the negative predictive value of CTPA initially but many studies now have shown a vanishingly small rate of PE of around 1% following a negative test. Unfortunately, the radiation dose to the female breast during the study is substantial and so there are arguments for limiting the use of CTPA to the more difficult and older cases and in particular to those where VQ imaging is clearly unlikely to be helpful.

There are a few cases where CTPA is more difficult such as kidney failure, gross obesity, and poor venous access but these are low in number.

10.4.7 Role of Ventilation/Perfusion Imaging

The recent decisive developments in CT technology have changed substantially the role of VQ imaging in the diagnostic algorithm [8]. Nuclear medicine can now concentrate its involvement in the question of suspected PE to those clinical scenarios where the technology has most to offer (i.e. mainly for the exclusion of PE). Firstly, VQ imaging with a normal chest X-ray can correctly exclude PE in the majority of patients with a low or medium pre-test probability at less than 7% (0.6 mSv from IRCP publications) of the radiation dose to the breast from MDCT (8–10 mSv from www.impactscan.org). Secondly, and again given a normal chest X-ray, VQ imaging can correctly pick up PE with a high probability scan in four out of five cases with proven PE, which accounts for 30–35% of all those presenting with proven PE. Clearly, the important factor in the success or otherwise of VQ scanning is the chest X-ray, which must be normal. Ideally, all patients in whom PE is suspected with an abnormal chest X-ray should have CTPA as the initial investigation. However, due to limited available time on most CT scanners, VQ imaging is often used as the first-line investigation, to exclude patients with normal or high probability of PE examinations from further investigation. Those with intermediate (indeterminate) findings on VQ imaging then undergo further investigation with CTPA.

The major weaknesses of VQ imaging must also be recognized. The pathology behind a perfusion abnormality can only be inferred and rarely confirmed without contrast studies. Secondly, it is usually non-diagnostic when the chest X-ray is abnormal unless there are mismatched perfusion abnormalities in the other lung, which is clear on chest X-ray. Thirdly, it may be very difficult to interpret in patients with chronic heart and lung disease. These latter groups can represent up to 40–50% of inpatients previously sent for VQ scanning in the UK. Finally, and unlike CTPA, VQ imaging rarely provides a credible alternative diagnosis for cases without PE.

Current wisdom therefore suggests that VQ imaging is the screening test of choice for suspected PE when the D-dimer is abnormal, the chest X-ray is normal, and when the pre-test clinical probability is low or medium [8]. This may be particularly the case for young females given the breast dose from MDCT. VQ imaging should be performed as soon as practical after the clinical suspicion is raised to enable its completion before the development of pulmonary infarction that complicates VQ image interpretation. Delay of more than 48 hours is considered unwise since diagnostic perfusion abnormalities can resolve within a few days.

It is hoped that VQ imaging in patients with normal chest X-rays can provide a post-test PE risk of 5% or less in more than two-thirds presenting at the department or a post-test risk of 90% or more in at least one-third of those with PE. If the post-test risk is more than 10% and less than 85% (i.e. diagnostic doubt), CTPA should be used to clarify and refine the risk further.

10.4.8 VQ Scan Interpretation

Unlike CTPA where pulmonary and segmental artery thrombus is usually visualized or not visualized, VQ imaging reveals normal pulmonary ventilation and perfusion or the effects of diverse diseases upon pulmonary ventilation and perfusion. In truth, all perfusion defects are non-specific since the pathological basis of the abnormality or abnormalities can never be forensically proven without further contrast studies. In reality though, perfusion defects that conform to segmental or lobar boundaries, particularly when multiple and bilateral with a normal accompanying ventilation, are highly correlated with acute or previous PE. Recognizing this relative non-specificity, most experienced reporters of VQ scans will use probability terms in their report [9]. A very low probability category scan is least likely to indicate acute PE while the high probability category is most likely. Many patterns of abnormality, however, are indefinite and are therefore quite unhelpful. These images are entitled indeterminate or intermediate

Table 10.7. Neoclassical criteria for VQ scan interpretation: modified PIOPED

High probability
Two or more moderate/large mismatched perfusion defects.*
Prior heart and lung disease probably requires more abnormalities (i.e. four or more).
Triple match in one lung with one or more mismatches in the other lung field.
Intermediate probability
Difficult to categorise or not described as very low, low or high, including all cases with a chest X-ray opacity, pleural fluid or collapse.
Single moderate VQ match or mismatch without corresponding radiograph abnormality.
Low probability
Large or moderate focal VQ matches involving no more than 50% of the combined lung fields with no corresponding radiograph abnormalities.
Small VQ mismatches with a normal chest X-ray.
Very-low probability
Small VQ matches with a normal chest X-ray.
Near-normal
Perfusion defects due to raised hemi diaphragm, cardiomegaly, enlarged hila or aorta.
Normal
No perfusion abnormalities.

*Large defects are >75% segment, moderate defects are 25–75% segment and small defects are <25% segment.

probability categories and the terms used clearly emphasize that these particular patterns lack any contribution to the diagnostic process. CTPA is always required for accurate diagnosis under these circumstances. Fortunately, abnormalities on the chest X-ray permit us to predict when VQ imaging will provide an indeterminate result and to move smartly to CTPA in the first instance if available.

Consistent and accurate interpretation of VQ images is easier now that CTPA takes the difficult cases but it remains a challenging cognitive task involving, firstly, the integration of the perfusion and ventilation images with the chest X-ray. The second step involves the assessment of the pre-test clinical probability of PE. The third step involves integration of the scan result with the pre-test clinical probability of PE to provide the final post-test diagnosis. The author favors a "neoclassical" approach to VQ scan analysis (Table 10.7) that recognizes that the low probability scan becomes less useful for diagnosis when the pre-test clinical risk is medium. This neoclassical approach uses the very-low category only to exclude PE in this important clinical group, the rest requiring CTPA if indicated. The only VQ category of value in the high clinical pre-test group is the normal scan excluding PE.

Several principles of lung scan interpretation can be recognized that permit a more accurate and reproducible categorization of the scans to guide those who currently provide a VQ scan service for clinical and radiological colleagues.

The *first principle* states that a normal perfusion scan (Figure 10.5) excludes PE for clinical purposes no matter the clinical presentation. This is by far the most valuable diagnostic finding in VQ scanning for those without PE and is of particular value in pregnancy where there is a need to limit further use of ionizing radiation. A near-normal perfusion scan is really just as valuable and reveals a widened mediastinum or raised hemi-diaphragm with clear lung fields on chest X-ray. These findings are totally reliable and can be followed immediately by a search for alternative pathology.

The *second principle* states that PE can present with any perfusion abnormality but the risk of acute PE will be dependent in part upon the pattern of that abnormality. For example, the smaller the perfusion abnormality or abnormalities, the more matched they are to concordant abnormal ventilation and the less numerous, the less the risk of PE (Figures 10.11, 10.12a and b). Conversely, the larger the perfusion abnormality, the more segmental its appearance and the more normal ventilation (mismatching), the greater the risk of PE becomes (Figure 10.13). Many patterns of VQ abnormality with a normal chest X-ray cannot be interpreted with sufficient accuracy and will always attract an intermediate or indeterminate label. Such patterns include extensive parenchymal disease with multiple and widespread ventilation and perfusion abnormalities throughout both lung fields (Figure 10.14), multiple matched and mismatched perfusion abnormalities (Figure 10.15), a single mismatched perfusion abnormality of whatever size (Figure 10.16), and possibly a single segmental matched defect (Figure 10.17). The author would add from personal experience, the group with multiple matched but clearly segmental perfusion defects (Figure 10.18). PE is known to cause matching of ventilation abnormalities in a small minority of cases so if the defects look segmental, even though matched, CTPA should be seriously considered as the most appropriate next investigation.

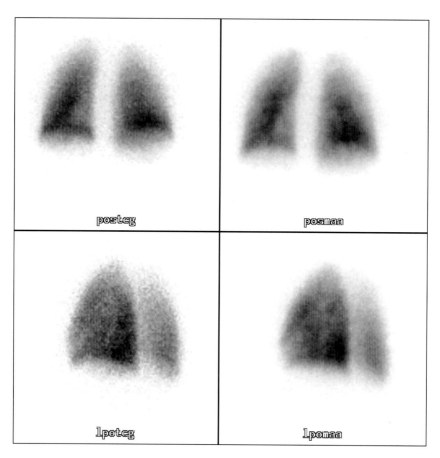

Figure 10.11. Almost normal Technegas ventilation (left) with minor matched perfusion abnormalities (<25% seg) on the perfusion image (right). Very low probability category scan for PE.

The *third principle* states that a good quality erect and contemporaneous chest X-ray is essential for accurate VQ scan interpretation and must be available when the decision about the need for VQ imaging is made. This is because any parenchymal abnormality on chest X-ray not only increases the risk of PE in an unquantifiable manner but also completely degrades the diagnostic potential of VQ imaging (Figure 10.19). VQ imaging can uncommonly be positive for PE in the presence of an abnormal chest X-ray but only when the triple-match of X-ray, perfusion, and ventilation abnormalities in one lung is associated with mismatches and a clear lung field on X-ray in the other lung (Figure 10.20). This occurs in only 5–7% of PE so VQ imaging is not recommended when the chest X-ray is abnormal. CTPA will almost certainly provide a diagnosis in up to 90% of cases.

The *fourth principle* states that the pre-test clinical probability of PE, that is the PE risk as determined by the clinical presentation, is itself an independent risk factor for PE along with the lung scan result and the D-dimer level (if normal). Bayes' theorem gives the mathematical expression for combining the pre-test clinical probability of PE and the probability of PE from the lung scan. This combination provides a more closely defined post-test probability of pulmonary embolism than either of the variables taken singly (Figure 10.21). The principle is only annulled by the presence of a normal perfusion scan where PE is excluded for clinical purposes whatever the history (Tables 10.8, 10.9, and 10.10).

The *fifth principle* states that the VQ scan and chest radiograph should be interpreted and its category determined whenever possible before becoming apprised of the clinical details of the

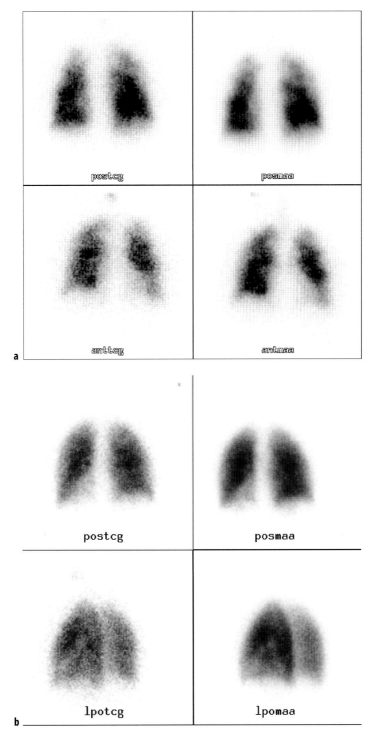

Figure 10.12. a Multiple small peripheral matched Technegas ventilation (left) and perfusion (right) abnormalities in a patient with a normal chest X-ray. Low probability category lung scan for PE. **b** Single matched VQ abnormality of the left lower lobe mainly in the areas of the lateral and anterior segments but not clearly segmental. Low probability category lung scan for PE. The CTPA was negative.

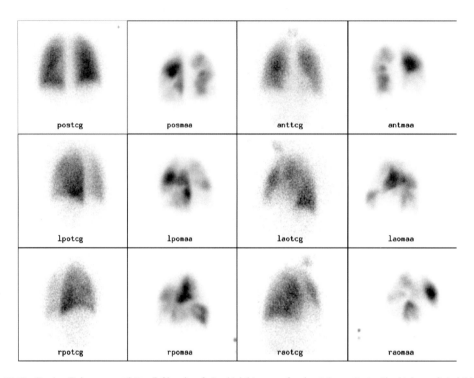

Figure 10.13. Six-view Technegas ventilation (left) and perfusion (right) images of each pair in a patient with a high pre-clinical risk of PE. Multiple segmental and lobar mismatched perfusion abnormalities with normal ventilation confirm a high probability category of lung scan for PE.

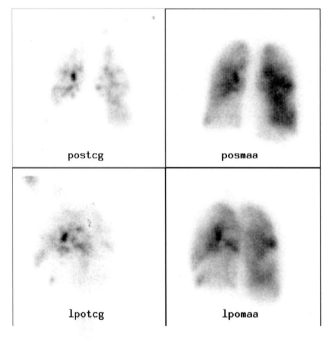

Figure 10.14. Technegas ventilation (left) and perfusion (right) in the posterior and left posterior oblique projection showing matching of small and large perfusion abnormalities extending over more than 50% of lung field. Indeterminate/intermediate lung scan category.

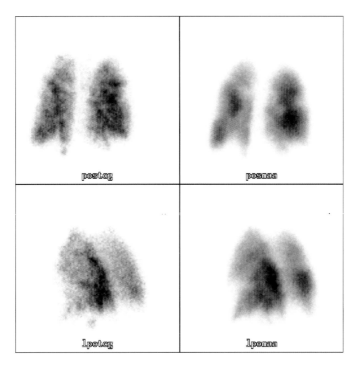

Figure 10.15. Technegas ventilation (left) and perfusion (right) in the posterior and left posterior oblique projection. Multiple matched and mismatched abnormalities are seen involving both lungs. Indeterminate/intermediate lung scan category.

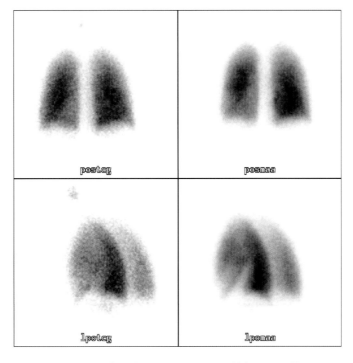

Figure 10.16. Technegas ventilation (left) and perfusion (right) in the posterior and left posterior oblique projection. A single mismatched segmental perfusion abnormality of the anterior segment of the left lower lobe is noted. Indeterminate/intermediate lung scan category.

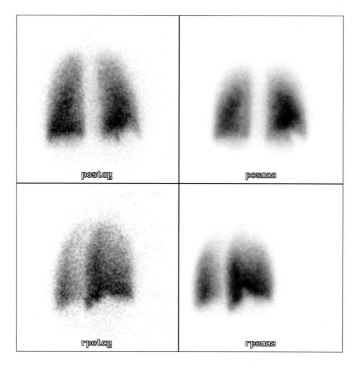

Figure 10.17. Technegas ventilation (left) and perfusion (right) in the posterior and right oblique projection. A matched VQ abnormality of the lateral segment of the right lower lobe is seen. Low probability category scan for PE but at the higher end of that risk.

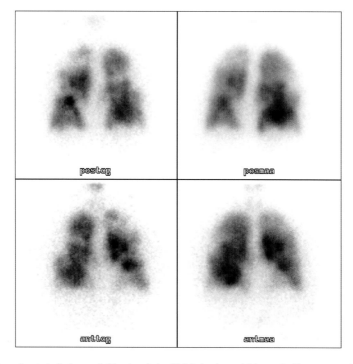

Figure 10.18. Anterior and posterior Technegas (left) and perfusion (right) showing multiple matched but segmental-looking abnormalities. Favors an indeterminate/intermediate category label.

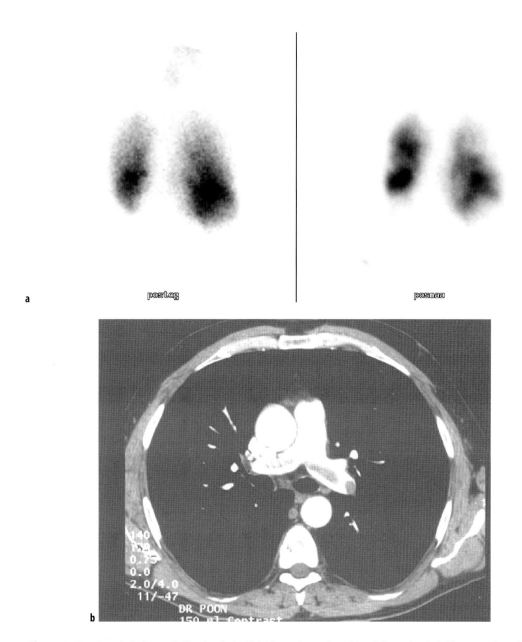

Figure 10.19. **a** Posterior Technegas (left) and perfusion (right) images in a patient with a triple match at the left base secondary to left basal consolidation on chest X-ray. Multiple mismatched perfusion abnormalities on the radiological normal right lung confirm a high probability category for PE. **b** PE confirmed by CTPA centrally.

patient's presentation. This ensures that the two independent variables, VQ scan and pre-test clinical probability of PE, remain independent during the analysis of the VQ study. Clearly, this can be difficult in practice if one has to assess a patient's suitability for VQ scanning in the first instance but it is an important point. British Thoracic Society guidelines agree and state that knowledge of the clinical probability should not influence the description of the VQ scan category, but is essential

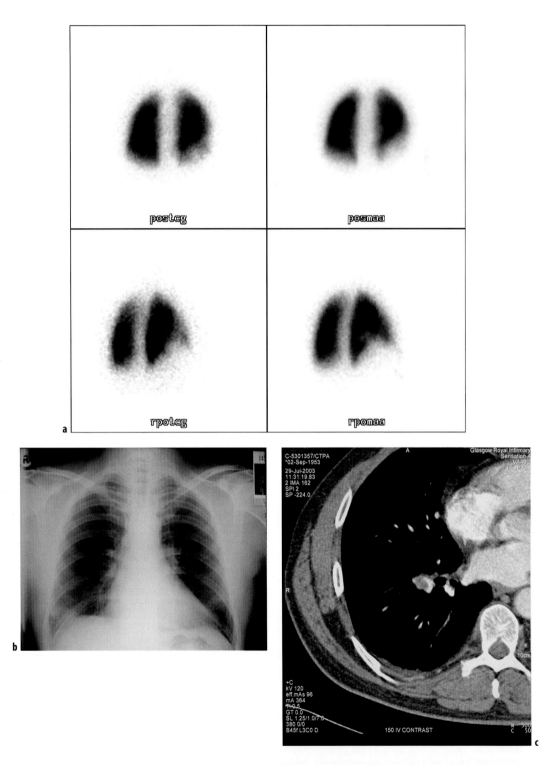

Figure 10.20. a Posterior and right posterior oblique Technegas and perfusion images showing a triple matched defect on the right confirming an indeterminate VQ scan category. **b** Chest X-ray showing right lower lobe consolidation matching the VQ abnormality. **c** PE confirmed by CTPA on the right.

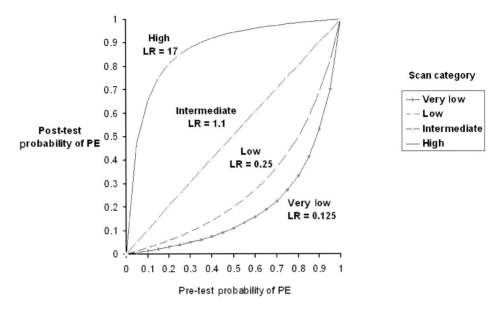

Figure 10.21. The conditional probability graph for PE diagnosis is constructed using the likelihood ratios (LR) calculated from the realigned PIOPED 1 data. The graph combines the clinical pre-test probability and the VQ categories into the post-test probability of PE.

for interpreting the report's meaning (i.e. for the derivation of the post-test risk of PE).

The *sixth principle* states that a D-dimer level below the upper limit of normal (<500 units) is an accurate method of excluding VTE and eliminating the need for VQ imaging or CTPA. The false negative rate is likely to be between 2 and 4% so one would consider further imaging with VQ scanning or CTPA after a negative D-dimer only if the clinical history was highly suggestive of PE.

A basic algorithm for the analysis of VQ lung scans is given in Figure 10.22.

10.4.9 Formation of a Post-test Diagnosis

Modification of the PIOPED (Prospective Investigation of Pulmonary Embolism Diagnosis) study data has permitted the development of neoclassical criteria for VQ image categorization that majored on augmenting the negative predictive value of VQ imaging. Using strict criteria and careful selection of cases with normal chest X-rays, an accurate post-test diagnosis can be provided for each clinical presentation and scan category combination (Tables 10.8, 10.9, 10.10). For example, no further investigation is required when a pa-

tient presents with a low clinical pre-test likelihood and a normal, very low probability or low probability category with matching defects since the ongoing risk of PE is so small. If risk factors for VTE are noted in the clinical history (medium pre-test), a normal scan eliminates PE, a very low probability scan makes it highly unlikely, while a high probability scan is almost diagnostic of PE. In cases with many risk factors or a DVT (high pre-test), a normal scan eliminates PE and a high probability is diagnostic. Clearly, most other clinical and VQ scan category combinations are non-diagnostic or unhelpful to varying degrees. In the author's institution, VQ imaging is usually diagnostic in up to three-quarters of cases with normal chest X-rays. Age and smoking history are the factors that prevent improvement on these statistics.

A new strategy will be required from each hospital/institution and imaging department concerning the algorithm that clinicians can use for further investigation of those cases with indecisive VQ scans. Most X-ray departments will already be coping with increasing numbers of primary requests for CTPA where chest X-rays have been found to be abnormal by the clinicians. Creative use of the resource allocation for routine and emergency provision of CTPA may be required for the foreseeable future.

This algorithm starts with a normal chest X-ray. Q = Perfusion and V = Ventilation

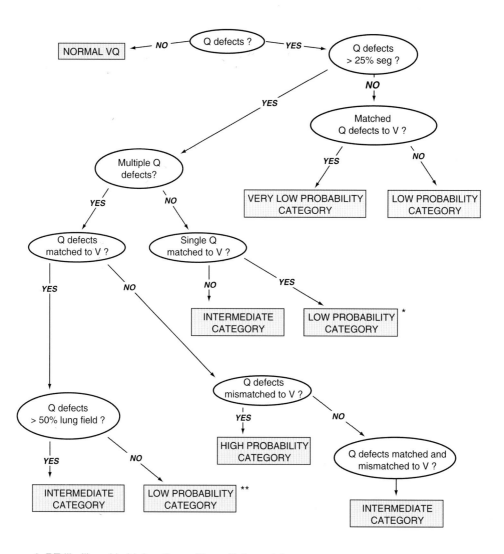

* PE likelihood is higher than with multiple matches.
** Multiple matched segmental abnormalities should raise suspicion of PE.

Figure 10.22. A basic algorithm for VQ scan interpretation.

10.4.10 Communicating the Risk of PE after VQ imaging

Communication of PE risk to clinicians can be difficult, given our probability jargon, and it is possible that the addition of a numerical estimate of risk along with the verbal report will clarify that risk for clinicians. Our policy, with others, is to communicate the post-test diagnosis on completion of the VQ scan providing both a verbal assessment and a percentage risk of PE, which was obtained from an analysis of the original PIOPED data (Figure 10.21). A two-way discussion may then permit

Table 10.8. Diagnosis of venous thromboembolism: the low clinical pre-test probability

Scan category	Description of abnormalities	PE risk, VQ and clinical	Post-test result
Normal	None	0%	PE excluded
Near normal	↑hemi-diaphragm:↔ mediastinum	0%	PE excluded
Very low	Multiple match; <25% seg	2%	PE highly unlikely
Low	Multiple match; >25% seg	3%	PE highly unlikely
	Single match; 25%<seg <100%	10%	Diagnosis uncertain
Indeterminate	Single mismatch; 25%<seg <100%	10–15%	Diagnosis uncertain
	Multiple match; <25% seg; <50% lung	10–15%	Diagnosis uncertain
	Multiple match and mismatch	10–15%	Diagnosis uncertain
High	Multiple mismatch; <2.5 segs	50–60%	Diagnosis uncertain
	Single match (chest X-ray and Q) with multiple mismatch other lung	50–60%	Diagnosis uncertain

Table 10.9. Diagnosis of venous thromboembolism: the medium clinical pre-test probability

Scan category	Description of abnormalities	PE risk, VQ and clinical	Post-test result
Normal	None	0%	PE excluded
Near normal	↑hemi-diaphragm:↔ mediastinum	0%	PE excluded
Very low	Multiple match; <25% seg	5%	PE highly unlikely
Low	Multiple match; >25% seg	10%	PE unlikely
	Single match; 25%<seg <100%	20%	Diagnosis uncertain
Indeterminate	Single mismatch; 25%<seg <100%	20–30%	Diagnosis uncertain
	Multiple match; >25% seg; >50% lung	20–30%	Diagnosis uncertain
	Multiple match and mismatch	20–30%	Diagnosis uncertain
High	Multiple mismatch; >2.5 segs	80–90%	PE likely
	Single match (chest X-ray and Q) with multiple mismatch other lung	80–90%	PE likely

Table 10.10. Diagnosis of venous thromboembolism: the high clinical pre-test probability

Scan category	Description of abnormalities	PE Risk, VQ and clinical	Post-test result
Normal	None	0%	PE excluded
Near normal	↑hemi-diaphragm:↔ mediastinum	0–5%	PE unlikely
Very low	Multiple match; <25% seg	10–20%	Diagnosis uncertain
Low	Multiple match; >25% seg	20–40%	Diagnosis uncertain
	Single match; 25%<seg <100%	20–40%	Diagnosis uncertain
Indeterminate	Single mismatch; 25%<seg <100%	40–70%	Diagnosis uncertain
	Multiple match; >25% seg >50% lung	40–70%	Diagnosis uncertain
	Multiple match and mismatch	40–70%	Diagnosis uncertain
High	Multiple mismatch; >2.5 segs	95%	PE highly likely
	Single match (chest X-ray and Q) with multiple mismatch other lung	95%	PE highly likely

the nuclear medicine doctor to clarify for the clinician the impact of the post-test result on the diagnostic strategy and whether or not further investigation is advisable. Tables 10.8, 10.9, and 10.10 provide the synthesis of categorical analysis, clinical presentation, and post-test risk with verbal and numerical risk outlined.

Role of Post-test VQ Investigations

In the author's experience of a teaching hospital, the analysis of VQ imaging in cases with a normal chest X-ray and its subsequent integration with the clinical pre-test probability of PE does provide definitive post-test results in over three-quarters of cases. Final diagnoses of "PE excluded", "PE highly unlikely", "PE likely", and "PE highly likely" all have sufficient diagnostic power to permit immediate decisions regarding no-treatment or treatment. On the other hand, patients with a "PE unlikely" have a PE risk of up to 10% and therefore may need a further diagnostic test to lower the risk to a more clinically useful range. Negative well-performed duplex ultrasound of both legs would likely reduce this probability of PE to 5–7%. Unfortunately, a negative ultrasound does not exclude calf vein thrombosis and a repeat test after 7 to 10 days might be necessary to reduce the number of false negative tests. Patients with "diagnosis uncertain" have a risk of PE of between 10 and 60%. CTPA is the only investigation at present that can confidently confirm or eliminate PE in this group of patients, apart from formal pulmonary angiography.

It is for each hospital or institution, the clinicians and imaging department, to formulate their individual imaging strategy for suspected PE. In particular, it will be necessary to decide whether an abnormal chest X-ray, a 5–10% clinical risk or 10% plus risk of PE following VQ imaging should be an agreed trigger for CTPA.

References

1. NHSBSP Publication 54. Review of Radiation Risk in Breast Screening, Feb. 2003.
2. Gray HW. The natural history of venous thromboembolism: Impact on ventilation/perfusion scan reporting. Semin Nucl Med 2002; 32:159–172.
3. Wells PS, Ginsberg JS, Anderson DR, et al. Use of a clinical model for safe management of patients with suspected pulmonary embolism. Ann Intern Med 1998; 129:997–1005.
4. Wicki J, Perneger TV, Junod AF, et al. Assessing clinical probability of pulmonary embolism in the emergency ward: A simple score. Arch Intern Med 2001; 161:92–97.
5. Perrier A. D-dimer for suspected pulmonary embolism: Whom should we test? Chest 2004; 125:807–809.
6. American College of Emergency Physicians. Clinical Policy. Critical issues in the evaluation and management of adult patients presenting with suspected pulmonary embolism. Ann Emerg Med 2003; 41:257–270.
7. Schoepf UJ, Costello P. CT angiography for diagnosis of pulmonary embolism: State of the art. Radiology 2004; 230:329–337.
8. British Thoracic Society guidelines for the management of suspected acute pulmonary embolism. Thorax 2003; 58:470-483.
9. Gray HW. The languages of lung scan interpretation. In: Freeman LM, ed. Nuclear Medicine Annual. Philadelphia: Lippincott Williams & Wilkins; 2001.

11

The Urinary Tract

Philip S. Cosgriff

11.1 Introduction

Despite recent technical advances in computed tomography, magnetic resonance, and ultrasound imaging, nuclear medicine (NM) has maintained its crucial role in the functional assessment of the urinary tract, particularly the kidneys.

Indeed, nuclear medicine techniques maintain "gold standard" status in the diagnosis of upper urinary tract obstruction and pyelonephritic scarring secondary to urinary tract infection (UTI). Importantly, all NM renal imaging techniques also provide an estimate of relative renal function. Absolute renal function (e.g. glomerular filtration rate (GFR) in ml/min) can also be measured by blood sample-based radionuclide methods that are superior in accuracy to routinely used indicators of renal function (e.g. serum creatinine). Finally, renographic techniques also play important roles in the diagnosis of renovascular hypertension, renal transplant complications, and some lower urinary tract disorders such as vesico-ureteric reflux.

The main imaging techniques in the investigation of the urinary tract are renography, which has numerous variants, and static DMSA imaging. The techniques and indications for these tests will be considered, along with their strengths and weaknesses. A test selection guide is given in Table 11.1.

11.2 Anatomy

The urinary tract comprises two kidneys, individually connected to the urinary bladder by ureters, and a urethra that connects the bladder to the external genitalia. The kidneys are situated in the lumbar region at a depth of about 6 cm from the surface of the back. They are positioned symmetrically about the vertebral column, their upper and lower poles lying between the 12th thoracic vertebra and the 3rd lumbar vertebra respectively. Each kidney is about 12 cm long, 6 cm wide, 3 cm thick and weighs approximately 150 grams.

A cross-section through the long axis of the kidney reveals that the renal parenchyma consists of a pale outer region, the cortex, and an inner darker region, the medulla. Unlike the cortex, which has a relatively homogeneous appearance, the medulla consists of radially striated cones called renal pyramids, the apices of which form papillae which project into the renal sinus and interface with a calyx (Figure 11.1). As the renal artery enters at the hilum it divides into several interlobar arteries which themselves branch to form arcuate ("bow-shaped") arteries which run along the boundary between medulla and cortex. Smaller interlobular arteries branch off at right angles from the arcuate arteries heading outwards into the cortex. Finally, the branches from the interlobular arteries, called afferent arterioles, supply blood to the glomerular capillaries.

Table 11.1. A test selection guide for the urologist/nephrologist. See text for details. Prerequisite: renal ultrasound. When MAG3 is mentioned it is the clearly preferred radiopharmaceutical. However, ^{99m}Tc-DTPA can be used as an alternative if renal function is good

Clinical question(s)	Procedure to request	Comment
Need accurate estimate of relative renal function	DMSA renal scan	In situations where accuracy is paramount (e.g. prior to planned nephrectomy) or where renographic estimate is likely to be technically difficult (e.g. in certain infants). No information is provided on the status of the outflow tract
Suspected renal scarring	DMSA renal scan	Estimate of relative renal function will be routinely provided.
Suspected PUJ (and/or ureteric) obstruction	Diuresis MAG3 renogram	Estimate of relative renal function will be routinely provided
Suspected renal scarring and suspected upper tract obstruction	Diuresis MAG3 renogram	Scarring may be apparent on the early MAG3 images. If not proceed to a DMSA scan
Suspected VUR (or UUR in duplicated systems)	Basic MAG3 renogram followed by Indirect radionuclide cystogram	Estimate of relative renal function will be routinely provided
Suspected VUR and suspected upper tract obstruction	Diuresis MAG3 renogram followed by indirect cystogram	If indirect cystogram negative for reflux, repeat the test without furosemide
Need accurate estimate of absolute GFR in ml/min	GFR measurement (^{51}Cr-EDTA)	Could also use ^{99m}Tc-DTPA
Need estimate of both relative and absolute GFR	Basic DTPA renogram with GFR	In principle, both can be measured by a single injection of ^{99m}Tc-DTPA. However, in children (or adults with compromised renal function) it is preferable to inject ^{99m}Tc-MAG3 and ^{51}Cr-EDTA simultaneously. Absolute GFR is measured by blood sampling

PUJ, pelvi-ureteric junction; VUR, vesico-ureteric reflux; UUR, ureter-to-ureter reflux.

The functional unit of the kidney, the nephron, consists of a glomerulus and its attached tubule (Figure 11.2). There are approximately 1 million nephrons in each kidney. The glomerulus is a tight cluster of specialized blood capillaries which serve to filter potential urinary excreta into the tubule, thereby forming a fluid called the glomerular filtrate. Under normal circumstances proteins and other large molecules are too large to pass through the filter and return to the systemic circulation via the efferent arteriole, perirenal capillaries, renal venules and, finally, the renal vein. The tubule originates as a blind sac, known as Bowman's capsule, which leads in turn to the proximal convoluted tubule, Henle's loop, the distal convoluted tubule and, finally, the collecting tubule (or duct). For functional reasons, the proximal convoluted tubule and Henle's loop are sometimes collectively referred to as the proximal tubule and the distal convoluted tubule and collecting duct as the distal tubule (or distal nephron).

The majority of nephrons (approximately 85%) have glomeruli situated in the outer two-thirds of the cortex and are known as cortical nephrons. In contrast, the juxtamedullary nephrons have glomeruli situated in the inner third of the cortex. These two populations of nephrons also differ with respect to the length of Henle's loop, juxtamedullary nephrons having relatively long loops which extend deep into the medulla, whereas cortical nephrons have short loops which extend only a short distance into the medulla (Figure 11.2).

11.3 Physiology

The main function of the kidneys is to conserve substances that are essential to life, and they should therefore be regarded as regulatory organs that help maintain the constancy of the extracellular fluid (ECF), in terms of both volume and composition. The importance of this lies in the fact that most body cells will only function properly if the concentration of solutes in the tissue fluid surrounding them is kept within quite narrow limits.

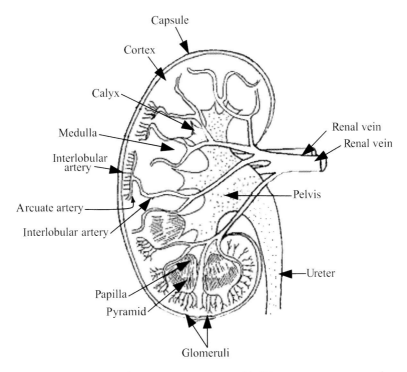

Figure 11.1. Gross anatomy of the kidney.

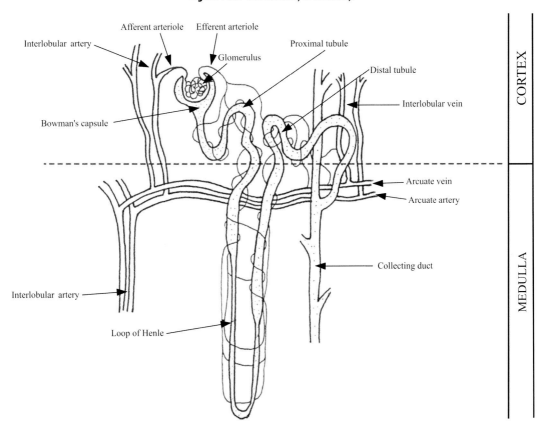

Figure 11.2. Anatomy of the nephron, showing main components (glomerulus and tubule) and associated blood vessels. The nephron illustrated has its glomerulus in the inner third of the cortex and is known as a juxtamedullary nephron, having a relatively long loop of Henle (see text).

The importance of the kidneys in human physiology can be gauged from the staggering fact that a pair of organs accounting for about 3% of body weight consume about 20% of all the oxygen used by the body at rest. Compared to other organs, a relatively high renal blood flow (RBF) of around 1100 ml/min (i.e. 20% of cardiac output) is thus required to (a) provide energy for the "blood cleansing" process, (b) provide basic oxygen and nutrients for the renal cells, and (c) maintain a net positive glomerular perfusion pressure (GPP) for filtration. Collectively, the glomeruli have a huge surface area, so only a modest GPP (about 8 mmHg) is required for filtration. However, a drop in GPP of only 15% stops filtration altogether. The maintenance of renal blood flow (RBF) is therefore critical and there is a unique mechanism to autoregulate it. Moreover, a "back-up" mechanism is triggered when a change occurs that cannot be corrected by autoregulation (see Section 11.5.7). Renal plasma flow (RPF), referring to the component of blood available for filtration, is around 600 ml/min ((1 − hematocrit) × RBF).

The first stage of the urine production process is glomerular filtration, whereby plasma water and its non-protein constituents (crystalloids) are passively separated from blood cells and protein macromolecules (colloids). Although the glomerulus is actually considerably more complex than a simple sieve, it behaves as if it were a filtering membrane containing pores of 7–10 nm diameter, excluding to a large extent any substance with a molecular weight of greater than about 60 000. Normal glomerular filtration rate (GFR) is about 120 ml/min, which means that the fraction of the plasma actually filtered (the filtration fraction, FF = GFR/RPF) is about 20%. The vast majority of this "ultrafiltrate" (over 99%) is subsequently reabsorbed (i.e. reclaimed) during its passage along the tubule, resulting in a final urine output of about 1 ml/min.

After the blood has passed through the glomerulus, it enters the efferent arteriole which leads to a second capillary network woven around the tubule (see Figure 11.2), an arrangement unique to the kidney. This provides the opportunity for selected materials (particularly salt and water) to be reabsorbed from the glomerular filtrate into the blood via the tubular cells, a process referred to as tubular reabsorption. The main site of all reabsorption is the proximal convoluted tubule, which accounts for about 90% of filtered sodium and 75% of filtered water. In addition to being partially filtered by the glomerulus, certain substances are also transported from the post-glomerular blood capillaries into the lumen of the proximal tubule. This process, which can be considered the reverse of tubular reabsorption, is called tubular secretion.

In summary, the functions of the kidney can be explained by studying the functions of an individual nephron, consisting of high pressure plasma filter (the glomerulus) and fine control device (the tubule).

11.4 Radiopharmaceuticals

The site of uptake of the main renal radiopharmaceuticals is shown in Figure 11.3.

The pharmokinetics of agents used in nuclear medicine are largely determined by their degree of protein binding in plasma (Table 11.2). The minimal protein binding of ^{99m}Tc-DTPA and ^{51}Cr-EDTA means that they rapidly diffuse into the extravascular space and are freely filtered at the glomerulus, which represents their only excretory pathway under normal circumstances. As neither agent is reabsorbed in the renal tubule, the plasma clearance of these agents is effectively the renal clearance, so either can be used to determine glomerular filtration rate (see Section 4.11).

Table 11.2. Properties and characteristics of commonly used renal radiopharmaceuticals

Radiopharmaceutical	Uptake mechanism	Protein binding	Extraction efficiency	ARSAC DRL (MBq)
^{99m}Tc-DTPA	GF	< 0.03	0.2	300
^{99m}Tc-MAG3	GF + TS	≈ 0.85	0.5	100
^{99m}Tc-DMSA	DTU + GF/TR	≈ 0.85	0.06	80
^{123}I-OIH	GF + TS	≈ 0.50	0.8	20
^{51}Cr-EDTA	GF	< 0.01	0.2	3

GF, glomerular filtration; TS, tubular secretion; TR, tubular reabsorption; DTU, direct tubular uptake.
DRL, diagnostic reference levels for injected activity in adults, as recommended by the UK Administration of Radioactive Substances Advisory Committee (ARSAC).
All the molecules listed above are relatively small in size (< 400 Da).

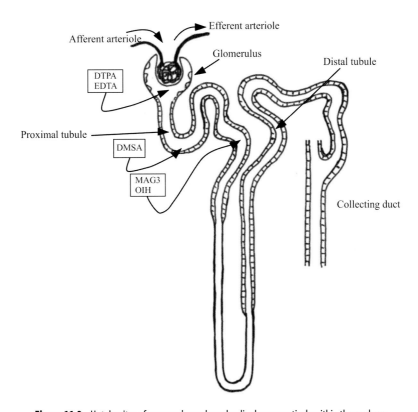

Figure 11.3. Uptake sites of commonly used renal radiopharmaceuticals within the nephron.

Strictly, an agent with an extraction efficiency of 1.0 is required to measure RPF but brief consideration of basic renal physiology shows that such an agent is impossible. The closest that can be achieved is about 0.9 and the best substance in this respect is the organic compound para-aminohippuric acid (PAH). In fact, it was considered such an important marker in renal physiology that a new physiological term, effective renal plasma flow (ERPF), was invented to describe its clearance. The substance used in nuclear medicine, ortho-iodohippurate (OIH), is a close relative of PAH, and has an extraction efficiency nearly as high. Over time, the clearance of OIH has itself become synonymous with ERPF.

Radiopharmaceuticals used for gamma camera renography include ^{99m}Tc diethylenetriamine-pentaacetic acid (DTPA), ^{123}I ortho-iodohippurate (OIH), and ^{99m}Tc mercaptoacetyl-triglycine (MAG3). ^{99m}Tc-MAG3 is the current agent of choice. Technetium-99m and iodine-123 have short physical half-lives (6 h and 13 h respectively), monoenergetic gamma ray emissions (140 keV and 159 keV respectively) and are both well suited to gamma camera imaging. ^{99m}Tc-

DMSA (2,3-dimercaptosuccinic acid) is used for static and SPECT imaging of the kidneys, and ^{51}Cr-EDTA is used for absolute measurement of GFR.

Although OIH, MAG3, DTPA, and DMSA are cleared from the blood by different renal mechanisms, and with different extraction efficiencies, all can, in general, be used to measure relative renal function from gamma camera imaging. The phenomenon responsible for this equivalence is glomerulo-tubular balance, which ensures that a change in GFR is paralleled by a change in proximal tubular reabsorption, i.e. the fractional tubular reabsorption is maintained essentially constant. This means that, although disease may cause the overall filtration fraction (FF) to vary, the FF for each kidney will be the same – explaining why either a glomerular or tubular agent may be used to determine relative renal function.

11.4.1 ^{99m}Tc-DTPA

Diethylenetriaminepenta-acetic acid (DTPA) is a physiologically inert compound that diffuses rapidly into the extravascular space following intravenous injection. Its molecular characteristics are such that it is cleared from the plasma purely by glomerular filtration. That is, the plasma clearance is the same as the renal clearance. Dynamic imaging with ^{99m}Tc-DTPA reveals rapid transit through the renal cortex with activity appearing in the collecting system within a few minutes. ^{99m}Tc-MAG3 is preferred for routine renography but DTPA is used when estimating individual kidney GFR (in ml/min) from the renogram (see Section 11.5.2). Some centers also use ^{99m}Tc-DTPA for blood-sample-based GFR measurement but ^{51}Cr-EDTA is generally preferred for this purpose (see Section 4.11).

11.4.2 ^{123}I-OIH

Ortho-iodohippurate (OIH) – also known as "Hippuran" – has a relatively high degree of protein binding and is cleared by a combination of glomerular filtration and, predominantly, tubular secretion. As a result, the extraction efficiency of OIH by the normal kidney (approximately 0.8) is much higher than that of DTPA (approximately 0.2). It is thus an excellent renal imaging agent but its use is severely limited by cost and, particularly, availability. The plasma clearance of ^{123}I-OIH can be used to estimate ERPF.

11.4.3 ^{99m}Tc-MAG3

While the renal extraction mechanism of MAG3 (mercaptoacetyltriglycine) is essentially the same as OIH, its clearance is only 50–60%. ERPF cannot be directly measured using MAG3, so a correction factor, based on correlation with OIH clearance, needs to be used.

Technetium-99m-MAG3 is now the agent of choice for all renographic procedures except absolute function renography (see Section 11.5.2). Its extraction efficiency is 2–3 times higher that ^{99m}Tc-DTPA but is lower than ^{123}I-OIH. Given the cost and supply problems associated with ^{123}I products, ^{99m}Tc-MAG3 currently represents the best compromise for routine dynamic imaging. It is a simple ^{99m}Tc kit, so can be made up at any time for urgent inpatient procedures. The advantage of using ^{99m}Tc-MAG3 over ^{99m}Tc-DTPA becomes more apparent as renal function deteriorates, but images will be of a generally higher contrast at all levels of renal function.

11.4.4 ^{99m}Tc-DMSA

^{99m}Tc-labeled DMSA (2,3-dimercaptosuccinic acid) is avidly taken up by cells of the proximal tubule, with about 35% of the injected activity being localized (bound) in the renal cortex by one hour. Renal uptake continues to rise, leveling off at about 6 hours post-injection, by which time about 50% of the injected dose can be accounted for. The remainder is cleared by other organs, primarily liver and spleen, but skeletal clearance is also a factor in infants.

As the degree of protein binding is still uncertain (probably somewhere in the range 75–90%) so is the exact renal uptake mechanism. Direct peritubular uptake of the bound fraction is probably the main effect but glomerular filtration/tubular reabsorption of the unbound fraction is also significant.

DMSA is subject to degradation due to oxidation and, if uncontrolled, will result in reduced renal uptake, increased background activity, and high liver uptake. For this reason, the radiopharmaceutical should be injected as soon as possible after reconstitution with ^{99m}Tc pertechnetate.

11.4.5 ^{51}Cr-EDTA

Like ^{99m}Tc-DTPA, ^{51}Cr ethylenediaminetetraacetic acid (EDTA) has very low binding to plasma proteins, is freely filterable at the glomerulus, and is not handled by the renal tubules. Extrarenal clearance is negligible and less than 1% remains in the body 24 hours after intravenous injection. The gamma radiation from ^{51}Cr can be easily measured in a well-type scintillation detector but the photon flux is too low for gamma camera imaging. In terms of radiochemical purity and stability ^{51}Cr-EDTA is slightly superior to ^{99m}Tc-DTPA and is the agent of choice for GFR determination in situations where renal imaging is not required. It is extremely well established and has been validated against inulin clearance (the ultimate substance for determination of GFR).

11.5 Renography

11.5.1 Basic Renography

In basic renography a contiguous series of 10 second duration digital images of the urinary tract

Table 11.3. Renography

Radiopharmaceutical	^{99m}Tc-MAG3
Application	Basic renography
Administered activity for adults	80 MBq (2.2 mCi)
Effective dose equivalent	0.6 mSv (60 mrem)
ARSAC DRL for adults	100 MBq (2.7 mCi)
Pediatric activity	Fraction of adult activity, based on body weight and subject to a minimum injected activity [1]
Patient preparation	Avoid dehydration; 500 ml oral fluid given 20–30 min before injection
Collimator	Low-energy general-purpose
Images acquired	Posterior dynamic study, 10 second frames for 30 minutes, to obtain renogram as described in Section 11.5.1. Acquired digital images summed every 2 minutes (15 images in all) to provide visual summary of the study
Radiopharmaceutical	^{99m}Tc-DTPA
Application	Basic renography
Administered activity for adults	150 MBq (4 mCi)
Effective dose equivalent	1 mSv (100 mrem)
ARSAC DRL for adults	300 MBq (8 mCi)
Pediatric activity	As for ^{99m}Tc-MAG3
Patient preparation	As for ^{99m}Tc-MAG3
Collimator	As for ^{99m}Tc-MAG3
Images acquired	As for ^{99m}Tc-MAG3

DRL, diagnostic reference level for injected activity (in adults) given in guidance notes issued by the UK Administration of Radioactive Substances Advisory Committee [2]. Lower activities should be used if practical (ALARP principle) and the activity quoted above for renography should be more than adequate using a modern gamma camera.

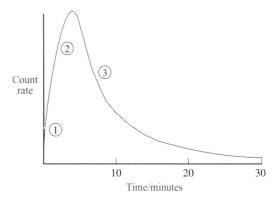

Figure 11.4. Normal renogram, showing first, second, and third phases.

11.4). The so-called "time–activity curve" (TAC) associated with an individual kidney is called a renogram.

As a pre-processing step, the extent of patient movement during the study is assessed by viewing the dynamic data in cine mode and, if necessary, corrected using special software. The renogram curves and associated images can be visually inspected to determine whether the drainage function from each kidney is normal or abnormal but, in this basic form, renography cannot determine the cause of any abnormal drainage.

Background Subtraction

The curve derived from a kidney ROI (i.e. the raw renogram) contains a "background" contribution from uptake in tissues over and underlying the kidney that must be removed prior to estimation of relative renal uptake/function. Indeed, the raw renogram can be thought of as a background curve on which the true renogram is superimposed. The background is composed of contributions from intravascular and extravascular activity. Furthermore, the intravascular component is itself composed of contributions from renal and non-renal blood vessels. Despite many years of research in this area, no single extrarenal ROI – or even combination of separate ROIs – has been found that contains intra- and extravascular components in exactly the same proportion as that found within the kidney ROI. Separate background ROIs placed perirenally (avoiding the pelvic area) or inferolaterally represent the best compromise of those tested (Figure 11.5).

As a result, this "simplistic" form of background subtraction tends to undercorrect the renogram

are recorded over a period of about 30 minutes following injection of a suitable radiopharmaceutical. The field of view should include the heart, kidneys, and at least part of the bladder. Details of the radiopharmaceuticals and their dosage levels are given in Table 11.3. Image processing is then performed using computer-generated regions of interest (ROI) in order to obtain graphs showing the variation of radioactive count rate with time within organs and tissues of interest (Figure

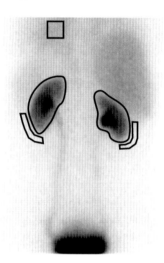

Figure 11.5. Summed images with regions of interest (ROI) superimposed. Separate background ROIs are shown for each kidney, placed infero-laterally. A heart region (square ROI) is also shown, which is used in the derivation of the output curve (see text).

for background activity, as it particularly underestimates the renal vascular component. As this effect can be asymmetric, it can occasionally lead to a significant error in the estimate of relative renal function (see below).

The quality of the background subtraction process can be crudely judged from the position of the y-axis intercept of the background subtracted renogram, a positive value indicating under-subtraction, and vice versa. Although simplistic background subtraction, when combined with the integral method (see below), will produce a good estimate of relative renal function in most cases, it is preferable to treat the intravascular and extravascular background components separately (see Rutland–Patlak method, below).

Estimation of Relative Renal Function

Although estimation of relative renal function is implicit in any renographic procedure, a renogram would not generally be performed if this were the only clinical requirement. In that case, a DMSA scan (Section 11.6) would be preferable as it is generally more accurate and certainly easier to perform. It should also be borne in mind particularly that renographic estimation of relative renal function (using posterior imaging only) is subject to significant systematic error in patients with conditions such as a pelvic kidney and nephroptosis,

where the kidneys can lie at markedly different depths and orientations. Despite these potential limitations, measurement of relative renal function is always an important part of any renogram report, even when, as is usually the case, the primary question relates to the underlying condition (e.g. obstruction, urinary reflux, etc.).

Integral Method

Up to the point at which excretion occurs, the relative uptake of glomerular or tubular agents is proportional to the individual renal clearance of the particular agent. The most straightforward method of estimating relative renal function therefore involves summing, or integrating, the counts under the respective background subtracted renogram curves (see above) between about 1 and 3 minutes after radiopharmaceutical injection. The relative function of the left kidney (LKF), for example, would be calculated as follows:

$$LKF(\%) = \frac{LKCC}{LKCC + RKCC} \times 100$$

where LKCC and RKCC are the integrated counts from the background corrected left and right renograms, respectively.

The starting point for integration corresponds to the end of the first phase of the renogram (Figure 11.4), by which time initial mixing within the renal vasculature is complete. Note that the point of inflection between the first and second phases may not always be seen, in which case the start point should be set at 1 minute. Elimination of activity from the kidney actually starts just before the peak of the renogram, so the endpoint for integration should be set at 30 seconds before the peak. The more normal kidney should always be used as the reference when setting the integration limits but a problem obviously arises when both renograms are abnormal (i.e. significantly delayed peaks, or no peak at all). In this case, a default integration period of 1–2.5 minutes should be used.

Rutland–Patlak Method

The so-called Rutland–Patlak (R–P) method was independently developed by the two named authors, but was popularized for renographic application by Rutland [3]. The method can appear obscure on first encounter but its importance derives from the way in which background activity is treated.

THE URINARY TRACT

Returning briefly to first principles, the observed ("raw") renogram derived from a kidney ROI can be thought of as a continuous function, $R'(t)$, which is simply the sum of the true renal activity and the tissue background activity. That is:

$$R'(t) = R(t) + B(t)$$

where $R'(t)$ = observed renogram, $R(t)$ = true renogram, and $B(t)$ = background curve.

The background term, $B(t)$, is composed of contributions from intravascular and extravascular activity, so:

$$R'(t) = R(t) + B_i(t) + B_e(t)$$

where $B_i(t)$ = intravascular background activity and $B_e(t)$ = extravascular background activity.

Furthermore, the intravascular component is itself composed of contributions from renal and non-renal blood vessels. Up to the time at which activity starts to leave the kidney (i.e. the minimum transit time, t_1) the kidney acts as a simple integrator with respect to its input function, $I(t)$. If the fraction of blood activity taken up per unit time is denoted as f_1 (known as the uptake constant), the pure renal activity will be equal to the total input up to time t_1:

$$R(t) = f_1 \int_0^{t_1} I(t) dt.$$

Ideally the blood input ROI should be placed over the renal artery but this is somewhat impractical and it is acceptable to use the left ventricle instead.

The intravascular background curve, $B_i(t)$, can be expressed as a given fraction, f_2, of the blood input curve itself, thus:

$$B_i(t) = f_2 . I(t).$$

Combining equations, we get:

$$R'(t) = f_1 \int_0^{t_1} I(t).dt + f_2 . I(t) + B_e(t).$$

The background subtraction process can thus be described by the following equation:

$$R(t) = R'(t) - [B_i(t) + B_e(t)].$$

It is convenient to deal with the background components separately, so background correction is a two-stage process. First, the extravascular component (mostly the result of uptake in the interstitial tissues) is removed by recourse to an appropriate (extrarenal) background ROI (see section on background subtraction, above).

We can thus define a renogram curve, $R''(t)$, that has been corrected for extravascular background activity, but not intravascular.

$$R''(t) = R'(t) - B_e(t) = f_1 \int_0^{t_1} I(t).dt + f_2 . I(t).$$

In fact, the "background ROI" method partially corrects the intravascular background (by virtue of the fact that a perirenal ROI contains a contribution from contained blood vessels) but it particularly underestimates the background contribution of intrarenal blood vessels.

However, if we divide both sides of the above equation by I(t) we obtain the so-called Rutland–Patlak equation:

$$\frac{R''(t)}{I(t)} = f_1 \cdot \frac{\int_0^{t_1} I(t) \cdot dt}{I(t)} + f_2.$$

The motivation for this seemingly arbitrary act is that plotting $R''(t)/I(t)$ against

$$\int_0^{t_1} I(t) \cdot dt / I(t)$$

yields a straight line of slope f_1 and y-intercept f_2. The key point is that the slope (f_1) is unaffected by the amount of vascular background activity present within the renal ROI, so a measurement of relative renal uptake (function) based on the respective f_1 values is automatically corrected for intravascular background. The amount of blood background present is in fact reflected in the f_2 intercept value. It is important to emphasize that this graphical method does not account for the extravascular component of the background signal, so this must be separately removed, as described above.

In practice we find that, even using MAG3, the R-P plot is non-linear over the first few minutes (Figure 11.6), due to early clearance of tracer from the kidney and accumulation of tracer in the extravascular space. To minimize the variability in measured slope (f_2), the curve fitting routine should be restricted to between 1 minute after injection and a full minute before the observed renogram peak. If a delayed peak is observed

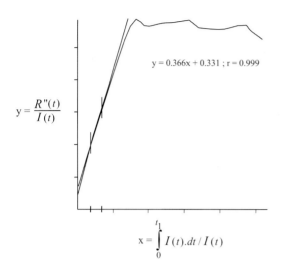

$$y = \frac{R''(t)}{I(t)}$$

$$y = 0.366x + 0.331 \; ; \; r = 0.999$$

$$x = \int_{0}^{t_1} I(t).dt / I(t)$$

Figure 11.6. Typical Rutland–Patlak (R-P) plot, derived from a normal background subtracted renogram ($R(t)$) and blood input (heart) curve ($I(t)$). The renogram data (R-P plot relates to right kidney) is shown in Figure 11.9B. The fitted line straight line is superimposed on the upslope part of the curve, starting at 1 minute after injection. The vertical marker lines on the curve indicate the portion of the curve over which the line was fitted, and the equation of the line is output. If the correlation coefficient is below 0.995 the derived renal function estimate will be subject to significant error and an alternative method (i.e. integral method) should be used.

(>5 minutes) a default fitting period of 1.0–2.5 minutes should be used [4]. Compared to the integral method, the R-P method only additionally requires an ROI to be placed over the heart, the time–activity curve from which is also required for the calculation of output efficiency (Section 11.5.4).

Interpretation

When interpreting the renogram it is important to bear in mind that it is a record of what is left behind in the kidney (not what is "coming out"), the amount of radiopharmaceutical left behind at any given time depending on rate of input and tubular transit time, as well as the rate of loss.

The normal renogram curve has three identifiable phases (Figure 11.4). The first and second phases represent, respectively, arrival of radiopharmaceutical in the kidney vasculature, followed by uptake and transit through the nephrons. The arrival of the first bolus of activity represents the largest "input" to the kidney. The successive ones, resulting from recirculation of non-extracted tracer, become progressively smaller due to the large fraction of the input that is

removed on each passage through the kidney, and general mixing within the circulation. Meanwhile, activity that has been "taken up" by the kidney (a phrase that covers glomerular filtration and/or tubular secretion) passes relatively slowly along the tubular lumen (transit time $\approx$ 2–3 minutes) before emptying into the collecting ducts and, subsequently, the renal pelvis. The net result of these simultaneous processes is that the radiopharmaceutical content of the kidney (i.e. the renogram) rises sharply after the initial arrival of the injection and then more slowly. The change in slope which is often seen at approximately 45 seconds after injection (marking the end of the first phase) is an artifact produced by a combination of a rapidly rising renal component and a rapidly falling background component.

When activity starts to be eliminated from the renal pelvis (into the ureter and bladder), a sharp fall in activity from the kidney area will be recorded which, following a rising second phase, therefore produces a peak. Excretion from the kidney is the dominant feature at this stage and the renogram falls sharply for a few minutes. The downslope thereafter becomes progressively less steep as smaller and smaller amounts of activity are excreted from the kidney. It is, however, important to remember that, even at this stage, the relatively small amount of radiopharmaceutical in the plasma which has thus far bypassed the renal extraction mechanism remains in circulation and continues to present an input to the kidney. The third phase of the renogram therefore reflects continuing input and tubular transit, as well as loss through excretion. With this model it is simple to explain how a prerenal disorder like renal artery stenosis can give rise to an impaired third phase, and it has nothing to do with "lack of excretion". Similarly, labeling the third phase as the "excretion phase" makes it impossible to explain the phenomenon whereby abrupt fluctuations in renal blood flow (caused by anxiety or pain) can produce "humps" in the latter stages of the renogram.

11.5.2 Absolute Function Renography

The most accurate and reliable way to estimate both absolute and relative renal function from a "single" study is to effectively combine a basic renogram with a standard (multi-sample) GFR measurement, the benefit for the patient being that both tests can be performed in a single visit using a single injection, usually ^{99m}Tc-DTPA. Although the renogram curves will be "noisy" when renal function is poor, relative renal function can still be estimated with acceptable accuracy down to a GFR level of about 20 ml/min. However, in such situations it is wise to calculate relative function using two different renographic methods (Section 11.5.1).

11.5.3 Indirect Radionuclide Cystography

Indirect radionuclide cystography (IRC) is effectively a combination of a basic renogram (i.e. without furosemide) and a subsequent relatively short dynamic study monitoring free voiding into a receptacle (voiding study). The purpose of this test is to detect vesico-ureteric reflux (VUR), which may be seen during physiological filling of the bladder (i.e. during the renogram) – so-called low pressure reflux – or, more commonly, just after the onset of voiding when the bladder pressure is high. VUR is an obvious source of upper urinary tract infection (UTI), which can lead to pyelonephritic scarring and hypertension (see Section 11.6).

At the completion of a 30-minute renogram at least 80% of the injected activity should be in the bladder. Clearly, the voiding phase has to be delayed until the patient (usually a child) feels able to void on demand, which limits the method to cooperative toilet-trained children. For younger children, a bladder catheter needs to be employed and radiographic micturating cystourethrography (MCU) is preferred over direct radionuclide cystography since it offers relevant anatomical information (e.g. posterior urethral valves, ureteric dilatation) as well as the detection and grading of reflux itself. However, the MCU is a distinctly unpleasant procedure for children with an attendant risk of infection and a relative high radiation dose. The IRC should therefore be employed whenever possible for children over the age of about 3 years, including follow-up patients first diagnosed using MCU.

Technique

For the voiding part of an indirect study, study girls are seated on an imaging chair/commode with their backs to the gamma camera and boys are stood, back to camera, holding a urine bottle. The computer is set up to acquire 5 second frames for approximately 5 minutes. At least 30 seconds worth of data should be acquired before the child is given the signal to void to allow establishment of baseline activity levels in both kidneys and bladder. Recording is continued for a couple of minutes after completion of micturition to assess natural bladder refilling. Finally, the volume of urine voided is measured and recorded.

Even if there is considerable residual activity in the renal collecting system (e.g. due to hydronephrosis) at the time when the child needs to void, the cystogram should still be recorded as it is possible to detect gross reflux despite the masking effect of this residual activity. In these circumstances, however, a negative study is inconclusive, so should be repeated when activity has cleared from the kidneys and the bladder has refilled naturally, possibly following further oral hydration.

Patients presenting with known/suspected upper tract dilatation, as well as suspected VUR, present a difficulty since, ideally, activity in the kidneys should be cleared before the cystogram starts. Administration of intravenous furosemide (frusemide) at 15 minutes (F + 15) will effectively eliminate activity from the renal pelvis in patients with non-obstructive dilatation, and this has been advocated [5], but there are two potential disadvantages to the use for furosemide in this setting. Firstly, in some patients with an already nearly full bladder, intravenous furosemide will bring on the urgent need to micturate and may even necessitate terminating the renography study early, possibly missing the chance to properly record the act of voiding. Secondly, and more importantly, it has been reported that furosemide can inhibit VUR in patients in whom it would otherwise occur [6]. For the present time, a reasonable strategy would be to administer furosemide, if clinically indicated, during the first appointment. If the subsequent indirect cystogram shows VUR even under conditions of increased urine flow, then no further study is needed. If, however, the cystogram is negative, it should be repeated without furosemide.

Interpretation

The renogram part of the study is processed in the usual manner (see Section 11.5.1) except that a bladder ROI is created in addition to the kidney ROIs. If the third phase of the renogram has a "saw-tooth" appearance, it may be due to either low pressure reflux or a peristaltic abnormality ("hesitancy"). To make a confident diagnosis of reflux, the renogram peaks and troughs should be out of phase with similar perturbations in the bladder curve (Figure 11.7).

For the cystogram study, a careful check for patient movement should be made prior to image processing. ROIs/time–activity curves are then created for the kidneys and the whole of the bladder. There is no need for background ROIs. A normal study shows no significant increase in renal activity in the period immediately before or after voiding. The bladder curve shows a sharp fall in activity corresponding to voiding itself, then levels off. An abnormal study is one that shows one or more "humps" in one or both kidney curves in the period after voiding, corresponding to a transient rise in renal activity due to reflux. The bladder may then refill with previously refluxed urine due to a "yo-yo" effect, which is a useful indicator of reflux (see Figure 11.8).

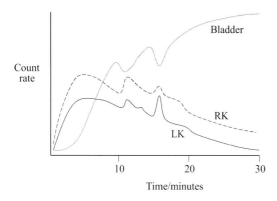

Figure 11.7. Renogram curves showing bilateral "low pressure" reflux during normal physiological filling of the bladder. Note how the peaks in the renogram curve correspond to troughs in the bladder curve, confirming retrograde flow of urine from bladder into the kidneys.

11.5.4 Diuresis Renography

Diuresis renography is the primary diagnostic tool for upper urinary tract obstruction in both adults and children, although there is still debate about the reliability of a positive test in infants with antenatally diagnosed hydronephrosis. An implicit assumption of the technique is that a true obstruction will be present at high and low urine flow rates, thereby justifying a technique which assesses the response of the kidney to flow rates that are well above the normal range. In fact, the

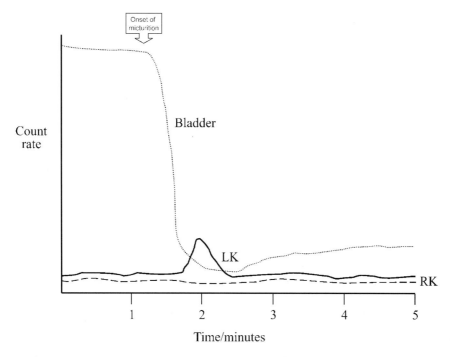

Figure 11.8. Voiding stage of an indirect radionuclide cystogram. The peak in the left kidney (LK) curve (bold line) indicates vesico-ureteric reflux occurring at the onset of micturition. The flat right kidney (RK) curve (- - line) is normal. The subsequent rise in the bladder curve (. . . line) indicates refilling from above (i.e. the left kidney), confirming the diagnosis of left-sided reflux.

maximal total diuresis produced by intravenous furosemide (0.5 mg/kg) in an adult patient with normal renal function is around 20 ml/min, which is about twenty times normal.

Technique

The method is essentially that for basic renography (Section 11.5.1), augmented by diuretic administration. Furosemide, the drug of choice, is rapidly injected at around 15 minutes after the radiopharmaceutical, which allows the effect of the drug on the renogram to be properly appreciated. If the renogram duration is 30 minutes the notation is $\{F + 15; t = 30\}$. The furosemide dosage is 1.0 mg/kg in infants (0–1 year) and 0.5 mg/kg in children and adults.

If activity remains in either renal collecting system at the end of the study, pre- and post-void static images should be acquired. As part of this process, both the time of micturition and voided volume are recorded, thus permitting the average urine flow rate to be calculated, which provides a useful assessment of the adequacy of diuresis.

The dynamic images should be processed as for basic renography, with the additional calculation of output efficiency (OE) for quantifying the effect of furosemide [7]. In order to use the normal range values given in Table 11.4, the measurement must be made at 30 minutes (OE_{30}), and the furosemide given at between 15 and 20 minutes. The hard copy output should include the input and output curves from which the OE measurement was derived (Figure 11.9).

Interpretation

The renographic response to furosemide depends on a number of factors, including individual renal function, baseline urine flow rate (hence hydration), flow rate induced by diuretic (hence furosemide dosage), renal pelvic volume at time of administration, elasticity of the wall of the renal pelvis, and degree of ureteric peristalsis. The central problem of interpretation therefore lies in deciding whether the rate of fall of the renogram following furosemide is appropriate for that kidney.

Total average urine flow rates measured after furosemide injection (0.5 mg/kg) are generally in the range 8–15 ml/min, although values above 20 ml/min are not uncommon. A value of less than 5 ml/min (in an adult) represents an inadequate diuresis (kidneys have not been sufficient stressed) and the associated furosemide responses should be interpreted with caution. The effect of voiding is assessed by comparison of the pre- and post-void static images. In some patients, the stasis in the renal pelvis will drain spontaneously immediately after voiding, thus excluding significant obstruction.

Obstructive and non-obstructive hydronephrosis have a characteristic appearance on the renogram post-furosemide (Figure 11.10) providing that the affected kidney GFR is above 15 ml/min. The renographic response to furosemide can then be called non-obstructive if the fall in the curve is rapid, substantial and has a concave slope [8]. A renogram curve which shows no (or very little) decline post-furosemide is classified as obstructive. Drainage patterns falling between these extremes represent an equivocal response, and will be seen in 10–15% of cases, usually the result of impaired (individual) renal function and/or gross renal pelvic dilatation. A fourth response (the so-called "Homsy sign") is sometimes seen where an initial positive renographic response to furosemide is followed by a premature leveling off or a rise (Figure 11.11), which is indicative of high flow or intermittent obstruction [9]. Output efficiency measurement is particularly useful in the assessment of equivocal responses and will reduce the rate to about 5%. Simple curve indices such as clearance half-times do not have sufficient discriminatory ability in this context [10].

The small group of patients whose results remain equivocal after output efficiency analysis should be retested, this time giving the furosemide at 15 minutes before the radiopharmaceutical $\{F - 15; t = 20\}$, based on the fact that furosemide produces its maximal effect about 15 minutes after injection [9]. Some centers use $F - 15$ renography as a first-line technique, but this does not permit a before and after assessment, and requires routine furosemide administration to all patients. With $F + 15$ renography, the decision to administer the drug can be delayed until the need is clear. Some pediatric centers give the

Table 11.4. Classification of output efficiency measured at 30 minutes (OE_{30}), with furosemide given at 15 minutes

OE_{30} (%)	Diagnosis
>78%	No obstruction
<70%	Obstruction
70–78%	Equivocal

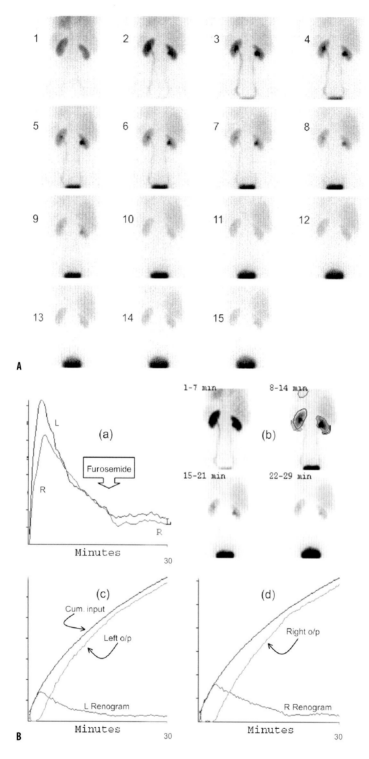

Figure 11.9. **A** Summarized image data from a 30-minute dynamic study in an adult, whereby 180 images are condensed down to 15; each new image thus representing 2 minutes of data. The study clearly demonstrates the normal passage of injected tracer (^{99m}Tc-MAG3) from blood to urine via the kidneys. There is also some hepatobiliary clearance of MAG3, hence the liver uptake.
B Curve data presentation for reporting, showing **a** the background subtracted renograms, **b** a selected of summed images covering the 30-minute study (with ROIs superimposed on one image), **c, d** the left and right output (o/p) curves (for calculation of output efficiency), derived from the respective renograms and the cumulative input curves (see Piepsz et al [4]). Relative renal function was calculated as: left = 63%, R = 37%, and output efficiency at 30 minutes (OE30) calculated as: left = 96%, right = 95%. The right kidney relative function was slightly below the lower limit of normal but the renogram shows no evidence of outflow tract obstruction. Furosemide was given at 16 minutes (prompting accelerated washout) but both renogram curves were already clearly descending at this point.

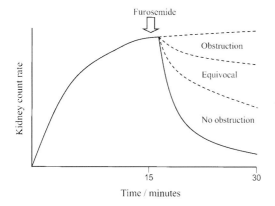

Figure 11.10. Possible renographic responses to furosemide injected 15 minutes after injection of the radiopharmaceutical {F + 15, t = 30} in a kidney with a dilated collecting system. A "washout" phenomenon is observed in non-obstructed systems, causing a rapid fall in the renogram curve.

furosemide immediately after the radiopharmaceutical (F + 0) in an attempt to keep the study duration to a minimum [11], but this has the same disadvantages as the F − 15 approach.

Renographic tests also have a useful role in the assessment of lower ureteric obstruction, particularly in excluding significant obstruction in patients with dilated ureters on IVU. Although diuresis renography was primarily designed to diagnose upper tract obstruction, the concept of furosemide-induced washout can also be applied to the ureter. It should be noted that the presence of lower tract disorders also has an important bearing on the interpretation of upper tract obstruction [12].

11.5.5 Transit Time Analysis

The main clinical application of renal transit times is in the diagnosis of upper urinary tract obstruction. Briefly, when upper tract obstruction occurs, the pressure gradient between the glomerulus and the obstruction site is altered (i.e. the pressure in the renal pelvis and the tubular lumen rises). The kidney responds by passively increasing the reabsorption of salt and water in the proximal tubule, triggered by the obstruction-associated pressure difference between the tubular lumen and the peritubular capillary. The net result is that any non-reabsorbable solute (like OIH, DTPA or MAG3) will be concentrated in a smaller volume of filtrate, thus prolonging its tubular (parenchymal) transit time.

Pelvic (and hence whole kidney) transit times will be prolonged in cases of obstructive and non-obstructive hydronephrosis, and will not therefore provide a differential diagnosis. In fact, the whole kidney mean transit time (WKMTT) is directly related to the patient's state of hydration and is therefore meaningless unless this is strictly controlled. The parenchymal mean transit time (PMTT) is unaffected by the state of hydration, but is dependent on urine flow rate, a first order correction for which is provided by subtracting the minimum PTT from the mean PPT to yield the corrected PPT (CPTT). In the absence of other conditions known to cause prolonged transit (e.g. renovasuclar hyptertension), a CPTT of greater than 4 minutes in a patient with renal pelvic dilatation indicates obstructive nephropathy.

Deconvolution Techniques

The shape of the renogram is dependent on the rate of tracer input, tubular transit time, and rate of loss. The fact that the input function varies with time is a further complicating factor since it is subject to physiological effects that are unrelated to renal function. Also, for a given input function, there will be a spread of transit times due to the fact that nephrons of a given type vary in length, and there are two different populations of nephrons within the kidney (see Section 11.2). The renogram is therefore a complex curve from which transit times cannot be directly measured. The renographic time-to-peak gives a crude estimate of parenchymal transit time, but a purer representation of renal transit is required for its accurate measurement. This purer function, "hidden" within the renogram, is called the renal retention function (RRF), and mathematical techniques are required to extract it.

The RRF can be thought of as an internal property of a particular kidney that determines how the input (blood curve) is converted into an output (i.e. the observed renogram) (Figure 11.12). Mathematically speaking, the input function is convolved with the retention function to produce the output function. The problem therefore is to deconvolve the input function from the output function to produce the retention function.

The convolution operation is represented by the following equation:

$$R(t) = \int_0^t I(\tau) \cdot H(t - \tau) d\tau$$

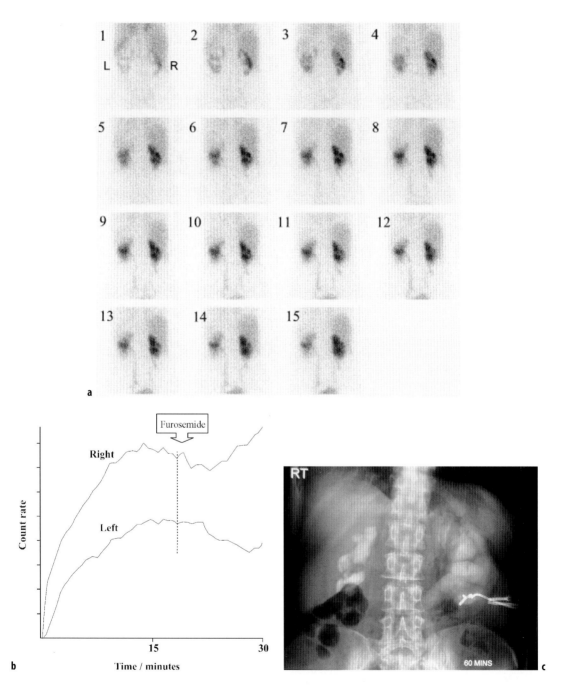

Figure 11.11. MAG3 renogram study in a 46-year-old female patient with a distal left ureteric stenosis and a blocked nephrostomy, showing **a** summary of dynamic images covering a period of 30 minutes, **b** renogram curves, and **c** contemporary IVU. The images **a** show a grossly hydronephrotic kidney with specific abnormality in the upper pole. There is evidently impaired drainage from both upper tracts. The curve data **b** show an equivocal response to furosemide on the left. The right kidney renogram shows the "Homsy sign" where an initial response to furosemide is followed by a pronounced rise. The IVU **c** shows the pigtail catheter in place in the lower pole of the left kidney, which is hydronephrotic. The left ureter is dilated. The right kidney also shows impaired drainage, as well as cortical thinning and scarring.

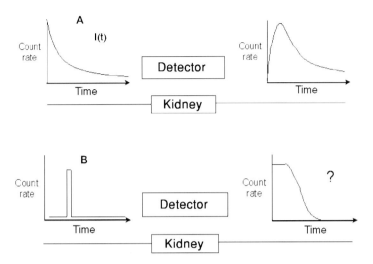

Figure 11.12. The kidney depicted as a linear system. Input is converted to output via the kidney's impulse response (or retention) function. Knowledge of the actual input and output functions **A** allows calculation, via deconvolution, of the retention function. This represents the response of the kidney (depicted as ?) to a simpler, idealized, input **B** .

where $R(t)$ = response of kidney to input, $I(\tau)$, $H(t)$ = retention function (also called the impulse response function or transfer function), and τ is a continuous variable representing time.

Solving the above equation for $H(t)$ is called deconvolution and several techniques are available, including the matrix method [13], transform methods [14], constrained optimization [15] and, most recently, a method based on differentiation of the Rutland–Patlak plot [16]. The matrix method of deconvolution is certainly the most widely used clinically, but is subject to a number of potential pitfalls.

The retention function, $H(t)$, represents the response of the system to a unit impulse, i.e. a rectangular ("delta") function having unit area but infinitesimally narrow width (see Figure 11.12). Such an input cannot be achieved in clinical practice but could be approximated by a rapid bolus injection given directly into the renal artery with no recirculation. The renal retention function, $H(t)$, can therefore be thought of as the renogram that would be produced if we could perform such an idealized injection. It therefore represents the simplest form of renogram imaginable and should provide a clearer insight into the pathophysiological processes affecting renal transport mechanisms than that derivable from the background subtracted renogram. The general shape of the normal retention function is shown in Figure 11.13.

The mean transit time, MTT, can be calculated according to the expression:

$$MTT = \frac{\int_{0}^{\infty} H(t)\, dt}{H(0)}.$$

$H(0)$, the amplitude of plateaued retention function at $t = 0$, will equal unity by definition since $H(t)$ is a fraction. The mean transit time is therefore simply the total area under the RF curve (up to the point at which it crosses the time axis) divided by the initial plateau height. Negative excursions of the retention function are non-physiological, and any data points giving rise to such variations should be set to zero.

The main assumptions made in the foregoing discussion are that the response of the kidney to a series of impulse inputs is simply the sum of the individual impulse responses. Since a continuous input function can be regarded as a series of impulse inputs, the corresponding output function (i.e. the renogram) can therefore be predicted by convolving the input function with the impulse response function. Secondly, that ERPF, GFR, and urine flow rate must all remain constant for the duration of the test. Normal physiological fluctuations in urine flow rate are such that they are effectively smoothed out using an acquisition frame time of 10–20 seconds and can usually be ignored. Fluctuations in renal blood flow can be minimized

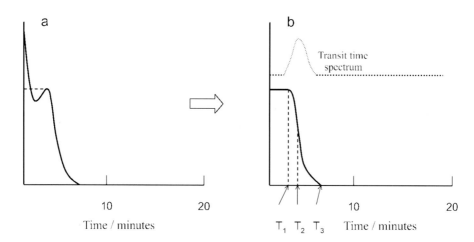

Figure 11.13. The normal retention function showing **a** the initial vascular spike, and **b** the "plateaued" version with vascular spike removed. The spread of transit times, illustrated by the superimposed transit time spectrum, gives rise to the gradual rather than the abrupt fall in the retention function. T_1 = minimum transit time, T_2 = mean transit time, and T_3 = maximum transit time, which refer to the renal ROI (either parenchymal or whole kidney) from which they were indirectly derived.

by ensuring that the patient is as relaxed and comfortable as possible, excellent injection technique (i.e. avoiding pain and anxiety), and conducting the study in a quiet environment. In short, the success of transit time analysis is dependent on attention to detail, and close adherence to published validated methods.

Comparison of Transit Time Analysis and Furosemide Response

The renographic response to furosemide (see Section 11.5.4) and parenchymal transit time measurement (Section 11.5.5) are complementary techniques, since they assess obstructive uropathy and the obstructive nephropathy, respectively. Although direct comparisons have shown that transit time measurement and furosemide response perform similarly in the diagnosis of upper tract obstruction, the furosemide test is regarded as the primary diagnostic tool as it provides a more direct assessment and is easier for urologists to comprehend. After relief of obstruction, urinary drainage from the renal pelvis will improve before any associated improvement in parenchymal function, so diuresis renography will therefore provide an earlier indication of surgical outcome.

It is perfectly feasible to derive transit time data from an F + 15 renogram (using data acquired before the administration of furosemide), so it

is helpful to do this routinely, thereby providing complementary information in all cases. Since a heart ROI/TAC is already required for the measurement of output efficiency (Section 11.5.4) and the Rutland–Patlak plot (Section 11.5.1), the only addition to the processing method is the definition of parenchymal ROIs.

11.5.6 Perfusion Renography

Perfusion renography describes a technique whereby a short (40 second) period of relatively rapid fast framing (frame rate = 1/s) precedes the basic renogram acquisition. The resultant "split-frame" study thus comprises a "perfusion phase" followed by a "function phase". The technique has been used in the context of renal transplantation (Section 11.5.8) and renovascular hypertension (RVH). For the latter, it was reasonably assumed that assessing the relative perfusion of the kidneys might hold the key to diagnosing renal artery stenosis (RAS), but clinical results (with and without ACE inhibition) have been disappointing. The technique is now of purely historical interest in this context, having been replaced by captopril renography.

11.5.7 Captopril Renography

The diagnosis of RVH (i.e. functionally significant RAS) is essentially retrospective, so the key question relates to prognosis: can renography reliably predict those patients who will benefit from revascularization, in terms of blood pressure response and/or improvement in renal function? To understand the role of captopril in this setting requires brief consideration of the renin-angiotensin system.

When a severe (>70%) narrowing of the renal artery causes a reduction in renal blood flow which cannot be "compensated" by the autoregulation system, the glomerular perfusion pressure falls. As a result, the kidney secretes an enzyme called renin that, in turn, acts on a plasma protein called angiotensinogen to form angiotensin I. Angiotensin converting enzyme (ACE) then acts on angiotensin I to produce angiotensin II, which is a potent vasoconstrictor at the arteriolar level, acting directly upon peripheral and intrarenal blood vessels to raise systemic and renal perfusion pressure. Captopril, a so-called ACE inhibitor, blocks the conversion of angiotensin I to angiotensin II, thereby removing the mechanism by which the affected kidney's perfusion pressure is maintained, causing individual kidney GFR to fall in patients with RVH.

Technique

In its conventional form, captopril renography actually comprises two separate renograms, one to act as baseline and another one hour after oral administration of 25 mg captopril. The order in which the studies are conducted varies between centers but both are routinely performed when the objective is to measure the change in renal function following ACE inhibition. If the baseline study is performed first, the whole test can be completed in one day without hospital admission.

The main intrarenal effect of ACE inhibition is on GFR and it is therefore logical to use a glomerular imaging agent such as ^{99m}Tc-DTPA in this context. However, the quality of the DTPA kidney image falls dramatically as renal function decreases, making changes in renal function difficult to detect in these patients. Tubular agents such as ^{123}I-OIH and ^{99m}Tc-MAG3 have better imaging properties but the observed renographic changes are sometimes more difficult to interpret.

Interpretation

Several renographic parameters have been tested in this setting. As a minimum, relative function (Section 11.5.1) should be estimated for both studies. A significant fall in the contribution of the affected kidney (after captopril) is taken as an indication of functionally significant unilateral RAS. A significant fall has been stated as a shift of >5% (i.e. 5 percentage points) to a value below 40% [17]. The use of relative function alone as a monitoring tool is of course subject to the fundamental disadvantage that an observed change may be due to improved function on one side or deterioration on the other. It would therefore appear advantageous to perform absolute function renography (Section 11.5.2) with and without captopril. Renographic time-to-peak and/or parenchymal mean transit time (Section 11.5.5) are also routinely calculated in some centers.

Disease prevalence is a key issue in this context, so it is essential to select only those hypertensive patients with a medium-to-high pre-test probability of RVH (e.g. moderate-to-severe hypertension in a young patient (25 years), sudden onset, sudden worsening of previously controlled hypertension, unresponsive to antihypertensive drug therapy).

Varying sensitivities and specificities have been reported for captopril renography in the diagnosis of RVH, largely explained by the varying prevalence of the disease in the populations studied, and differences in scintigraphic methodology. A pooled average of recent reports (for ^{99m}Tc-DTPA) gives a sensitivity of 76% and specificity of 90%, based on changes in renographic parameters. Analogous results for the post-captopril study alone were 92% and 66% respectively [18]. Generally, the sensitivity of the test falls as the level of function in the affected kidney decreases.

Captopril renography is less reliable in the evaluation of bilateral RAS. Apart from the fact that changes in renographic parameters expressed as left-to-right ratios become difficult to interpret, RVH arising from bilateral RAS is much less renin dependent than unilateral RAS. As a consequence, the effect of ACE inhibition on renal function is less marked, and sensitivity of the captopril test is therefore reduced. In bilateral disease, the test will only tend to identify the more stenosed kidney as abnormal, and angioplasty on this side alone may not ameliorate the hypertension.

11.5.8 Transplant Renography

Transplant renography is simply perfusion renography (Section 11.5.6) applied to the renal transplant. The gamma camera is positioned anteriorally over the allograft, usually located in the iliac fossa (Figure 11.14).

For the perfusion phase, ROIs are created for the transplant itself, a background area, and adjacent iliac artery. The "perfusion index" (PI) is derived from the associated time–activity curves (Figure 11.15). For the function phase, the transplant ROI is used with the background ROI to generate a transplant renogram. The typical renogram from a functioning transplant is similar in shape to that derived from a normal native kidney but often has a delayed/flattened peak due, in part, to prolonged parenchymal transit of tracer.

An isolated PI value will not reliably differentiate the main acute medical complications of transplantation (acute rejection and acute tubular necrosis). Repeating the renogram every 2–3 days during the early transplant period is more useful (sudden fall in the PI trend can predict impending rejection) but the fall may only precipitate the rise in serum creatinine by 24 hours, and performing frequent renograms on all transplant patients is a huge undertaking, even for a well-resourced nuclear medicine department. In both Europe and the USA, routine transplant renography thus became perceived as a high cost/small benefit procedure and was already in slow decline when a new breed of immunosuppressive agents appeared in the early 1980s, prompting a further fall in popularity due the fact that (a) acute rejection became less frequent and more controllable and (b) the associated mild nephrotoxity associated with ciclosporin A made diagnosis of rejection based on PI even more difficult. The more routine use of renal biopsy and developments in other imaging modalities techniques (especially Doppler ultrasound) means that transplant renography is now rarely used to diagnose rejection. It is, however, still used to investigate suspected surgical and urological complications (Figure 11.16).

11.6 Static and SPECT Renal Imaging Using ^{99m}Tc-DMSA

The uptake mechanism of DMSA was discussed in Section 11.4. Clearly, a renal agent that is effectively fixed in the renal cortex provides an ideal means of estimating relative function without interference from overlying pelvicalyceal activity. The two main indications for ^{99m}Tc-DMSA imaging are thus accurate measurement of relative renal function (in various clinical settings) and the diagnosis of renal scarring in the presence of urinary tract infection (UTI). Indeed, the DMSA scan is regarded as a reference technique in both areas.

UTI is associated with vesico-ureteric reflux and pyelonephritic scarring. The detection of VUR was discussed in Section 11.5.3. In this section we consider the effect of urinary reflux on the kidney (reflux nephropathy), which is investigated primarily using renal ultrasound and ^{99m}Tc-DMSA imaging. The aim is to detect renal scarring, which has prognostic implications for the development of hypertension and end-stage renal failure, although the latter is very rare. About 10% of children with UTI will develop scars, usually as a result of the first episode and, of these, about 10% will develop consequential hypertension in later life.

SPECT imaging of the kidneys should theoretically improve the detection of renal scars but there is no consensus on the clinical usefulness of SPECT imaging in children. SPECT studies invariably detect more defects than planar imaging but doubt remains as to the true clinical significance of these additional "abnormalities", particularly as there are more normal variants to consider. Predictably, inter-observer variability is higher than for static imaging, although this may represent a "learning curve problem". The addition of SPECT imaging obviously extends the total imaging time considerably so will be resisted in pediatric circles until such time as the clinical benefits are clearer. In summary, SPECT imaging of the kidneys is not currently recommended for routine clinical use.

11.6.1 Static Imaging Technique

General and child-specific procedure guidelines have been developed [19, 20]. High-resolution images should be obtained in the anterior, posterior, and posterior oblique projections. Details of the acquisition protocol are shown in Table 11.5. The basic relative uptake measurement is simple to perform but must be corrected for both background activity and for differences in kidney depth. The latter correction is less important in children than adults but is recommended for all patients. The correction is achieved by simply calculating the geometric mean of the anterior and posterior count rates for each kidney and expressing the result as a ratio. If a dual-head gamma camera is used the anterior and posterior views can be acquired simultaneously.

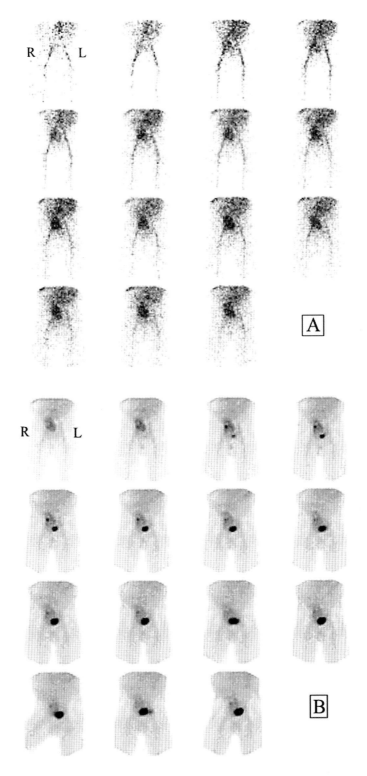

Figure 11.14. Normal anterior perfusion images **A**, acquired at 7 days post-transplant showing aortic bifurcation, iliac arteries, and renal transplant. The 15 3-second images were derived from the acquired dataset of 45 1-second images, initiated a few seconds after bolus injection of ^{99m}Tc-DTPA. The summarized function phase **B** show uptake in the transplant and prompt excretion into the adjacent bladder. The 15 1.3-minute frames were derived from an acquired dataset of 60 20-second frames. (Images courtesy of Dr M. Keir, Royal Victoria Infirmary, Newcastle.)

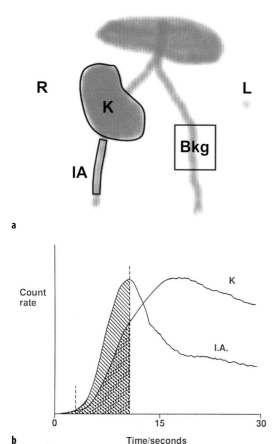

a

b

Figure 11.15. Processing of the perfusion part of a transplant renogram showing **a** position of whole kidney (K), background (Bkg) and iliac artery (IA) ROIs and **b** associated normal time–activity curves. The kidney curve is background subtracted. After area normalization of the kidney and iliac artery curves, the perfusion index (PI) is defined as the ratio of areas under the two curves (iliac artery/kidney) up to the peak of the iliac artery curve. In this example, the PI is 1.3.

The contribution of the left kidney to total renal function is thus calculated using the formula:

$$LKF(\%) = 100 \times LKGM/(LKGM + RKGM).$$

LKGM and RKGM are the geometric means of anterior and posterior counts from the left and right kidneys, after background subtraction.

Right kidney relative function (RKF) can be independently calculated using an analogous expres-

Table 11.5. Renal imaging

Radiopharmaceutical	^{99m}Tc-DMSA
Application	Static renal imaging for assessment of relative renal function and pyelonephritic scarring
Administered activity for adults	80 MBq (2.2 mCi)
Effective dose equivalent	0.7 mSv (70 mrem)
Pediatric activity	As for ^{99m}Tc-MAG3
Patient preparation	None
Collimator	ow-energy, high-resolution
Images acquired	Images should be acquired at approximately 3 hours post-injection, and include anterior, posterior, left and right posterior oblique views. Use appropriate acquisition (hardware) zoom for children

sion, but is most easily calculated as:

$$RKF(\%) = 100 - LKF.$$

DMSA imaging is thus technically simple to perform, allows a wide time window in which the images can be acquired (2–6 hours post-injection), and only requires the patient to keep still for 2–3 minutes at a time. It provides a more accurate measurement of relative renal function than that obtained from renography (Section 11.5.1), particularly when renal function is severely impaired and/or when a kidney is rotated or in an unusual position. Multicenter audit studies have shown that measurement of relative renal function measurement from DMSA images is highly reproducible [21, 22].

Interpretation

DMSA uptake within the kidney reflects the distribution of functioning renal cortical tissue. A modern gamma camera fitted with a high-resolution collimator will visualize some of the internal architecture of the kidney, so normal uptake is not generally uniform. Calyces will often be seen, particularly if dilated, as may the columns of Bertin (Figure 11.17). Extrinsic compression of the lateral aspect of the left upper pole by the spleen is often seen (Figure 11.18) and fetal lobulation may be

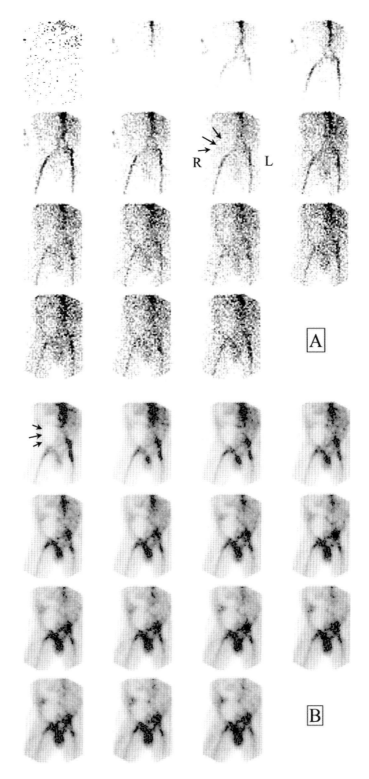

Figure 11.16. Perfusion **A** and function **B** images showing a non-perfused, non-functioning graft (photopenic area overlying the right iliac artery) due to early postoperative infarction. (Images courtesy of Dr M. Keir, Royal Victoria Infirmary, Newcastle.)

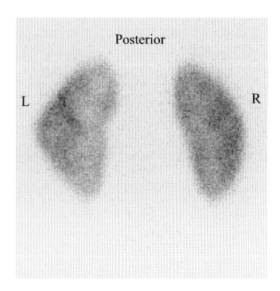

Figure 11.17. Normal DMSA image in an 8-year-old girl with history of UTI. The lateral aspect of the mid pole of the left kidney shows prominent columns of Bertin.

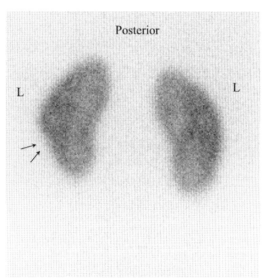

Figure 11.19. Normal DMSA image in a 3-year-old girl with history of UTI. The lower pole outline of the left kidney (arrowed) shows segment of concavity typical of fetal lobulation, which is a normal variant. The mid pole appears to bulge slightly as a result.

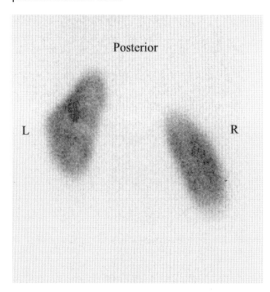

Figure 11.18. Normal DMSA image in an adult, showing extrinsic compression by the spleen in the left upper pole. The left kidney also shows prominent calyces (photopenic area) in the mid and lower poles, which are also normal variants.

seen in young children (Figure 11.19). It is clearly important to recognize these normal variants in order to avoid false positives. Indeed, visual interpretation of static DMSA images is subject to significant inter-observer variability and has led to the production of guidelines [20].

A pyelonephritic scar is generally manifest as a segmental area of reduced uptake. Other space-occupying lesions (e.g. cyst, tumor) produce areas of reduced uptake but will usually be of different shape, and should be identifiable on renal ultrasound or CT. The DMSA scan is certainly the "gold standard" for diagnosis of scarring, but renal ultrasound plays a pivotal role in the general management of patients with febrile UTI. The DMSA scan may show a patchy appearance during the inflammatory stage of acute UTI, which will either resolve or progress to focal areas of reduced uptake. In turn, focal parenchymal defects may disappear or degenerate into permanent scars (Figure 11.20). It is therefore important to be aware of the clinical history (i.e. date of last UTI) when interpreting DMSA images. Although the presence of segmental cortical defects on an "acute" DMSA scan indicates a high (approximately 80%) probability of permanent renal damage, the defect should not be called a "scar" unless it is still evident at 6-month follow-up.

Although the measurement of relative DMSA uptake is clearly useful in this setting (for baseline assessment and monitoring), there is no clear correlation between relative renal function and presence or extent of scarring. Indeed, up to 35% of patients with unilateral scarring will have evenly

THE URINARY TRACT

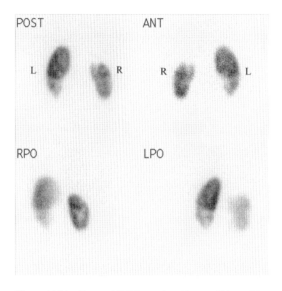

Figure 11.20. Abnormal DMSA scan in a 13-year-old boy with a history of UTIs and bilateral grade 4 reflux. The relatively small right kidney shows a wedge-shaped defect in the upper pole that is typical of renal scarring. There is also an area of significantly reduced uptake in the lower pole of the left kidney – best seen on left posterior oblique (LPO) view – that also represents scarring. Relative renal function was measured as: L = 61%, R = 39%.

divided renal function [23]. The normal range for relative function measurement, applicable to both DMSA static imaging and renography, is 42–58%.

References

1. Paediatric Task Group of the European Association of Nuclear Medicine. Eur J Nucl Med 1990; 17:127–129.
2. ARSAC Notes for guidance. Nucl Med Commun 2000; 21: S1–S95.
3. Rutland MD. A comprehensive analysis of renal DTPA studies I: Theory and normal values. Nucl Med Commun 1985; 6:11–30.
4. Piepsz A, Kinthaert M, Tindeur M, Ham HR. The robustness of the Patlak-Rutland slope for the determination of split renal function. Nucl Med Commun 1996; 17:817–821.
5. Meller ST, Eckstein HB. The value of renal scintigraphy in reduplication. In: Joekes AM, Constable AR, Brown NJG, Tauxe WN, eds. Radionuclides in Nephrology. London: Academic Press; 1982: 229–236.
6. Cremin BJ. Observations on vesico-ureteric reflux and intrarenal reflux: A review and survey of material. Clin Radiol 1979; 30:607–621.
7. Jain S, Turner DTL, Cosgriff PS, Morrish O. Calculating the renal output efficiency as a method for clarifying equivocal renograms in adults with suspected upper tract obstruction. BJU Int 2003; 92:485–487.
8. O'Reilly PH. Nuclear medicine in urology. Contrib Nephrol 1987; 56:215–224.
9. O'Reilly PH. Urinary dilatation and obstruction in the adult. In: Peters AM, ed. Nuclear Medicine in Clinical Diagnosis. London: Martin Dunitz; 2003: 181–188.
10. Cosgriff PS, Gordon I. Diuretic renogram clearance half-times in the diagnosis of obstructive uropathy (letter to the Editor). Nucl Med Commun 2003; 24:1255–1257.
11. Wong DC, Rossleigh MA, Farnsworth RH. F+0 diuresis renography in infants and children. J Nucl Med 1999; 40:1805–1811.
12. Jones DA, Lupton EW, George NJR. Effect of bladder filling on upper tract urodynamics in man. Br J Urol 1990; 65:492–496.
13. Lawson RS. Mathematics. In: O'Reilly PH, Shields RA, Testa HJ, eds. Nuclear Medicine in Urology and Nephrology, 2nd edn. London: Butterworths; 1987: 247–270.
14. Carlson O. Direct deconvolution algorithms based on Laplace transforms in nuclear medicine applications. Nucl Med Commun 2000; 21:857–868.
15. Sutton DG, Kempi V. Constrained least squares restoration and renogram deconvolution: a comparison by simulation. Phys Med Biol 1992; 37:53–67.
16. Rutland MD. Database deconvolution. Nucl Med Commun 2003; 24:101–106.
17. Fommei E, Ghione S, Hilson AJW, et al. Captopril radionuclide test in renovascular hypertension: a European multicentre study. Eur J Nucl Med 1993; 20:617–623.
18. Prigent A. The diagnosis of renovascular hypertension: the role of captopril renal scintigraphy and related issues. Eur J Nucl Med 1993; 20:625–644.
19. BNMS quality guidelines for renal cortical scintigraphy. (DMSA). www.bnms.org.uk/bnms_dmsa.html. Last revised: Feb 2003.
20. Piepsz A, Colarinha P, Gordon I, et al. Guidelines on ^{99m}Tc-DMSA scintigraphy in children. Eur J Nucl Med 2001; 28:BP37–41.
21. Fleming JS, Cosgriff PS, Houston A, et al. UK audit of relative renal function measurement using DMSA scintigraphy. Nucl Med Commun 1998; 19:989–997.
22. Tondeur M, Melis K, De Sandeleer C, et al. Inter-observer reproducibility of relative ^{99}Tc^m-DMSA uptake. Nucl Med Commun 2000; 21:449–453.
23. Smellie JM, Shaw PJ, Prescod NP, Bantock HM. ^{99m}Tc dimercapto-succinic acid (DMSA) scan in patients with established radiological renal scarring. Arch Dis Child 1988; 63:1315–1319.

12

The Brain, Salivary and Lacrimal Glands

Alison D. Murray

12.1 Introduction

Brain imaging is most often carried out with X-ray computed tomography (CT) or magnetic resonance imaging (MRI). CT is fast, widely available, and has made conventional nuclear medicine ^{99m}Tc pertechnetate brain imaging obsolete. MRI has the advantages of lack of ionizing radiation and superior soft tissue resolution. However, in an expanding number of clinical situations, brain single photon emission computed tomography (SPECT) or occasionally positron emission tomography (PET) may be the investigation of choice or provide complementary information to structural imaging. Virtually all nuclear medicine applications in the brain involve SPECT and there is rarely a role for planar imaging. It is important to understand the strengths and limitations of brain imaging in nuclear medicine so that these techniques are used appropriately alongside other methods of brain imaging. New methods of imaging neurotransmitter receptors and transporters have been developed and offer expanded roles for brain SPECT. Nuclear medicine can make valuable contributions to the diagnosis and follow-up of patients with dementia, cerebrovascular disease, movement disorders, brain tumors, and other neurological diseases.

This chapter will be divided into sections covering normal anatomy and physiology, technical aspects of brain SPECT, clinical applications of regional cerebral blood flow SPECT (rCBF SPECT), dopamine transporter and receptor imaging in movement disorders, and applications in brain tumor imaging. Where appropriate, the role of positron emission tomography (PET) will be indicated in the relevant sections. The only nuclear medicine application in the spine is bone scintigraphy, which is dealt with in Chapter 8.

12.2 Anatomy and Physiology

Anatomically the brain is a largely symmetrical structure, composed of cerebral hemispheres, cerebellum, and brainstem. The basic cell of the brain is the neuron, which has a cell body containing the nucleus and an axon of variable length. In addition there are supporting glial cells, which form structural and metabolic "scaffolding" for the neurons. In the cerebral hemispheres and cerebellum the cell bodies lie in the outer layers and form the gray matter. The axons have an "insulating" myelin sheath, transmit impulses between neurons in different parts of the brain and spine, and form the more centrally placed white matter. Within the cerebral hemispheres are deeply placed gray matter structures called the basal ganglia. Brain anatomy is illustrated in Figure 12.1a and b.

The blood supply to the brain is from four arteries in the neck: the two internal carotid arteries anteriorly, which divide into the anterior and middle cerebral arteries bilaterally; and the two vertebral arteries posteriorly. These join in front of the brainstem to form the basilar artery, which then divides into two posterior cerebral arteries. There are variable communications (anastomoses) between the cerebral arteries called the "circle

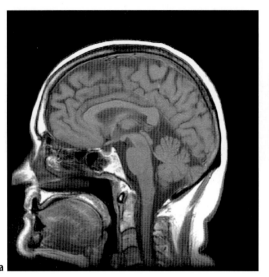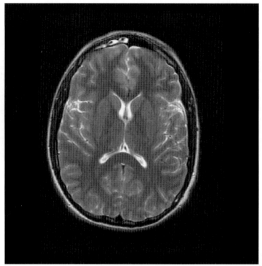

Figure 12.1. T1 sagittal midline **a** and T2 axial **b** MRI of the brain.

of Willis" and the arterial anatomy is shown in Figure 12.2. Blood flow to the gray matter is approximately 80 ml/min/100 g of tissue and is considerably greater than to the metabolically less active white matter, which receives 20 ml/min/100 g. The venous drainage of the brain is into deep and superficial veins and then into venous sinuses, which are invaginations of the dura, a fibrous layer around the brain. The venous sinuses drain into the internal jugular veins bilaterally.

The metabolic substrate of the brain is glucose and high uptake is seen in the brain on [18]FDG PET in Figure 12.3, particularly in the gray matter. The

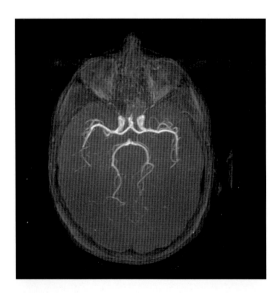

Figure 12.2. Magnetic resonance angiogram of the arteries supplying the brain.

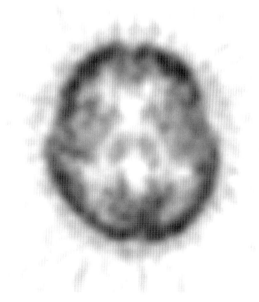

Figure 12.3. Axial [18]FDG PET image of the brain.

brain is unique, compared with other tissues in the human body, in having virtually no means of storing energy. Because of this it is entirely dependent on maintaining cerebral blood flow, as a means of delivering glucose and oxygen, and varying this in response to the metabolic requirements of neurons, a process known as autoregulation. Oxygen is required for metabolism of glucose and there is close coupling of neuronal activity and blood supply, a feature that is exploited in brain activation studies with $H_2^{15}O$ PET, functional MRI, and occasionally activation studies with rCBF SPECT.

Conversely, reduced function of part of the brain will result in a reduction in regional cerebral blood flow, although such hypofunctioning areas may appear anatomically normal on structural imaging with CT or MRI. This ability of rCBF SPECT to reflect brain function is its key strength and it should be regarded as a complementary method of investigation to structural imaging methods.

12.3 Regional Cerebral Blood Flow SPECT

12.3.1 Technical Aspects

The physics of single photon emission computed tomography is covered in Chapter 2. Image quality depends on several factors, including the compromise between sensitivity and image resolution, the presence of free pertechnetate, patient motion and, perhaps most crucially, the radius of rotation of the gamma camera heads.

Patients undergoing rCBF SPECT should be injected with the radiopharmaceutical (RP) in a quiet, darkened environment, to avoid excessive neuronal stimulation that might affect RP distribution. Dose and data acquisition parameters are given in Table 12.1. Hexamethyl propylene amine oxime (HMPAO) and ethylene cysteine dimer (ECD) are lipophylic and are taken up on first-pass cerebral perfusion. Both reach a steady state after a few minutes and remain bound for between two (ECD) and six (HMPAO) hours. This property allows delayed imaging, which can be useful in certain clinical situations. ECD has similar properties to HMPAO but importantly reflects cellular metabolism, rather than blood flow. The two agents may thus behave differently in certain clinical situations (see below).

Table 12.1. SPECT imaging of regional cerebral blood flow

Radiopharmaceutical (RP)	^{99m}Tc hexamethyl propylene amine oxime (HMPAO)
Activity administered	500 MBq (14 mCi)
Effective dose equivalent	5.0 mSv (500 mrem)
Patient preparation	Patient rests in quiet, darkened room for 10 min before and after RP injection
Collimator	Low-energy, high-resolution (LEHR)
Images acquired	Start acquisition 30 min post-injection SPECT: 128 views acquired over 30 min, dual-headed gamma camera, 128 × 128 matrix, 1.3 zoom

12.3.2 Clinical Applications

Clinical applications of rCBF SPECT include diseases that alter brain function, with secondary perfusion changes, such as dementias and epilepsy, and those that primarily affect brain perfusion, such as cerebrovascular disease.

Dementias

Alzheimer's Disease

Alzheimer's disease (AD) is the commonest primary dementia, accounting for over 50% of all cases. The prevalence of AD is 0.3% in 60–69-year-olds, rising to 10.8% in 80–89-year-olds, and is predicted to rise dramatically over the next few decades. Patients present clinically with deficits in memory and other cognitive domains. Neuropathologically AD is characterized by intracellular neurofibrillary tangles, containing abnormal hyperphosphorylated tau. Extracellular plaques composed of β-amyloid are also considered characteristic of AD but do not correlate with disease severity or duration. The disease begins in the entorhinal cortex of the medial temporal lobes, then extends posteriorly to involve the posterior temporal and parietal regions and later the frontal lobes. Characteristic posterior temporoparietal perfusion defects are seen on rCBF SPECT and are illustrated in Figure 12.4a and b. Although both ECD and HMPAO are useful in the diagnosis of AD, they do not give identical patterns of perfusion loss, with ECD showing relatively greater uptake in the occipital cortex and HMPAO in the hippocampus [1].

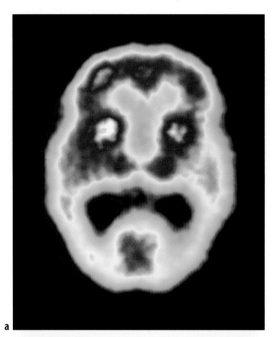

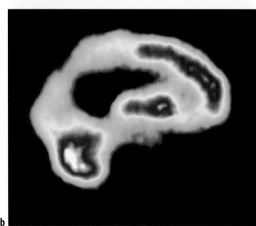

Figure 12.4. Axial **a** and sagittal **b** ^{99m}Tc-HMPAO SPECT of the brain in Alzheimer's disease showing posterior temporoparietal defects.

The predictive value of rCBF SPECT in the diagnosis of AD varies from 60 to 96% [2, 3], which is no better than clinical diagnosis based on detailed neuropsychological testing using NINCDS-ADRDA (National Institute of Neurological and Communicable Disease and Stroke/Alzheimer's Disease and Related Disorders Association) criteria. However, such detailed assessment is not routinely used and, in clinical practice, rCBF SPECT is useful in distinguishing AD from other types of dementia. Given a clinical diagnosis of probable or possible AD using a well-validated method, rCBF SPECT improves the correlation with neuropathology [4]. The primary motor, sensory, and visual cortex are spared in AD and involvement of the latter has been suggested as one of the distinguishing features between AD and dementia with Lewy bodies. It is important to recognize that the perfusion defects observed reflect dysfunction of the underlying brain and are disproportionate to any atrophy on structural imaging early in the disease process.

Various quantitative methods have been applied to analysis of rCBF SPECT data in AD, including region of interest analysis, volume of interest (VOI) analysis [5], and statistical parametric mapping (SPM) [6]. Such methods are useful in the context of research, allowing comparison between subject and control groups or comparison within any one subject over time or in different environmental or pharmacological circumstances, such as monitoring the effect of treatment.

Both [18]FDG and H_2 [15]O PET have been studied in AD and demonstrate metabolic and perfusion defects respectively in the typical posterior temporoparietal areas. The advent of PET/CT systems will have the advantage of providing structural and functional data in one examination.

Other methods of imaging cerebral blood flow, such as MR dynamic susceptibility contrast perfusion imaging, have shown similar appearances to rCBF SPECT and similar predictive values.

Newer radiopharmaceuticals have been developed for use in AD with the aim of having better specificity than perfusion agents. [123]I iomazenil binds to benzodiazepine receptors and shows larger areas of reduced uptake than ^{99m}Tc-HMPAO [7]. More recently Pittsburgh Compound B, a PET tracer, has been developed to bind to amyloid deposits in the brain [8].

Dementia with Lewy Bodies

Dementia with Lewy bodies (DLB) is thought to be the second most common primary dementia after AD and may be as common as vascular dementia. The clinical presentation is characterized by dementia with fluctuation in confusion, attentional deficit, and psychotic symptoms, typically visual hallucinations. Parkinsonian features are also common and there is overlap both clinically and neuropathologically between DLB and idiopathic Parkinson's disease. Many patients with Parkinson's disease become demented and the

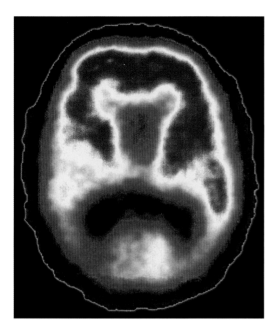

Figure 12.5. Axial ^{99m}Tc-HMPAO SPECT of the brain in dementia with Lewy bodies showing posterior perfusion defects with involvement of the occipital cortex.

distinction between DLB and Parkinson's disease dementia is arbitrary, with the latter term used if motor symptoms predate the onset of dementia by 10 years or more. Both diseases are characterized by accumulation of Lewy bodies, containing α-synuclein, in the brainstem and cerebral cortex. Regional CBF SPECT can show similar appearances to AD with posterior perfusion defects. However, more global reductions are reported in DLB using HMPAO, with involvement of the frontal lobes [9]. Global and visual cortical involvement has also been found in DLB using FDG PET [10]. Figure 12.5 shows posterior perfusion defects on HMPAO SPECT in a patient with DLB demonstrating involvement of the visual cortex.

Frontotemporal Dementias

Frontotemporal dementia (FTD) is a primary dementia resulting in severe frontal and anterior temporal atrophy and accounts for 5–10% of all dementia cases. It comprises three subtypes: frontal variant FTD, semantic dementia, and progressive non-fluent dysphasia. Frontal variant FTD is the commonest and clinically patients present with personality change, emotional and behavioral problems, and social conduct im-

pairment. Compared with AD, memory problems are less severe.

Neuropathologically, as in AD, accumulation of abnormal tau has been found. Functional imaging in FTD demonstrates anterior perfusion defects involving the frontal and anterior temporal lobes, with preserved perfusion posteriorly, as

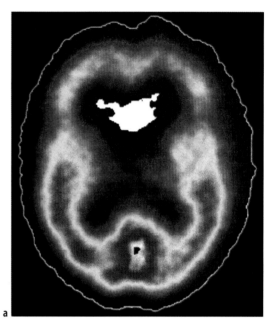

a

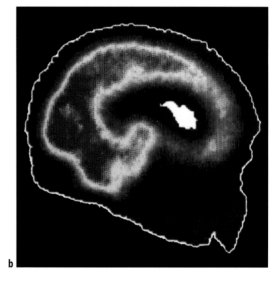

b

Figure 12.6. Axial **a** and sagittal **b** ^{99m}Tc-HMPAO SPECT of the brain in frontotemporal dementia showing anterior perfusion defects – contrast this pattern of defects with Figure 12.4.

shown in Figure 12.6a and b. Reduced frontal perfusion is not specific to FTD and can occur in a variety of other diseases including schizophrenia, depression, Creutzfeldt–Jakob disease, HIV encephalopathy, vascular dementia, and some cases of AD. However, in a demented patient, rCBF SPECT is useful in distinguishing between FTD and AD [11]. Similarly [18]FDG PET has shown widespread hypometabolism, most severe in the frontal and anterior temporal lobes [12].

Vascular Dementia

This is the second most common form of dementia and may coexist with Alzheimer's disease [13] or other dementias, so-called "mixed dementias". It has been suggested that if mixed dementias are included, vascular dementia may be the commonest type of dementia in the elderly [14]. The presence of coexisting cerebrovascular disease increases the rate of decline in elderly patients with AD [15]. Vascular dementia is secondary to inadequate or absent perfusion of parts of the brain due to atheroma usually of the internal carotid arteries or middle cerebral arteries and hypertension is the main clinical risk factor. Traditionally it has been associated with a stepwise deterioration clinically and the presence of one or more supratentorial infarcts on structural imaging. It is increasingly recognized that white matter ischemia, in the absence of cortical infarcts, is also associated with cognitive impairment [16] but, being largely a gray matter imaging technique, rCBF SPECT is less sensitive for perfusion abnormalities in the white matter.

HMPAO SPECT may demonstrate multiple patchy perfusion defects or reduced perfusion in one or more arterial territories, as in Figure 12.7. Basal ganglia perfusion defects are characteristic. Reflecting the prevalence of mixed Alzheimer's and vascular dementia, HMPAO SPECT may show both posterior temporoparietal defects and reduced perfusion in one or more vascular territories.

Cerebrovascular Disease

Acute Ischemic Stroke and Cerebral Ischemia

The aim of imaging in acute stroke is to demonstrate brain which has reduced perfusion, but which has not yet undergone irreversible infarction (the "ischemic penumbra") and exclude intracranial hemorrhage. Regional CBF SPECT will demonstrate a perfusion defect immediately in

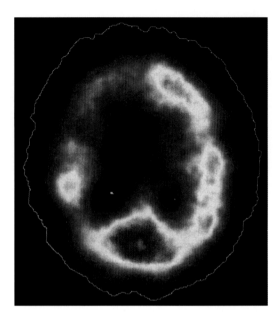

Figure 12.7. Axial ^{99m}Tc-HMPAO SPECT of the brain in vascular dementia showing multiple patchy perfusion defects, with generally reduced perfusion in the right internal carotid territory.

acute ischemic stroke and this method has been used to select acute stroke patients for intervention with thrombolysis. However, in acute stroke, structural imaging is also required to exclude intracranial hemorrhage prior to thrombolysis. Recent advances in MRI with diffusion and perfusion imaging, and more recently with CT perfusion imaging, are readily available methods of demonstrating the ischemic penumbra and predicting response to thrombolysis. A newer SPECT method of demonstrating the ischemic penumbra using ^{99m}Tc ethylene dicysteine metronidazole compares favorably with diffusion weighted MRI and shows good correlation with clinical outcome [17] but does not address the issue of excluding intracranial hemorrhage in the acute stroke setting. rCBF SPECT has also been used to assess the risk of progression to stroke following a transient ischemic attack [18] and to detect irreversible ischemia following acetazolamide stress [19]. Cardiac bypass surgery frequently results in cognitive deficits postoperatively and rCBF SPECT has predictive value in identifying patients at greatest risk of this preoperatively [20].

PET is the most accurate method of quantifying changes in cerebral hemodynamics.

H_2 ^{15}O studies have been used to measure CBF and cerebral blood volume and $C^{15}O$ oxygen extraction fraction. PET has been used to study acute stroke and cerebral hemodynamics before and after carotid surgery. Although valuable in a research context, PET is unlikely to have widespread use in clinical management of acute stroke due to limited current availability.

Epilepsy

Epilepsy is a common disorder and most patients do not require localization of the epileptogenic focus. However, in around 10% of patients seizures are refractory to medical therapy and surgery is of potential benefit. Methods of localizing the epileptogenic focus preoperatively are electroencephalography (EEG), MRI, and rCBF SPECT and SPECT is indicated when there is discordance between EEG and MRI. During an epileptic seizure, neuronal activity in part of the brain is increased and there is associated increase in local blood flow. This can be demonstrated on ictal rCBF SPECT where the radiopharmaceutical (RP) is injected during or shortly after a seizure. Because of RP fixation, imaging can take place a few hours later, up to six in the case of HMPAO, and ictal SPECT has been shown to have a >95% sensitivity and specificity for demonstrating the epileptogenic focus [21]. Interictal SPECT, carried out between seizures, may show hypoperfusion at the epileptogenic focus and subtraction of interictal from ictal images can maximize detection of this [22]. PET with FGD or ^{11}C flumazenil has also been used in epilepsy. Both SPECT and PET are better at detecting temporal foci than extratemporal foci. Increased uptake in the thalamus on ictal SPECT has been reported to be an additional localizing sign and appears to follow lateralization of cortical foci [23].

Infection

Encephalitis

Acute encephalitis is most often due to herpes simplex virus and typically affects the temporal lobe. Despite marked clinical abnormality in acute encephalitis, there is often very little abnormality on structural imaging with CT or MRI. However, rCBF SPECT will show increased perfusion, reflecting brain inflammation, early in the disease process. This will often precede changes on structural imaging and more accurately reflect the extent of clinical abnormality.

Cerebral Abscess

Cerebral abscess may occur due to spread of infection from adjacent air spaces in the skull, as a complication of sinusitis or mastoiditis, or as hematogenous spread from a septic focus distant from the brain. Usually the diagnosis is obvious in a clinically unwell patient with a ring-enhancing lesion demonstrated on CT or MRI. However, if the diagnosis is in doubt on standard imaging, ^{99m}Tc-HMPAO-labeled white cell scintigraphy will show increased uptake in a cerebral abscess.

Brain Death

Brain death is the term used when cardiopulmonary function is maintained, usually in an intensive care unit setting, but where there is no evidence of brain activity. Confirmation of brain death is usually a clinical diagnosis. However, formal clinical tests may be unreliable in the presence of centrally acting drugs and the diagnosis of brain death then relies on demonstrating absence of intracranial perfusion. Traditionally this is done using catheter angiography but more recently rCBF SPECT has been accepted as a reliable method of confirming brain death [24]. Figure 12.8 illustrates absence of intracranial perfusion, confirming brain death, in a young woman following a recreational drug overdose.

12.4 Receptor Imaging in Movement Disorders

Movement disorders include Parkinson's disease and other parkinsonian syndromes that present clinically with resting tremor, rigidity, and slowness of voluntary movement (bradykinesia). Idiopathic Parkinson's disease (IPD) is the commonest movement disorder and affects 2–3% of the population over 50 years of age. It is due to degeneration of the presynaptic neurons projecting from the substantia nigra, in the midbrain, to the putamen and caudate nucleus, which form part of the basal ganglia. Neuropathologically, IPD is characterized by Lewy bodies, which contain α-synuclein. Other parkinsonian syndromes, such as progressive supranuclear palsy and multiple

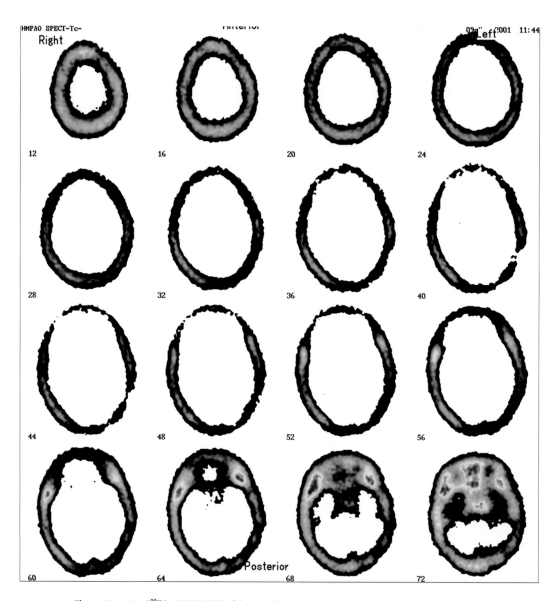

Figure 12.8. Axial ^{99m}Tc-HMPAO SPECT of the brain following brain death. There is no intracranial perfusion.

system atrophy, involve degeneration of pre- and postsynaptic neurons. Like AD, PSP is associated neuropathologically with intracellular accumulation of abnormal tau, while MSA is characterized by accumulation of α-synuclein. The clinical diagnosis of IPD is obvious in most cases. However, in around 20% of patients the diagnosis will not be clear and functional imaging is useful in appropriate selection of patients for expensive disease-modifying drug therapy [25].

12.4.1 Dopamine Receptor Imaging

^{123}I-IBZM binds to postsynaptic D_2 receptors and should demonstrate increased binding at these in IPD due to upregulation in a failing dopaminergic system, to maximize use of available dopamine in the synapse. Conversely, in other parkinsonian syndromes, binding at postsynaptic D_2 receptors is reduced. Radiopharmaceutical dose and image acquisition parameters are shown in Table 12.2.

THE BRAIN, SALIVARY AND LACRIMAL GLANDS

Table 12.2. SPECT imaging of D_2 receptors

Radiopharmaceutical	[123]I iodobenzamine (IBZM)
Activity administered	185 MBq (5 mCi)
Effective dose equivalent	6.3 mSv (630 mrem)
Patient preparation	Block thyroid
	Stop medication[a]
Collimator	Low-energy, high-resolution (LEHR)
Images acquired	Start acquisition 90–120 min post-injection
	SPECT: 128 views acquired over 30 min, dual-headed gamma camera, 128 × 128 matrix, 1.3 zoom
	Consider removing safety pads to minimize radius of rotation
	No attenuation correction

[a] Drugs containing L-dopa may interfere with IBZM uptake and should be discontinued 12 hours before injection.

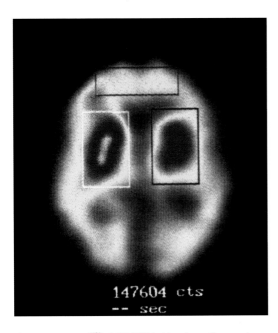

Figure 12.9. Axial ^{123}I-IBZM SPECT with regions of interest drawn around the basal ganglia (BG) bilaterally and the frontal cortex (FC) to allow calculation of the BG:FC ratio.

Images cannot be visually interpreted alone and region of interest (ROI) analysis is usually employed, producing a ratio of uptake in the basal ganglia, compared with the frontal lobes, the basal ganglia to frontal cortex (BG:FC) ratio as illustrated in Figure 12.9 [26]. A high BG:FC ratio is found in early IPD, compared with other parkin-

sonian syndromes, where the BG:FC ratio is reduced. In clinical practice each center needs to determine its own normal range and threshold of cut-off between IPD and other parkinsonian syndromes. While differences may be found on group comparison, we have not found ^{123}I-IBZM SPECT particularly useful in the investigation of an individual patient. PET using ^{18}F-dopa and ^{11}C raclopride has also been used to study binding at D_2 receptors.

12.4.2 Dopamine Transporter Imaging

^{123}I-FP-CIT is a cocaine analogue that binds to dopamine transporters and is an indicator of presynaptic dopaminergic integrity. FP-CIT uptake is reduced in the posterior part of the putamen early in IPD, progressing to involve the head of the caudate nucleus later in the disease process [27]. Radiopharmaceutical dose and image acquisition parameters are shown in Table 12.3. FP-CIT images can be interpreted by visual analysis with reduction in uptake in the posterior putamen classified as grade 1, activity confined to the caudate as grade 2, and reduced or absent uptake in the caudate as grade 3 [28]. Examples of a normal study and the three grades of abnormality are shown in Figure 12.10a–d. FP-CIT SPECT will be abnormal

Table 12.3. SPECT imaging of dopamine transporters

Radiopharmaceutical	[123]I ioflupane (FP-CIT)
Activity administered	185 MBq (5 mCi)
Effective dose equivalent	4.35 mSv (435 mrem)
Patient preparation	Block thyroid
	Stop drugs that may interfere with FP-CIT binding[a]
Collimator	Low-energy, high-resolution (LEHR)
Images acquired	Start acquisition 3–4 h post-injection
	SPECT: 128 views acquired over 30 min, dual-headed gamma camera, 128 × 128 matrix, 1.3 zoom
	Consider removing safety pads to minimize radius of rotation
	No attenuation correction

[a] The following categories of drugs may interfere with FP-CIT binding: antidepressants (particularly SSRIs and tricyclics); psychostimulants; opiate analgesics; neuroleptics. More information can be found at the following website: www.fpcit.net.

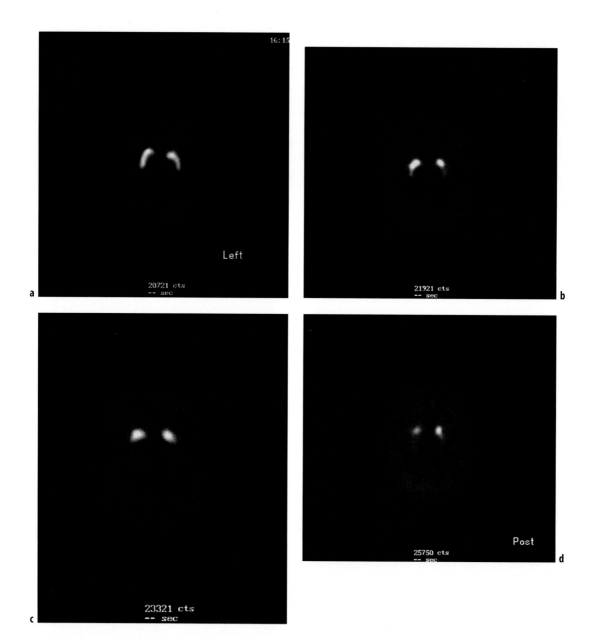

Figure 12.10. a–d. Axial ^{123}I-FP-CIT. **a** Normal example showing symmetrical uptake in the putamen and heads of caudate bilaterally; **b** grade 1 abnormality showing reduced uptake in the tail of the left putamen; **c** grade 2 abnormality showing activity confined to the heads of the caudate bilaterally; **d** grade 3 abnormality showing reduced uptake in the heads of caudate, worse on the right.

in IPD and other parkinsonian syndromes as both involve degeneration of presynaptic dopaminergic neurons. The clinical indication for ^{123}I-FP-CIT SPECT is to distinguish between a parkinsonian disorder and essential tremor, in which dopamine transporter uptake is normal. FP-CIT SPECT is able to detect subclinical IPD as patients with unilateral clinical symptoms have been found to have bilateral reductions in uptake.

Similar results have been found with other dopamine transporter agents, such as ^{123}I-βCIT and ^{99m}Tc-TRODAT-1 and more recent studies have suggested that quantitative analysis can distinguish between IPD and MSA, with greater asymmetry in the former [29].

12.5 Intracranial Tumors

Intracranial tumors are divided into intra-axial, that is those arising within the brain, and extra-axial, arising from the layers around the brain. Gliomas are the commonest intra-axial tumors and range from relatively benign low-grade tumors to the highly malignant glioblastoma multiforme. The commonest extra-axial tumor is the meningioma.

12.5.1 Gliomas

The diagnosis of glioma is not usually ambiguous on structural imaging with CT or MRI. Tumor size and contrast enhancement are a guide to tumor grade but in most cases excision or biopsy will be carried out and a histologic diagnosis made. In the occasional instances when non-invasive tumor grading is helpful, ^{201}Tl chloride SPECT, ^{99m}Tc sestamibi SPECT or ^{18}FDG PET have all been used and will show increased uptake relative to brain in high-grade gliomas and reduced uptake in low-grade gliomas. Quantitative evaluation of ^{201}Tl chloride SPECT, using early and late imaging, is useful in distinguishing benign from malignant lesions and predicting grade of malignancy [30].

^{123}I α-methyl tyrosine SPECT and PET using either ^{11}C methionine or ^{18}F α-methyl tyrosine are accurate at showing tumor extent and distinguishing this from surrounding edema but do not distinguish between high- and low-grade gliomas [31–33]. Preoperative planning of resection of gliomas potentially involving eloquent areas of brain is aided by functional cortical mapping and both fMRI and H_2 ^{15}O PET have been used to identify language areas so that these may be avoided during neurosurgery (Figure 12.11).

The diagnosis of tumor recurrence following radiotherapy, chemotherapy, and/or surgical resection is inaccurate on structural imaging and it is impossible to reliably distinguish between the effects of treatment and tumor recurrence. Nuclear medicine and PET are more useful in this context and both ^{201}Tl chloride SPECT and ^{11}C methionine or ^{18}F α-methyl tyrosine PET will show increased uptake in recurrent tumor (Figure 12.12).

12.5.2 Meningiomas

These have typical imaging characteristics on CT and MRI and there is little role for SPECT in the initial diagnosis. Following surgery, however, structural images can be difficult to interpret and ^{111}In octreotide SPECT is useful in demonstrating residual or recurrent tumor.

12.6 Other Nuclear Medicine Applications in the Head

12.6.1 Anatomy of the Salivary Glands

The largest salivary glands are the parotid glands, which lie around the posterior margin of both mandibular rami. Each gland is divided into larger superficial and smaller deep lobes, with branches of the facial nerve lying in the deep lobe. On structural imaging, the superficial and deep lobes are divided by the retromandibular vein (Figure 12.13). The saliva produced by the glandular tissue of the parotid glands drains into multiple small ducts that join to form the main parotid duct (Stensen's duct). The orifice of the main parotid duct lies in the cheek at the level of the second upper molar tooth.

The smaller submandibular glands lie in the floor of the mouth, medial to both sides of the body of the mandible and inferior to the myohyoid muscles. They drain via the submandibular duct (Wharton's duct), which passes around the posterior margin of the myohyoid muscles to open in the floor of the mouth, on either side of the frenulum of the tongue.

There are sublingual and other smaller salivary glands but these are not large enough to be seen on scintigraphy.

12.6.2 Sialoscintigraphy

The function and drainage of the parotid and submandibular salivary glands can be assessed simultaneously using ^{99m}Tc pertechnetate. Radiopharmaceutical dose and image acquisition parameters are given in Table 12.4. The examination is divided into an initial dynamic phase to assess function and drainage, then a static phase to assess

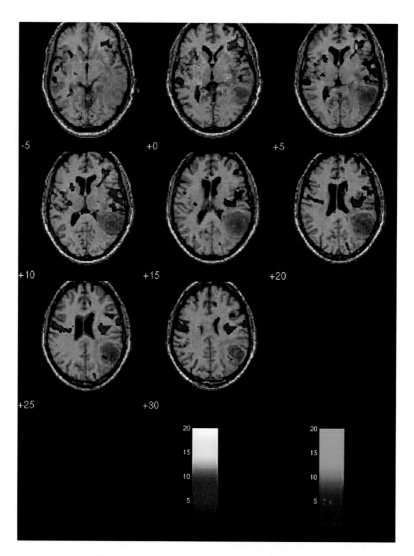

Figure 12.11. Language activation H_2 ^{15}O study in a patient with a left hemisphere glioma. Activation during articulation (red) and verb generation (blue) is anterior to the tumor and a posterior neurosurgical approach was adopted.

glandular size, shape, and the presence of any focal abnormalities. The salivary glands show rapid uptake of ^{99m}Tc pertechnetate following intravenous injection and uptake will also be seen in the thyroid. After 10 minutes, the patient is given a sialogogue, such as Carbex liquid or lemon juice, to stimulate saliva secretion and assess drainage (Figure 12.14). In the static phase generalized or focal increased or decreased uptake may be seen. Generalized reduction in activity occurs in connective tissue diseases, such as Sjögren's syndrome, and generalized increase is seen with infectious and inflammatory disorders, such as sarcoidosis. Focal abnormalities are usually photopenic and may be due to cysts or tumors. Focal increases occur with infections, abscesses and the less common benign adenolymphoma.

Most structural abnormalities of the salivary glands are best diagnosed on imaging with ultrasound or MRI. Obstruction of the main parotid or submandibular ducts, due to stricture or calculus, is diagnosed by contrast sialography. However, if routine investigations are unhelpful, sialoscintigraphy is useful and is the first line investigation

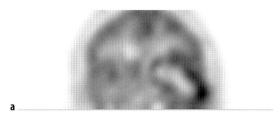

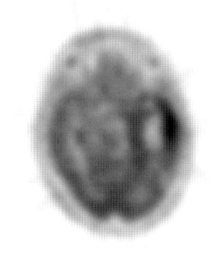

Figure 12.12. Coronal **a** and axial **b** [11]C methionine PET in a patient with recurrent glioma in the left temporal lobe. There is increased ^{11}C methionine uptake around the periphery of the photopenic operative defect.

Table 12.4. Sialoscintigraphy

Radiopharmaceutical (RP)	[99m]Tc pertechnetate
Activity administered	150 MBq (4 mCi)
Effective dose equivalent	1.4 mSv (140 mrem)
Patient preparation	None
Collimator	Low-energy, high-resolution (LEHR)
Images acquired	60 × 20 s anterior dynamic frames
	Carbex after 10 min
	Static anterior and both lateral obliques at 20 min

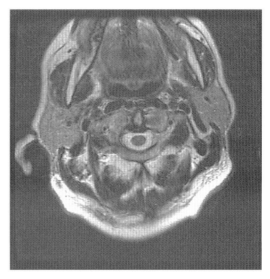

Figure 12.13. Axial T2 weighted MRI of the parotids. The deep and superficial lobes are divided by the retromandibular vein.

for some abnormalities, such as Sjögren's syndrome.

12.6.3 Anatomy of the Lacrimal System

The lacrimal glands are small and lie in the upper outer aspect of the orbits, superolateral to the globe. Tears secreted by the lacrimal glands wash over the conjunctiva and drain via the lacrimal apparatus to the nasal cavity. The lacrimal apparatus consists of superior and inferior canaliculi, the openings of which lie at the medial end of the eye lids, common canaliculus, lacrimal sac, and nasolacrimal duct.

12.6.4 Dacryoscintigraphy

Obstruction of any part of the lacrimal drainage system results in epiphora (a watery eye), which is the only clinical indication for investigation of

the lacrimal system. Dacryoscintigraphy is a noninvasive method of assessing lacrimal drainage, following insertion of ^{99m}Tc pertechnetate eye drops in normal saline. Serial static images are acquired, with the patient sitting in front of the gamma camera, as radioactivity drains from the conjunctival sac to the nose and the level of any obstruction can be readily identified (Figure 12.15). Radiopharmaceutical dose and image acquisition parameters are shown in Table 12.5.

Alternative methods of investigating the lacrimal system include contrast dacryocystography using fluoroscopy or CT, which are invasive, and MRI dacryocystography, which has the advantage of avoiding both radiation and cannulation of the lacrimal system.

The commonest cause for lacrimal obstruction is stenosis due to fibrosis following infection.

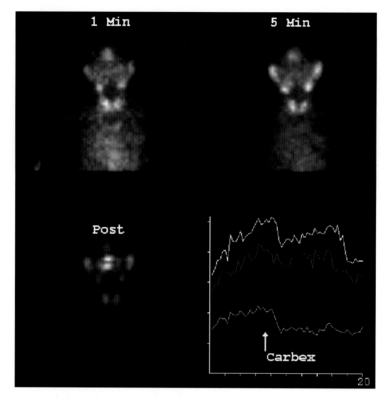

Figure 12.14. Sialoscintigram showing dynamic images at 1 and 5 minutes, then appearances after Carbex with activity in the mouth. Time–activity curves show the submandibular glands superiorly and the parotid glands inferiorly with a reduction in activity after Carbex.

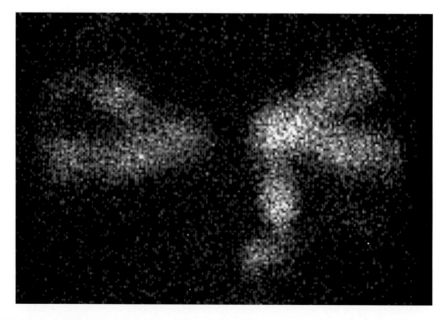

Figure 12.15. Dacryoscintigram showing normal drainage from the left eye but no drainage from the right eye, in keeping with obstruction at the level of the common canaliculus.

Table 12.5. Dacryoscintigraphy

Radiopharmaceutical (RP)	^{99m}Tc pertechnetate
Activity administered	2–4 MBq (50–100 μCi)
Radiation dose to the lens	0.02–0.04 mGy (2–4 mrad)
Patient preparation	Patient seated with head immobilized in front of gamma camera
Collimator	2 mm pinhole
Images acquired	Static anterior images at 5, 10, 15, and 20 min

Obstruction can also occur following facial trauma, due to tumors in adjacent sinuses or be congenital.

References

1. Koulibaly PM, Nobili F, Migneco O, et al. ^{99m}Tc-HMPAO and ^{99m}Tc-ECD perform differently in typically hypoperfused areas in Alzheimer's disease. Eur J Nucl Med Mol Imaging 2003; 30:1009–1013.

2. O'Brien JT, Eagger S, Syed GM, Sahakian BJ, Levy R. A study of regional cerebral blood flow and cognitive performance in Alzheimer's disease. J Neurol Neurosurg Psychiatry 1992; 55:1182–1187.

3. Jobst KA, Barnetson LP, Shepstone BJ. Accurate prediction of histologically confirmed Alzheimer's disease and the differential diagnosis of dementia: the use of NINCDS-ADRDA and DSM-III-R criteria, SPECT, X-ray CT, and Apo E4 in medial temporal lobe dementias. Oxford Project to Investigate Memory and Aging. Int Psychogeriatr 1998; 10:271–302.

4. Jagust W, Thisted R, Devous MDS, et al. SPECT perfusion imaging in the diagnosis of Alzheimer's disease: a clinical-pathologic study. Neurology 2001; 56:950–956.

5. Staff RT, Gemmell HG, Shanks MF, Murray AD, Venneri A. Changes in the rCBF images of patients with Alzheimer's disease receiving Donepezil therapy. Nucl Med Commun 2000; 21:37–41.

6. Staff RT, Venneri A, Gemmell HG, et al. HMPAO SPECT imaging of Alzheimer's disease patients with similar content-specific autobiographic delusion: comparison using statistical parametric mapping. J Nucl Med 2000; 41:1451–1455.

7. Fukuchi K, Hashikawa K, Seike Y, et al. Comparison of iodine-123-iomazenil SPECT and technetium-99m-HMPAO-SPECT in Alzheimer's disease. J Nucl Med 1997; 38:467–470.

8. Klunk WE, Engler H, Nordberg A, et al. Imaging brain amyloid in Alzheimer's disease with Pittsburgh Compound-B. Ann Neurol 2004; 55:306–319.

9. Defebvre LJ, Leduc V, Duhamel A, et al. Technetium HMPAO SPECT study in dementia with Lewy bodies, Alzheimer's disease and idiopathic Parkinson's disease. J Nucl Med 1999; 40:956–962.

10. Mirzaei S, Knoll P, Koehn H, Bruecke T. Assessment of diffuse Lewy body disease by 2-[18F]fluoro-2-deoxy-D-glucose positron emission tomography (FDG PET). 2003. http://www.biomedcentral.com/1471-2385/3/1.

11. Nagao M, Sugawara Y, Ikeda M, et al. Heterogeneity of cerebral blood flow in frontotemporal lobar degeneration and Alzheimer's disease. Eur J Nucl Med Mol Imaging 2004; 31:162–168.

12. Ishii K, Sakamoto S, Sasaki M, et al. Cerebral glucose metabolism in patients with frontotemporal dementia. J Nucl Med 1998; 39:1875–1878.

13. Whalley LJ, Murray AD. Vascular dementia. Br J Cardiol (Heart & Brain) 2003; 10:HB8–HB14.

14. Roman GC. Vascular dementia may be the most common form of dementia in the elderly. J Neurol Sci 2002; 203/204:7–10.

15. Mungas D, Reed BR, Ellis WG, Jagust WJ. The effects of age on rate of progression of Alzheimer disease and dementia with associated cerebrovascular disease. Arch Neurol 2001; 58:1243–1247.

16. Leaper SA, Murray AD, Lemmon HA, et al. Neuropsychologic correlates of brain white matter lesions depicted on MR images: 1921 Aberdeen Birth Cohort. Radiology 2001; 221:51–55.

17. Song HC, Bom HS, Cho KH, et al. Prognostication of recovery in patients with acute ischemic stroke through the use of brain SPECT with technetium-99m-labeled metronidazole. Stroke 2003; 34:982–986.

18. Bogousslavsky J, Delaloye-Bischof A, Regli F, Delaloye B. Prolonged hypoperfusion and early stroke after transient ischemic attack. Stroke 1990; 21:40–46.

19. Hattori N, Yonekura Y, Tanaka F, et al. One-day protocol for cerebral perfusion reserve with acetazolamide. J Nucl Med 1996; 37:2057–2061.

20. Hall RA, Fordyce DJ, Lee ME, et al. Brain SPECT imaging and neuropsychological testing in coronary artery bypass patients: single photon emission computed tomography Ann Thorac Surg 1999; 68:2082–2088.

21. Devous MDS, Thisted RA, Morgan GF, Leroy RF, Rowe CC. SPECT brain imaging in epilepsy: a meta-analysis. J Nucl Med 1998; 39:285–293.

22. Spanaki MV, Spencer SS, Corsi M, et al. Sensitivity and specificity of quantitative difference SPECT analysis in seizure localization. J Nucl Med 1999; 40:730–736.

23. Sojkova J, Lewis PJ, Siegel AH, et al. Does asymmetric basal ganglia or thalamic activation aid in seizure foci lateralization on ictal SPECT studies? J Nucl Med 2003; 44:1379–1386.

24. Facco E, Zucchetta P, Munari M, et al. ^{99m}Tc-HMPAO SPECT in the diagnosis of brain death. Intensive Care Med 1998; 24:911–917.

25. Whone AL, Watts RL, Stoessl AJ, et al. Slower progression of Parkinson's disease with ropinirole versus levodopa: The REAL-PET study. Ann Neurol 2003; 54:93–101.

26. Hertel A, Weppner M, Baas H, et al. Quantification of IBZM dopamine receptor SPET in de novo Parkinson patients before and during therapy. Nucl Med Commun 1997; 18:811–822.

27. Booij J, Habraken JB, Bergmans P, et al. Imaging of dopamine transporters with iodine-123-FP-CIT SPECT in healthy controls and patients with Parkinson's disease. J Nucl Med 1998; 39:1879–1884.

28. Benamer TS, Patterson J, Grosset DG, et al. Accurate differentiation of parkinsonism and essential tremor using visual assessment of [^{123}I]-FP-CIT SPECT imaging: the [^{123}I]-FP-CIT study group. Mov Disord 2000; 15:503–510.

29. Lu CS, Weng YH, Chen MC, et al. ^{99m}Tc-TRODAT-1 imaging of multiple system atrophy. J Nucl Med 2004; 45:49–55.
30. Sun D, Liu Q, Liu W, Hu W. Clinical application of ^{201}Tl SPECT imaging of brain tumors. J Nucl Med 2000; 41:5.
31. Woesler B, Kuwert T, Morgenroth C, et al. Non-invasive grading of primary brain tumours: results of a comparative study between SPET with ^{123}I-alpha-methyl tyrosine and PET with 18F-deoxyglucose. Eur J Nucl Med 1997; 24:428–434.
32. Inoue T, Shibasaki T, Oriuchi N, et al. ^{18}F alpha-methyl tyrosine PET studies in patients with brain tumors. J Nucl Med 1999; 40:399–405.
33. Ogawa T, Inugami A, Hatazawa J, et al. Clinical positron emission tomography for brain tumors: comparison of fludeoxyglucose F 18 and L-methyl-11C-methionine. Am J Neuroradiol 1996; 17:345–353.

13

Thyroid, Parathyroid, and Adrenal Gland Imaging

William H. Martin, Martin P. Sandler, and Milton D. Gross

13.1 The Thyroid

13.1.1 Anatomy

The thyroid is a bilobed structure evolving from the fourth and fifth branchial pouches. It is initially attached to the ventral floor of the pharynx by the thyroglossal duct. Thyroid tissue may be found anywhere between the base of the tongue and the retrosternal anterior mediastinum (Figure 13.1). The fetal thyroid gland begins to concentrate iodine and synthesize thyroid hormones by approximately 10.5 weeks, which is pertinent when the administration of ^{131}I to fertile women is contemplated. The two ellipsoid lobes of the adult thyroid are joined by a thin isthmus. Each lobe is approximately 2 cm in thickness and width and averages 4–4.5 cm in length. The thyroid gland, averaging approximately 20 grams in weight, resides in the neck at the level of the cricoid cartilage. A pyramidal lobe is present in approximately 30–50%, arising from either the isthmus or the superomedial aspect of either lobe; it undergoes progressive atrophy in adulthood but may be prominent in patients with Graves' disease. Although the right lobe tends to be somewhat larger than the left lobe, there is a great deal of variability in both size and shape of the normal gland.

13.1.2 Physiology

An appreciation of thyroid physiology and pathophysiology is essential for the optimal management of thyroid disorders. The function of the thyroid gland includes the concentration of iodine, synthesis of thyroid hormones, storage of these hormones as part of the thyroglobulin (Tg) molecule in the colloid, and their secretion into the circulation as required. Over 99% of circulating thyroid hormones are bound to plasma proteins, primarily thyroxine-binding globulin (TBG). Only the unbound fraction of thyroid hormone is metabolically active and, for this reason, accurate assays of free thyroid hormone, "free T_4" and "free T_3", have been developed.

Dietary sources of iodine include seafood, milk, eggs, and iodized products such as salt and bread. Approximately one-third of the absorbed dietary iodide is trapped by the thyroid, the remainder being excreted in the urine. Although gastric mucosa, salivary glands, and the lactating breast may also trap iodide, none of these organify it. The concentration of iodide by the thyroid gland, synthesis, and release of thyroid hormones are under the regulatory control of the hypothalamic-pituitary-thyroid axis. Thyroid stimulating hormone (TSH) from the pituitary plays the major role in regulating thyroid function and this, in turn, is

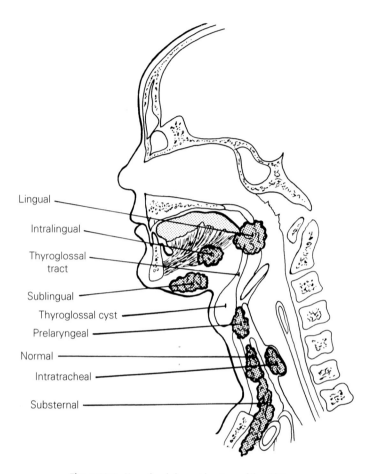

Figure 13.1. Normal and aberrant locations of thyroid tissue.

under the control of hypothalamic thyrotropin-releasing hormone (TRH) secretion. The present third generation assay for circulating TSH is highly sensitive and represents the most sensitive biochemical indicator of both hypothyroidism and hyperthyroidism; the serum TSH is elevated to above 5 mIU/l with even subclinical primary hypothyroidism and is suppressed usually to undetectable levels with hyperthyroidism. Numerous exogenous factors such as systemic illness, nutritional status, thionamides, beta blockers, steroids, iodide, lithium, amiodarone, and anticonvulsants, may affect thyroid hormone secretion and metabolism.

13.1.3 Clinical Applications

Radionuclide imaging and the measurement of thyroid radioactive iodine uptake (RAIU) both play an important role in the investigation of patients with thyroid disorders, especially those with thyroid nodules. RAIU is discussed in Section 4.12.

Thyroid Scintigraphy

With the development of fine needle aspiration biopsy (FNA) for evaluation of nodular disease combined with the exquisite anatomic detail provided by sonography, CT, and MRI, the use of thyroid scintigraphy has decreased appropriately. However, it will continue to play an important role in the functional evaluation of a variety of thyroid disorders as well as the detection of metastatic thyroid cancer. Technetium-99m pertechnetate is the most readily available radionuclide employed for thyroid imaging. Pertechnetate ions (TcO_4^-) are trapped by the thyroid in the same manner as

THYROID, PARATHYROID, AND ADRENAL GLAND IMAGING

Table 13.1. Thyroid scintigraphy

Radiopharmaceutical	[^{99m}Tc]pertechnetate	[^{123}I]sodium iodide
Activity administered	80–370 MBq (2–10 mCi) Intravenous	20 MBq (500 μCi) Oral or intravenous
Effective dose equivalent	1–5 mSv (200–400 mrem)	4 mSv (400 mrem)
Patient preparation	Withdrawal of thyroid medication, avoidance of foodstuffs with high iodine content	Withdrawal of thyroid medication, avoidance of foodstuffs with high iodine content
Collimator	Pinhole; low-energy, high-resolution parallel-hole; low energy converging	Pinhole; low-energy, high-resolution parallel-hole; low energy converging
Images acquired	Imaging started 15 min post-injection Anterior, right and left anterior oblique views, 600 second exposure per image or 200 kcounts/image	Imaging started 1–2 h post-injection if intravenous or 24 h if oral Anterior, right and left anterior oblique views

iodine through an active iodine transporter, but pertechnetate ions are not organified. ^{123}Iodine is both trapped and organified by the thyroid gland, allowing overall assessment of thyroid function. Since ^{123}I is cyclotron-produced and has a relatively short half-life of 13.6 hours, it is more expensive and advance notice is necessary for imaging. Because of its inferior image quality and the high thyroid and total body radiation dose from its β-emission, ^{131}I is not used for routine thyroid imaging other than for metastatic thyroid cancer assessment. Due primarily to less background activity, ^{123}I imaging provides somewhat higher quality images than ^{99m}Tc, but the diagnostic information provided by each is roughly

equivalent [1]. ^{123}I imaging is used in specific situations, such as retrosternal goiter. The protocol for thyroid imaging is given in Table 13.1.

The normal thyroid scintigram is shown in Figure 13.2. High-resolution images are obtained by using a pinhole collimator, thus permitting the detection of nodules as small as 5 mm in diameter. The oblique views permit detection of small nodules obscured by overlying or underlying physiological activity. Pinhole SPECT has been used to better detect subtle abnormalities. The radionuclide is distributed homogeneously throughout the gland with some increase seen centrally due to physiological thickness of the gland there; activity within the isthmus is variable and must

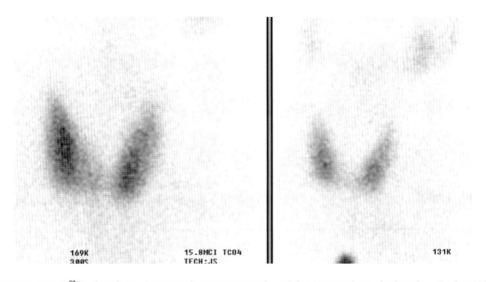

Figure 13.2. Normal ^{99m}Tc thyroid scan. Symmetric, homogeneous uptake with less intense salivary gland uptake and only mild background uptake. The inferior activity is due to a ^{57}Co marker at the suprasternal notch.

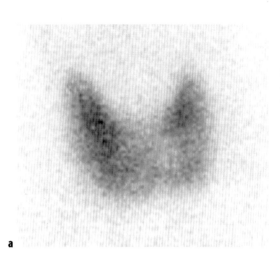

a

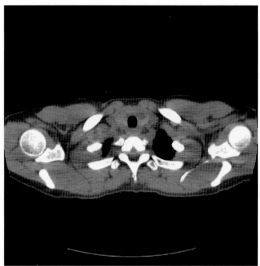

b

Figure 13.3. Subtle cold nodule. ^{99m}Tc pertechnetate anterior view **a** demonstrates a subtle hypofunctioning left lower pole nodule extending into the isthmus, confirmed on a subsequent contrast-enhanced CT **b** to be a thyroid cyst.

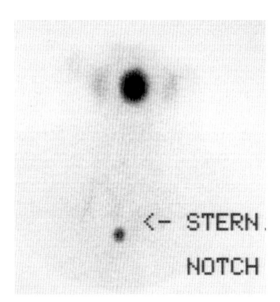

Figure 13.4. Lingual ectopic thyroid. An anterior ^{99m}Tc pertechnetate image demonstrates a focus of activity at the base of the tongue in this neonate. Cervical thyroid uptake is absent.

be correlated with physical examination and/or other imaging (Figure 13.3). With pertechnetate, salivary glands, gastric mucosa, esophagus, and blood pool background are seen in addition to thyroid activity. Due to delayed imaging, salivary gland activity is often absent with ^{123}I imaging.

In the euthyroid gland, thyroid activity should be greater than that of the salivary glands. Anatomic variations are relatively frequent and may include agenesis, hemiagenesis, and ectopia (Figure 13.4) as well as mere asymmetry. Ectopia is typically associated with hypothyroidism. Significant concavity of the lateral margin should be considered suspicious of a hypofunctioning nodule, and exaggerated convexity is often seen with diffuse goiters. The pyramidal lobe, a remnant of the distal thyroglossal duct, is identified in less than 10% of euthyroid patients, but is visualized in as many as 43% of patients with Graves' disease (Figure 13.5). Extrathyroidal accumulation of the radiopharmaceutical usually represents ectopic thyroid tissue or metastatic thyroid carcinoma if gastroesophageal and salivary gland activity can be excluded.

Multinodular Goiter

The patient with multinodular goiter (MNG) may present with what seems to be a solitary thyroid nodule, diffuse enlargement of the gland, or hyperthyroidism. Development of MNG is related to cycling periods of stimulation followed by involution and may be idiopathic or occur as a result of endemic iodine deficiency. Over time the gland enlarges and evolves into an admixture of fibrosis, functional nodules, and non-functioning involuted nodules. Scintigraphically, the MNG

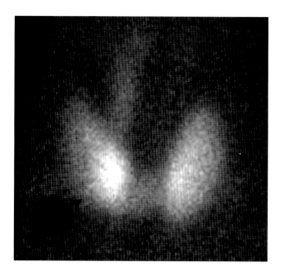

Figure 13.5. Graves' disease. ^{99m}Tc thyroid scan shows a pyramidal lobe emanating from the medial aspect of the right lobe. Note the convex contour of the gland and the diminished background activity.

is a heterogeneously-appearing, asymmetrically enlarged gland with multiple cold, warm, and hot areas of various sizes (Figure 13.6). The incidence of thyroid carcinoma in MNG is low at 1–6%, but a dominant or enlarging cold nodule should be

biopsied. The differential diagnosis includes autoimmune Hashimoto's thyroiditis, multiple adenomas, and multifocal carcinoma. Further characterization of the gland with ultrasound, CT, or MRI does not appreciably aid clinical diagnosis.

Thyroid Nodules

The management of patients with a solitary thyroid nodule remains controversial, related to the high incidence of nodules, the infrequency of thyroid malignancy, and the relatively low morbidity and mortality associated with differentiated thyroid cancer (DTC) [2]. Thyroid nodules may contain normal thyroid tissue, benign hypofunctioning tissue (solid, cystic, or complex), hyperplastic or autonomously functioning benign tissue, or malignant neoplasm. The evaluation of the patient with a solitary thyroid nodule is directed towards differentiating benign from malignant etiologies. Autopsy series have demonstrated a 50% incidence of single or multiple thyroid nodule(s), only 4% of which are malignant. Ultrasonography detects single or multiple thyroid nodules in 40% of patients with no known thyroid disease. The incidence of thyroid nodules increases with advancing age, and is more frequent

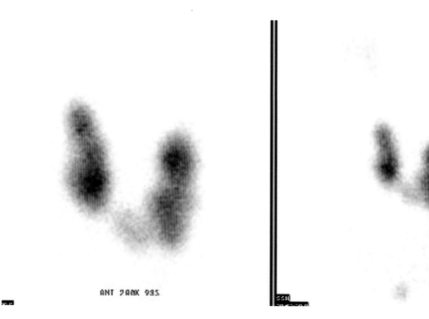

ANT 2ANX 93S

Figure 13.6. Multinodular goiter. An anterior ^{99m}Tc pertechnetate view demonstrates asymmetric enlargement of the gland with multiple areas of increased, decreased, and normal activity. The decreased background activity and faint salivary gland activity is compatible with the clinical impression of toxic multinodular goiter.

in females and in patients with a prior history of neck or facial irradiation.

Hypofunctioning ("cold") nodules concentrate less radioisotope relative to the remainder of the thyroid gland (see Figure 13.3). Eighty-five to ninety percent of thyroid nodules are hypofunctioning, but only 10–20% of cold nodules are malignant [2]. The remaining hypofunctioning nodules consist of degenerative nodules, nodular hemorrhage, cysts, thyroiditis, infiltrative disorders such as amyloid, and non-thyroid neoplasms. Clinical features that suggest thyroid cancer include male gender, a prior history of radiation exposure up to 15 Gy (1500 rad), a family history of medullary or papillary thyroid carcinoma, and relative youth. Local fixation of the nodule or palpable adenopathy is also suggestive. Recent rapid enlargement of a nodule is more often related to hemorrhage into a cyst or nodule rather than carcinoma.

Although ultrasound and MRI are sensitive for the detection of thyroid nodules, specificity for malignancy is poor. Similarly, sensitivity for detection of thyroid cancer is approximately 90% with scintigraphy, but specificity is poor at 15–20%. If extrathyroidal activity is seen in the neck on thyroid scintigraphy in a patient with a solitary thyroid nodule, metastatic thyroid carcinoma is likely. Some investigators have recommended the use of serum thyroglobulin and calcitonin determinations to improve the accuracy of clinical assessment and scintigraphy.

A hot or warm (hyperfunctioning) nodule concentrates the radioisotope to a greater degree than the normal thyroid gland and represents 10–25% of palpable nodules in patients. In over 99% of cases, a hot thyroid nodule is benign and biopsy is unnecessary. Although a functioning thyroid nodule in the euthyroid patient may represent hyperplastic (sensitive to TSH stimulation) tissue, most are autonomously functioning thyroid nodules (AFTN) arising independently of TSH stimulation. Biochemical hyperthyroidism, often subclinical, is present in 74% of patients at presentation, although overt hyperthyroidism is less common. Over a period of 3 years after detection, 33% of AFTNs enlarge in patients not receiving definitive therapy, and 24% of euthyroid patients develop hyperthyroidism [3]. In euthyroid patients, surrounding extranodular thyroid tissue will be visible (Figure 13.7a), thyroid function studies will be normal, and these patients can be followed on an annual basis. If hyperthyroidism

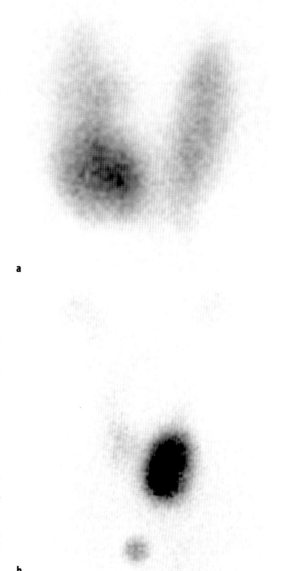

a

b

Figure 13.7. Autonomously functioning thyroid nodule. **a** An anterior ^{99m}Tc thyroid image reveals a focus of increased uptake in the lower pole of the right lobe consistent with a hyperfunctioning nodule. The normal extranodular thyroid activity is indicative of euthyroidism. **b** A focus of markedly increased activity in the lower pole of the left lobe accompanied by virtual complete suppression of extranodular activity and decreased background and salivary gland activity is consistent with toxic adenoma, subsequently confirmed by an undetectable serum TSH.

exists, the surrounding normal thyroid tissue will be suppressed, and the TSH level will be undetectable (Figure 13.7b). Spontaneous cystic degeneration occurs in 27%, manifested by central photopenia; there is little concern for malignancy.

Discordant thyroid imaging is a dissociation between trapping and organification, measured respectively with ^{99m}Tc pertechnetate and ^{123}I. It occurs in only 2–8% of thyroid nodules and is not specific for malignant disease. A nodule that traps ^{99m}Tc (hot) but is unable to organify iodine (cold) is much more likely to be benign than malignant. If it is assumed that 8% of hot nodules with ^{99m}Tc are cold with ^{123}I, and if 10% of those are malignant, then less than 1% of hot nodules seen with ^{99m}Tc imaging are malignant. Additional radioiodine imaging of hot nodules identified on a ^{99m}Tc scan should probably be reserved for patients deemed at higher risk for malignancy.

Hyperthyroidism

Hyperthyroidism is a clinical syndrome of tachycardia, weight loss, and hypermetabolism resulting from supraphysiological circulating levels of thyroid hormones, leading to suppression of TSH secretion. Most cases of hyperthyroidism are due to increased endogenous synthesis and secretion of thyroid hormones from the thyroid. Other less common etiologies are shown in Table 13.2. Clinical assessment combined with circulating hormone and thyroid autoantibody measurements, thyroid scintigraphy, and RAIU usually allow identification of the various disease processes that may be responsible.

Graves' disease (autoimmune diffuse toxic goiter) is due to the presence of thyroid-stimulating immunoglobulins and is associated with autoimmune exophthalmos and pretibial myxedema. Although it occurs primarily in young women, it may also occur in children and in the elderly. Radioiodine uptake will usually be elevated at 4 hours and/or 24 hours, and the gland will reveal diffuse enlargement in most cases with increased thyroid activity and minimal background and salivary gland activity (Figure 13.5). Hyperplasia of the pyramidal remnant is seen as increased paramedial activity in as many as 43% of Graves' patients. Occasionally, the gland will appear normal size. The low RAIU (usually ≤5%) of hyperthyroid patients with subacute thyroiditis, postpartum thyroiditis, silent thyroiditis, and surreptitious thyroid hormone administration is easily differentiated from the normal RAIU seen in the occasional patient with Graves' disease (Table 13.2). Although ultrasound demonstrates an enlarged homogeneously hypoechoic gland with prominent vascularity on color-flow Doppler imaging ("thyroid inferno"), it is usually unnecessary for diagnosis clinically. The thyroid scan should easily be able to distinguish toxic nodular goiters from Graves' disease. The clinical importance of this is that many patients with toxic nodular goiter will require a higher dose of ^{131}I for therapy than will Graves' disease patients.

Radioiodine Therapy of Hyperthyroidism

Graves' disease and toxic nodular goiter may be treated successfully with ^{131}I therapy. Radioiodine was first used for the treatment of hyperthyroidism in 1941 and has since evolved to the treatment modality of choice for the majority of adult patients, particularly in the USA. Antithyroid drug therapy achieves a permanent remission in only 10–40% of patients, but is used initially in many patients, particularly in Europe and Asia. Although subtotal thyroidectomy is effective and complications are infrequent, thyroidectomy is used only occasionally at present. It is normally limited to patients in whom radioiodine is unsuitable, such as women who may be pregnant, or who have extremely large goiters with compressive symptoms. Radioiodine therapy is effective, practical, inexpensive, and available on an outpatient basis.

Table 13.2. Classification of hyperthyroidism

Etiology	Radioiodine uptake
A. Thyroid gland (95%)	
Diffuse toxic goiter (Graves' disease)	↑
Toxic nodule goiter:	
multinodular (Plummer's disease)	↑
solitary nodule	↑
Thyroiditis (subacute/chronic)	↓
B. Exogenous thyroid hormone/iodine (4%)	
Iatrogenic	↓
Factitious	↓
Iodine-induced (Jod–Basedow)	↓
C. Rarely encountered causes (1%)	
Hypothalamic-pituitary neoplasms	↑
Struma ovarii	↓
Excessive HCG production by trophoblastic tissue	↑
Metastatic thyroid carcinoma	↓

Prior to initiation of therapy, the diagnosis of hyperthyroidism must be confirmed by elevation of thyroid hormone levels and suppression of circulating TSH. An elevated RAIU confirms that endogenous thyroidal secretion is the source of the hyperthyroidism and aids in excluding other etiologies of hyperthyroidism, such as silent thyroiditis, subacute thyroiditis, postpartum thyroiditis, iodine-induced hyperthyroidism, and factitious hyperthyroidism, all of which are associated with a low RAIU (Table 13.2). Rarely, clinical hyperthyroidism with diffuse goiter and elevated RAIU may be related to excessive secretion of human chorionic gonadotropin (HCG) by a trophoblastic tumor or by inappropriate secretion of TSH by a functioning pituitary adenoma. The presence of exophthalmos, pretibial myxedema, and diffuse goiter on physical examination confirms Graves' disease as the etiology. Otherwise, thyroid scintigraphy is useful to differentiate diffuse involvement due to Graves' disease from localized disease due to AFTN.

The patient must be counseled prior to therapy regarding the advantages and disadvantages of alternative therapies. Because iodide readily crosses the placenta, ^{131}I may not be administered during pregnancy so a pregnancy test is mandatory prior to administration. Exposure of the fetus to ^{131}I after the 10th week of gestation may result in severe fetal hypothyroidism.

The effectiveness of radioiodine treatment for hyperthyroidism is due to radiation-induced cellular damage resulting from high-energy beta emission, the magnitude of which is directly proportional to the radiation dose received by the thyroid gland. The major effect of radiation is impairment of the reproductive capacity of follicular cells. The radiation dose to the thyroid is related to (1) the amount of radioiodine administered, (2) the fraction deposited in the gland (uptake), (3) the duration of retention by the thyroid (biologic half-life), and (4) the radiosensitivity of the irradiated tissue. Administered dose is usually calculated with the goal of administering approximately 70–120 Gy (7000–12 000 rad) to the thyroid gland [4]. Some practitioners have adopted a fixed dose administration, usually approximately 370 MBq (10 mCi) with perhaps 300 MBq (8 mCi) for a small gland and 440–520 MBq (12 to 14 mCi) for a large gland. In the UK, a relatively larger fixed dose of 550 MBq (15 mCi) is given to the majority of adult patients [5]. Other practitioners will calculate a dose of 3–4.4 MBq (80 to 120 µCi)

per gram of thyroid tissue for the usual patient with Graves' disease. Even higher dosages of up to 7.4 MBq (200 µCi) per gram will be used to produce a more rapid response in patients with severe hyperthyroidism. The calculation is made as follows: administered microcuries = µCi/g desired × gland weight (g) × 100 ÷ percent uptake (24 hours). A higher dose may also be required for patients with toxic nodular goiter, in patients previously treated with antithyroid medications, patients with extremely large glands, patients with rapid iodine turnover (a 4 h/24 h RAIU ratio >1), and in patients with renal insufficiency. Although estimation of thyroid size is relatively accurate for glands weighing less than 60 grams, the degree of inaccuracy increases in larger glands. Ultrasound may provide an accurate estimation of size, but the increase in accuracy of thyroid radiation dose determination is limited.

The complications of radioiodine therapy include rare exacerbation of hyperthyroidism, possible exacerbation of existing Graves' orbitopathy, and post-therapeutic hypothyroidism. It is estimated that less than 10% of patients require retreatment, and this is rarely undertaken before 3–4 months following therapy. Most practitioners will give at least 20–30% more radioiodine on a second treatment. Pretreatment with antithyroid medications is advisable in elderly patients, in patients with known cardiac disease, and in patients with large thyroid glands, particularly multinodular goiters. These medications should be discontinued 48–72 hours prior to administration of ^{131}I, and it is preferable to wait several days before reinitiation of therapy. The administration of beta blockers before or after therapy serves only to ameliorate peripheral manifestations of hyperthyroidism and will not affect therapeutic efficacy of radioiodine.

The incidence of early post-^{131}I hypothyroidism varies from 10% to 50% according to the dose administered. Subsequently, there is an additional incidence of hypothyroidism at a relatively constant rate of 2–3% per year. A similar incidence of hypothyroidism occurs following surgery. Some degree of hypothyroidism may be a natural consequence of the autoimmune process of Graves' disease, since a small percentage of patients treated only with antithyroid medications will become hypothyroid during long-term follow-up after remission.

Although radiation exposure of more than 500 mGy (50 rad) is reported to increase the

THYROID, PARATHYROID, AND ADRENAL GLAND IMAGING

occurrence of leukemia, with a peak incidence at approximately 6 years after exposure, a single ^{131}I treatment delivers only 80–160 mGy (8–16 rad) to the blood and has not been associated with any increased incidence of leukemia, thyroid cancer, infertility, or congenital malformations. Although the desire for subsequent pregnancy is not a contraindication to radioiodine therapy for hyperthyroidism, patients are usually advised to avoid conception for 6 months in case retreatment is required.

Following radioiodine therapy, the patient should be advised to have serum thyroid hormone and TSH levels checked within 2 to 3 months. Patients may be symptomatically improved within 4 to 6 weeks, but clinically significant hypothyroidism rarely occurs before 2 to 3 months. Hypothyroidism is only a problem if not adequately treated, and many practitioners will initiate thyroxine replacement therapy at the earliest indication of post-therapy hypothyroidism.

Thyroiditis

Thyroiditis may be classified as acute, subacute, chronic/autoimmune, and other miscellaneous types; these different types of thyroiditis are unrelated to each other (see Further Reading). Acute suppurative thyroiditis is rare and is caused by hematogenous spread of infectious organisms. This is usually defined clinically and evaluated by CT and/or sonography; scintigraphy is only rarely performed.

Subacute (de Quervain's) thyroiditis is a benign, self-limited transient inflammatory disease of the thyroid, presumed to be of viral etiology. It may affect the gland diffusely or focally and usually presents as a tender gland in a patient with mild systemic symptoms and an elevated erythrocyte sedimentation rate. Serum thyroglobulin (Tg) is elevated and antithyroid antibodies are only marginally increased. A short-lived destruction-induced thyrotoxicosis is followed by several months of hypothyroidism, usually subclinical. Thyroid scintigraphy will show poor thyroid visualization with increased background activity and an RAIU of <5% (Figure 13.8). Most patients are eventually left with a normal thyroid gland, both histologically and functionally. Symptoms respond to non-steroidal or steroidal anti-inflammatory agents and beta blockade.

A second variety of thyrotoxic subacute thyroiditis is termed silent lymphocytic thyroiditis and is similar in presentation to de Quervain's thyroiditis except for the absence of pain, tenderness, and prodromal systemic symptoms. The etiology is thought to be an exacerbation of underlying autoimmune thyroid disease. Thyroid autoantibodies are present in high titers, but often diminish as the thyrotoxic phase resolves. A destruction-induced hyperthyroidism

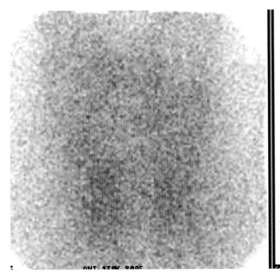
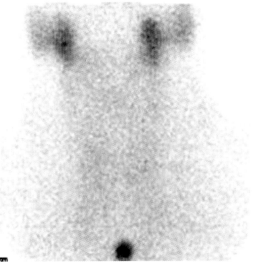

Figure 13.8. Subacute thyroiditis. An anterior ^{99m}Tc image reveals markedly reduced activity in the thyroid bed as compared to background and salivary glands. Serum TSH was undetectable.

is accompanied by markedly suppressed RAIU and mild thyromegaly, all of which resolve over months. This entity presents more frequently in postpartum women (termed postpartum thyroiditis) and tends to recur with subsequent pregnancies. Many of these women will eventually develop permanent hypothyroidism.

Chronic Hashimoto's autoimmune lymphocytic thyroiditis is the most common cause of hypothyroidism in the Western world and usually presents in women with a small to moderately-enlarged firm goiter, elevated antithyroglobulin and/or antimicrosomal (antiperoxidase) antibodies, and rarely any tenderness. Patients may be euthyroid or hypothyroid and rarely hyperthyroid. Scintigraphy reveals inhomogeneous activity throughout the gland in 50%, though a pattern of multinodular goiter, solitary hot nodule, or solitary cold nodule as well as a normal scan may occur. RAIU may be normal, low, or elevated. Biopsy is rarely necessary for diagnosis, and most patients are treated with thyroid hormone supplementation.

Iodine-induced thyrotoxicosis occurs most frequently in patients with pre-existing thyroid disease via the Jod–Basedow phenomenon. Patients with autonomously functioning thyroid adenoma(s), previously treated Graves' disease, and colloid goiter are most susceptible. Scintigraphy usually reveals a pattern of MNG, and RAIU is diminished. On the other hand, the patient with iatrogenic or factitious hyperthyroidism will exhibit only background activity on thyroid scintigraphy and may not have a palpable goiter. RAIU will be very low.

Mediastinal Goiter

The most common neoplasms of the anterior mediastinum are thymomas, lymphomas, and germ cell tumors. Although retrosternal thyroid accounts for only 7–10% of all mediastinal masses, the non-invasive demonstration of radioiodine uptake within a mediastinal mass is useful as it avoids more invasive tissue diagnosis. Retrosternal thyroid tissue is usually the result of inferior extension of a cervical goiter, but may be related to enlargement of ectopic mediastinal thyroid tissue. Continuity between the cervical and intrathoracic components of a mediastinal goiter may consist of only a narrow fibrous band and may not be demonstrable by CT or ultrasound. If goiter is considered, thyroid scintigraphy should be performed prior to CT imaging to avoid interference

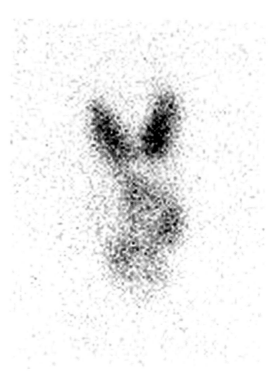

Figure 13.9. Mediastinal goiter. An anterior ^{123}I image demonstrates a relatively normal appearing cervical thyroid accompanied by heterogeneous irregular uptake within the superior mediastinum.

by administration of iodinated contrast media, the most common cause of false negatives.

Due to high background activity related to surrounding blood pool activity, ^{99m}Tc images are suboptimal and difficult to interpret. Iodine-123 is the radionuclide of choice for imaging retrosternal thyroid masses. ^{123}I scintigraphy yields high-quality images of thoracic goiters, even when uptake is relatively decreased (Figure 13.9). Despite the fact that clinically significant thyroid cancer occurs in only 4% of mediastinal goiters, the majority of patients with significant mediastinal goiters eventually undergo surgical resection [6]. However, ^{131}I treatment, sometimes augmented by administration of recombinant human TSH (rhTSH), can be used to reduce the size of the mass and alleviate tracheal compression in appropriate patients.

Neonatal Hypothyroidism

Congenital hypothyroidism (CHT) has an incidence of 1 per 2500–5000 births, and most infants do not exhibit signs or symptoms of hypothyroidism at birth. A delay in the institution of thyroxine replacement therapy beyond 6–8 weeks of life is likely to be associated with measurable impairment of intellectual function (cretinism). Since the institution of newborn screening programs for CHT by measuring serum TSH and/or T_4 levels, the intellectual impairment of CHT has been eradicated in developed countries.

Thyroid dysgenesis (agenesis, hypoplasia, ectopia) is the most common cause of neonatal hypothyroidism in the industrialized world and USA. ^{99m}Tc pertechnetate thyroid scintigraphy is performed immediately after CHT is confirmed. It can easily detect eutopic and ectopic thyroid tissue as well as assess degree of thyroidal uptake [7]. Using a pinhole collimator, a close-up and a more distant view (to include the face and chest) in the anterior projection as well as a lateral view are acquired 20–30 minutes after intravenous injection of 18 MBq (0.5 mCi). A normal image is seen in cases of false positive screening results. A small focus of relatively faint uptake cephalad to the thyroid cartilage is consistent with ectopia and indicates the need for lifelong thyroxine therapy (see Figure 13.4). A eutopic enlarged gland with increased uptake, usually marked, is most consistent with dyshormonogenesis; a small proportion of these are due to transient immaturity of the iodine organification process and will be normal at reassessment after age 3 years. Non-visualization of the thyroid on scintigraphy is due to agenesis in over 90% of cases, the remainder being due to the presence of maternal transmission of TSH-receptor blocking antibodies; these latter patients will be euthyroid at reassessment when these maternal antibodies have cleared. Patients with a non-visualized gland or patients with images suggesting dyshormonogenesis are all re-evaluated at age 3–4 years to exclude transient CHT; patients with ectopia are not reassessed.

Therefore, thyroid scintigraphy in the neonate is indispensable in the proper diagnostic work-up of congenital hypothyroidism, because it (1) provides a more specific diagnosis, (2) is cost-effective for selecting patients for subsequent reassessment to uncover transient CHT and allow discontinuation of thyroid hormone replacement therapy, and (3) defines dyshormonogenesis, which is familial and requires genetic counseling [7].

Detection of Thyroid Carcinoma and Metastatic Thyroid Carcinoma

Thyroid carcinoma accounts for 90% of all endocrine malignancies and 1.5% of all malignancies, with approximately 19 000 new cases occurring annually in the USA; but it constitutes only 1200 cancer deaths per year, resulting in a relatively high prevalence of disease with almost 200 000 patients living in the USA having undergone thyroidectomy for thyroid cancer and requiring regular assessment. Although 80% of thyroid malignancies are DTCs (papillary and follicular), medullary carcinomas (7%), lymphomas (5%), and undifferentiated anaplastic carcinomas (<5%) present specific challenges in imaging.

Differentiated Thyroid Carcinoma

Differentiated thyroid cancers (DTC), which constitute 80% of thyroid carcinomas, grow slowly, occur in young people, and are frequently responsive to therapy (90% 15-year survival). Eighty percent of DTCs are of the papillary or mixed papillary/follicular histology and the remaining are follicular. The behavior of the two tumor types differs, with papillary typically metastasizing to locoregional nodes and the lungs and follicular disseminating hematogenously to the bones. DTC usually maintains the capacity to trap and organify iodine and to synthesize and release Tg. These characteristics of DTC allow post-thyroidectomy treatment of iodine-avid disease with high-dose ^{131}I and the monitoring of therapy using (1) radioiodine scintigraphy and (2) serum Tg. However, dedifferentiation occurs to a variable extent with both types of DTC with loss of the iodide symporter and/or loss of Tg expression, thus presenting challenges for imaging and monitoring these patients. Other less differentiated thyroid malignancies have characteristics (such as calcitonin expression or increased glucose metabolism) that permit specific imaging and post-therapy monitoring.

The traditional methods of follow-up for patients with DTC are whole body radioiodine scintigraphy (RIS) and serum Tg monitoring. Optimal ^{131}I uptake by neoplastic tissue is TSH-dependent, so RIS is performed under conditions of TSH stimulation, either endogenous via thyroid hormone withdrawal or by exogenous administration of rhTSH. Adequate endogenous TSH levels of greater than 30 mIU/l can be attained 10–14 days after the discontinuance of exogenous tri-iodothyronine (T_3) (liothyronine) or 1–4 weeks after the discontinuance of thyroxine (T_4) therapy [8]. Recombinant human TSH (rhTSH) administration as a method of stimulating RAIU (and Tg release) is now available for use in patients maintained on thyroid hormone therapy.

Thyroglobulin is a complex iodinated glycoprotein synthesized and released by both benign and malignant thyroid cells but no other tissues. Circulating Tg, normally 1–25 ng/ml, should be undetectable in the absence of functioning thyroid tissue. An elevated serum Tg determination (>2 ng/ml) in post-thyroidectomy patients with DTC after ^{131}I ablation of the normal remnant is a highly sensitive and specific indicator of residual or metastatic thyroid carcinoma. TSH-stimulated Tg determinations are more sensitive for the detection of metastases than are levels done in patients on suppressive therapy. Traditionally, RIS in combination with TSH-stimulated serum Tg measurements are performed due to reports of recurrent disease occurring in the absence of TSH-stimulated Tg elevation.

Whole body RIS is first performed several weeks after thyroidectomy. Due to its potentially adverse effects on a fetus, exclusion of pregnancy is mandatory prior to administering scanning doses of [131]I. Following the oral administration of 2–5 mCi of ^{131}I, static whole body images are acquired at 48 to 72 hours. A low iodine diet may significantly increase RAIU into metastatic lesions. Although the specificity of ^{131}I scanning is 95%, one must not confuse the normal physiological activity in the salivary glands, nose, gastric mucosa, urinary bladder, bowel, and lactating breast with metastatic disease. Due to hepatic catabolism of iodothyronines, diffuse liver uptake is seen physiologically if there is benign or malignant functioning thyroid tissue present. Typically, ^{131}I uptake is not seen in Hürthle cell, medullary, or anaplastic tumors.

The sensitivity of ^{131}I scintigraphy for the detection of persistent or metastatic thyroid carcinoma is 50–70%, dependent in part on the dose administered. Imaging 3–7 days after a therapeutic dose of 3.7–5.4 GBq (100–200 mCi) of ^{131}I may increase the detection of metastatic lesions by up to 45% [9]. The combination of RIS and serum Tg determination augments the detection of metastatic disease to 85–100% [10, 11].

A schedule of follow-up examinations at 6–12 month intervals is recommended until the serum Tg is undetectable and RIS demonstrates no pathologic uptake. Scanning at 2–3 year intervals can then be instituted, remembering that 50% of DTC recurrences occur more than 5 years after initial treatment.

Stunning is the phenomenon in which the initial diagnostic dose of ^{131}I, 75–185 MBq (2–5 mCi), reduces trapping of the subsequently administered treatment dose. The frequency of this effect and its clinical significance is controversial, but quantitative uptake studies seem to confirm a 30–50% reduction of therapeutic radioiodine uptake as compared to the diagnostic dose. Many investigators now advocate utilizing ^{123}I scintigraphy with 37–185 MBq (1–5 mCi) partly to avoid ^{131}I-induced stunning but also because of the superior image quality. In most reports, there is little if any difference in the sensitivity for detection of thyroid remnant and metastases using ^{123}I versus post-therapy high-dose ^{131}I imaging, and SPECT acquisitions with or without CT fusion can be performed with diagnostic ^{123}I imaging when deemed appropriate [12].

Other DTC-avid radiopharmaceuticals such as ^{201}Tl, ^{99m}Tc-MIBI, and [18]FDG (^{18}F-fluoro-deoxyglucose) are most importantly used in the cohort that is ^{131}I scan-negative but serum Tg-positive, which constitutes about 10–15% of patients with negative diagnostic RIS. These alternative radiopharmaceuticals should not be used instead of RIS unless the patient is known from earlier studies to be ^{131}I-negative. Although skeletal metastases of DTC are mostly osteolytic, ^{99m}Tc diphosphonate scintigraphy is often positive in patients with bone metastases (64–85%) but may not accurately demonstrate the extent of disease.

Thallium-201 whole body scintigraphy has a sensitivity of 60–90% for the detection of metastatic DTC, including ^{131}I-negative, Tg-positive metastases, and SPECT may increase the sensitivity for the detection of small metastatic foci. False positive findings may be seen with non-thyroidal tumors, vascular structures, and salivary glands. ^{99m}Tc-MIBI is highly sensitive for the detection of cervical and mediastinal lymphadenopathy, but is less useful for detection of pulmonary metastases. In a large multicenter trial comprising 222 patients, sensitivity of [18]FDG PET was 85% for the patients with negative RIS and was significantly higher for [18]FDG than for ^{201}Tl or ^{99m}Tc-MIBI [13]. In a review of 14 studies, [18]FDG PET exhibited a consistently high sensitivity for detection of recurrent tumor in patients with elevated serum Tg and negative RIS [14]. The higher the serum Tg, the higher the sensitivity for detection of tumor (50% for Tg 10–20 ng/ml and 93% for Tg >100 ng/ml), but [18]FDG PET reportedly detects 70% of cervical nodes less than

1 cm in diameter. Furthermore, there is preliminary evidence that ^{18}FDG PET may have prognostic importance with 3-year survival of only 18% in patients with a high volume of ^{18}FDG-avid disease versus 96% survival in those with less bulky disease [15]. Patients whose metastases are ^{18}FDG-negative have a good prognosis, and ^{18}FDG-positive lesions tend to be resistant to ^{131}I therapy. There is accumulating evidence that TSH stimulation may increase sensitivity for ^{18}FDG PET detection of metastatic disease by up to 30%, with a 63% increase in tumor-to-background ratio. Many institutions now perform ^{18}FDG PET for thyroid cancer utilizing rhTSH administration or exogenous hormone withdrawal.

Seventy-five percent of patients with recurrent DTC will have positive ^{131}I scans. When treated with high-dose ^{131}I therapy, many of the remaining RIS-negative patients demonstrate positive post-therapy scans, indicating that their DTC is to some degree iodine-avid. Although the long-term success of ^{131}I therapy in RIS-negative/Tg-positive patients is controversial in regard to outcome, many do demonstrate a post-therapy reduction in serum Tg. Interestingly, 89% of patients with negative diagnostic RIS and elevated serum Tg but no radiographic evidence of tumor experience a significant reduction in serum Tg over prolonged follow-up, 68% down to undetectable levels, without ^{131}I or any other treatment [16]. Therefore, the extent of disease and advisability for surgical management in some of these patients with positive post-therapy scans and elevated serum Tg may better be demonstrated by ^{18}FDG PET combined with conventional cross-sectional imaging. Those patients with elevated serum Tg and negative RIS after ^{131}I therapy are best evaluated with ^{18}FDG PET, resulting in a change in management in over 50%. In fact, the possibility of the coexistence of iodine-negative and iodine-positive lesions and the discordance in localization of iodine-positive and ^{18}FDG-positive lesions are clinical challenges that may further increase the clinical utility of ^{18}FDG PET even in the presence of iodine-positive disease.

In summary, most patients who are RIS negative but serum Tg positive will have RIS performed after a therapeutic dose of ^{131}I. If no metastases are identified with the post-therapy RIS, the patient will be followed using a combination of conventional imaging including chest X-ray, neck ultrasound, and cross-sectional imaging with or without the use of alternative radiopharmaceuti-

cals. ^{18}FDG PET seems to be the radiopharmaceutical of choice and would be expected to be more sensitive than ^{99m}Tc-MIBI or ^{201}Tl for small volume disease.

Medullary Thyroid Carcinoma

Medullary thyroid carcinoma (MTC), representing approximately 3–5% of all thyroid cancers, is an intermediate grade malignancy occurring in both a sporadic (80%) and a familial (20%) form. Nearly 50% of patients have metastatic cervical adenopathy at presentation. Five-year survival is 94% in patients with metastatic lymphadenopathy but only 41% in those with extranodal disease. Typically, MTC does not concentrate iodine, so RIS is not useful and ^{131}I treatment results in no improvement in survival or recurrence rate.

Although numerous scintigraphic modalities including ^{123}I/^{131}I-MIBG, ^{99m}Tc-(V)-DMSA, ^{111}In octreotide, ^{201}Tl and ^{99m}Tc-MIBI imaging have been successfully utilized to a varying degree, ^{18}FDG PET is evolving into the primary modality for detection of MTC with a sensitivity of 73–94% in patients with MTC and elevated calcitonin levels [17].

Somatostatin receptors are present on the cell surface of medullary carcinomas, and many MTC metastases can be visualized using ^{111}In-labeled somatostatin receptor scintigraphy (SRS). In patients with recurrent MTC, ^{111}In octreotide imaging detects 44–65% of metastatic lesions, but it is not sensitive for detection of hepatic involvement due to its physiological liver uptake.

In summary, the early detection of recurrent MTC and the localization of the metastases is important because microdissection offers the chance for long-term remission for up to 40% of patients, improvement in symptomatology, reduction in the occurrence of distant metastases, and possibly the prolongation of survival. No single diagnostic modality is able to reliably demonstrate the full extent of disease in these patients, but the combination of cross-sectional radiography (US, CT, MR) with scintigraphy using ^{18}FDG PET or ^{111}In octreotide is recommended.

Thyroid Lymphoma and Anaplastic Carcinoma

Primary lymphoma of the thyroid, which accounts for less than 5% of all thyroid malignancies, presents as a rapidly enlarging goiter usually in an elderly patient with preexisting autoimmune lymphocytic thyroiditis. ^{99m}Tc and ^{131}I scintigraphy as well as ^{18}FDG, ^{201}Tl, and ^{99m}Tc-MIBI imaging are of little utility in differentiating thyroid lymphoma from thyroiditis. ^{18}FDG, ^{201}Tl, and ^{99m}Tc-MIBI activity is increased in lymphoma, so these modalities may be useful in the detection of extrathyroidal lymphoma and its response to therapy.

The rare undifferentiated or anaplastic carcinoma of the thyroid presents as a rapidly enlarging goiter in an elderly individual; survival is extremely poor. ^{99m}Tc and ^{123}I scintigraphy will demonstrate non-specific areas of diminished activity. Preliminary reports indicate that ^{18}FDG PET, ^{201}Tl, or ^{99m}Tc-MIBI imaging may be useful in evaluating recurrent anaplastic carcinoma, especially if CT/US findings are equivocal.

13.2 The Parathyroid Glands

13.2.1 Introduction

The diagnosis of hyperparathyroidism is made biochemically by the presence of both hypercalcemia and elevated parathyroid hormone (PTH) levels in the serum. The major contribution of imaging techniques is the localization of the source of abnormal PTH production in patients with hyperparathyroidism. Whereas the use of imaging techniques for localization in individuals

undergoing re-exploration for persistent or recurrent hyperparathyroidism is well accepted, substantial controversy surrounds the efficacy and cost effectiveness of localization procedures used prior to initial surgery.

13.2.2 Anatomy

In most cases, there are four parathyroid glands located posterior to the lateral lobes of the thyroid measuring approximately 5 mm in length and weighing about 35 mg each. Three percent of individuals have only three glands, and in approximately 10–13%, there are a variable number of supernumerary glands, most frequently a fifth gland in a thymic location (Figure 13.10).

The superior parathyroids originate from the fourth branchial pouch and migrate in close association with the posterior portion of the thyroid lobes, so only <10% of superior glands are ectopically placed. The inferior parathyroids arise from the third branchial pouch and descend along with the thymus toward the mediastinum. Variable location of the inferior glands is related to their migration, with only approximately 60% of them being found in the region of the inferior poles of the thyroid. Up to 39% may be found in the superior pole of the thymus, 2% in the mediastinum, and another 2% ectopically located

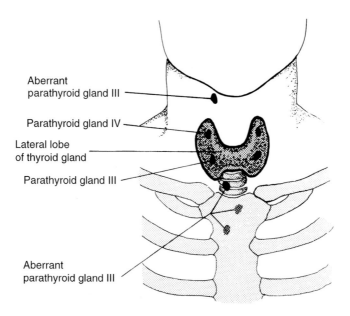

Figure 13.10. Normal and aberrant distribution of the parathyroid glands.

anywhere from the angle of the jaw to the level of the aortic arch. Intrathyroidal parathyroid adenomas may be found in 2–5% of cases. The arterial and venous anatomy supplying the parathyroid glands are variable depending upon the location of the gland, the presence of vascular variance, and previous neck surgery. Knowledge of the venous drainage is a prerequisite for successful diagnostic venous sampling for PTH.

13.2.3 Pathophysiology

Routine automated screening of the general population for serum calcium has resulted in earlier detection of patients with hyperparathyroidism. More than 80% of patients now are asymptomatic or have non-specific symptoms with less than 15% of patients presenting with renal stones. Primary hyperparathyroidism results from a solitary adenoma in over 80% of cases with multiple adenomas, diffuse hyperplasia, or rarely carcinoma accounting for the rest (Table 13.3). Treatment is usually surgical with a success rate of 90–95% without preoperative localizing procedures. Recurrent and persistent hyperparathyroidism is usually related to aberrant or ectopically located glands or recurrent hyperplasia. Re-exploration is technically difficult with a higher morbidity and poorer success rate than initial surgery. Preoperative non-invasive localization improves the cure rate of second surgery from 50–60% up to 90%. Diffuse hyperplasia accounts for approximately 15% of the cases of primary hyperparathyroidism, and a substantial proportion of these may occur in association with the multiple endocrine neoplasias. Secondary hyperparathyroidism in association with chronic renal failure is also related to diffuse hyperplasia, and may require surgical therapy due to progressive bone disease. Total parathyroidectomy plus autotransplantation of remnant tissue into upper extremity musculature is the conventional therapy for this group of patients.

Table 13.3. Pathologic classification of parathyroid lesions in patients with primary hyperparathyroidism

Class	Type	Percentage
Adenomas	Single	80
Hyperplasia	Chief cell	15
	Clear cell	1
Carcinoma		4

13.2.4 Parathyroid Scintigraphy

Both thyroid and parathyroid tissue take up ^{201}Tl, whereas only thyroid tissue will trap ^{99m}Tc pertechnetate. Beginning in 1983, this principle was exploited for the localization of parathyroid adenomas in patients with primary hyperparathyroidism using combined ^{99m}Tc/^{201}Tl subtraction imaging. (Table 13.4). Although this technique has a relatively high sensitivity and specificity for the detection of parathyroid adenomas, it is not sensitive for the detection of hyperplasia or for smaller adenomas. Patient motion during the acquisition of the two sets of images may cause misregistration of data, resulting in both false positive and false negative interpretations [18].

^{99m}Tc-MIBI has been found to accumulate in a wide variety of neoplasms including parathyroid adenomas. ^{99m}Tc-MIBI is distributed in proportion to blood flow and is sequestered intracellularly within the mitochondria. The large number of mitochondria present in the cells of most parathyroid adenomas, especially oxyphil cells, may be responsible for the avid uptake and slow release of ^{99m}Tc-MIBI seen in parathyroid adenomas compared to surrounding thyroid tissue. Physiological thyroid ^{99m}Tc-MIBI activity gradually washes out with a half-life of 60 minutes, whereas parathyroid activity is stable over 2 hours, thus explaining the better visualization of parathyroid adenomas at 2–3 hours post-injection. Due to its simplicity and the better imaging characteristics of ^{99m}Tc, the detection and localization of parathyroid adenomas with ^{99m}Tc-MIBI is now the universally preferred nuclear medicine technique.

Typically ^{99m}Tc-MIBI parathyroid scintigraphy is performed as a double-phase study. Following injection with 740 MBq (20 mCi) ^{99m}Tc-MIBI, two sets of planar images of the neck and mediastinum are obtained using a low-energy high-resolution collimator (Table 13.4). The initial set of images acquired at 10–15 minutes post-injection corresponds to the thyroid phase and a second set acquired at 2–3 hours post-injection to the parathyroid phase. A focus of activity in the neck or mediastinum that either progressively increases over the duration of the study or persists on delayed imaging in contrast to the decreased thyroidal activity on the delayed imaging is interpreted as differential washout consistent with parathyroid adenoma (Figure 13.11).

Table 13.4. Parathyroid imaging

Radiopharmaceutical	^{99m}Tc pertechnetate and ^{201}Tl	^{99m}Tc sestamibi
Activity administered	80 MBq (2 mCi) ^{201}Tl; 370 MBq (10 mCi) ^{99m}Tc	925 MBq (25 mCi)
Effective dose equivalent	4.6 mSv (460 mrem)	5 mSv (500 mrem)
Patient preparation	As for thyroid scanning	None
Collimator	Converging or low-energy, high-resolution, parallel-hole	Low-energy, parallel-hole, high-resolution
Images acquired	Inject Tl first and acquire 15-min 100 000 count view of neck and mediastinum. Then acquire similar Tc images without moving patient. Subtract Tc data from Tl after normalization to equal count densities	Anterior (and oblique) views at 15 min and at 2–3 h; SPECT as needed

This double-phase technique for the detection of abnormal parathyroid glands was reported to be successful in 671 of 803 (84%) patients who had adenomas and was successful in 59 of 93 (63%) patients with multiglandular disease or hyperplasia [19]. Because of the lower sensitivity for detection of very small adenomas and hyperplasia, a "normal" ^{99m}Tc-MIBI scan, in the context of hyperparathyroidism, should be interpreted with due caution. The mean sensitivity and specificity of preoperative ^{99m}Tc-MIBI imaging for the detection of a solitary adenoma is reported to be 91% and 99% respectively [20]. Although the parathyroid pathology is usually best visualized on the delayed images, an adenoma is occasionally best seen on the initial images due to rapid washout from the adenoma (Figure 13.12). As with ^{201}Tl imaging, thyroid pathology and lymphadenopathy may contribute to false positive findings with ^{99m}Tc-MIBI imaging, although specificity is generally reported to be in the range of 95%. In the patient with known thyroid pathology, a dual radioisotope technique may be preferable; ^{99m}Tc pertechnetate or ^{123}I subtraction has been used with reported sensitivities of 80–100% and improved specificity. SPECT may sometimes detect abnormalities not seen on the planar views, and SPECT/CT fusion imaging is promising for improved localization. Both ^{201}Tl subtraction imaging and positron emission tomography using ^{18}FDG may sometimes detect a parathyroid adenoma not identified using ^{99m}Tc-MIBI scintigraphy.

There is universal agreement on the need for accurate preoperative imaging for localization in patients undergoing reoperative parathyroid exploration and in patients undergoing parathyroid surgery after previous thyroidectomy. With accurate preoperative localization, reoperation is successful in over 90% of patients probably due to the fact that ectopia is 3–5 times higher and multiglandular disease is twice as high as in patients undergoing initial surgery. In the evaluation of patients with recurrent or persistent hyperparathyroidism, most surgeons prefer correlative imaging with at least two and sometimes three modalities, scintigraphy and at least one cross-sectional technique. Using high-frequency transducers, sonography can reliably detect eutopic enlarged parathyroid glands. Although CT scanning has been used successfully, its use is compromised by artifacts from metallic clips and the anatomic distortion related to post-surgical scarring. Magnetic resonance imaging (MRI) with a variety of echo sequences is highly accurate in the detection of aberrant glands in the neck, thoracic inlet, and mediastinum. Recent reports indicate that MRI is approximately 82–88% sensitive and ^{99m}Tc-MIBI scintigraphy is approximately 79–85% sensitive for the accurate localization of parathyroid pathology in patients with recurrent or persistent hyperparathyroidism [21]. The combination of these two modalities has provided a substantial improvement in the sensitivity and positive predictive value in the range of 89–94% for localizing the offending gland(s) in patients with recurrent/persistent hyperparathyroidism.

13.2.5 Conclusions

In summary, parathyroid imaging may not be necessary in the initial preoperative evaluation of patients with primary hyperparathyroidism. Exceptions to this may be patients

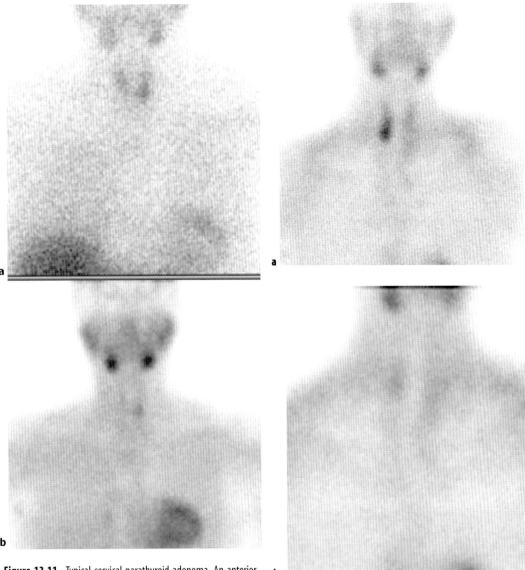

Figure 13.11. Typical cervical parathyroid adenoma. An anterior immediate ^{99m}Tc-MIBI image **a** demonstrates physiological thyroid activity with some prominence at the left lower pole. The 2-hour delayed image **b** shows a persistent focus of activity in the left neck after washout of the thyroid activity, consistent with an inferior left adenoma.

Figure 13.12. Atypical parathyroid adenoma. An anterior immediate ^{99m}Tc-MIBI image **a** demonstrates a focus of increased activity at the lower pole of the right lobe of the thyroid. A 2-hour delayed image **b** reveals washout of physiological thyroid activity as well as the focal increased activity at the right superior thyroid pole. Despite the atypical findings, a large 1600 mg inferior right parathyroid adenoma was resected with postoperative resolution of hypercalcemia.

with prior thyroid surgery, severe hypercalcemia, or severe concurrent medical problems. However, because of the high sensitivity and specificity of ^{99m}Tc-MIBI scintigraphy, routine preoperative localization is becoming a standard practice. In the assessment of patients with recurrent or persistent hyperparathyroidism, localization procedures prior to re-exploration are mandatory.

13.3 The Adrenal Glands

13.3.1 Introduction

The evaluation of adrenal disorders has been simplified by the development of sensitive and specific biochemical tests and by the availability of high-resolution CT and MR imaging. On the other hand, the exquisite spatial resolution of these imaging modalities has produced the diagnostic conundrum of the adrenal incidentaloma. The scintigraphic assessment of disorders of the adrenal cortex, such as Cushing's syndrome, primary aldosteronism, and adrenal hyperandrogenism, is only infrequently required, whereas the ability to survey the whole body for extra-adrenal disease in patients with pheochromocytoma has resulted in an expanding clinical role for adrenal medullary imaging.

13.3.2 Anatomy

Each adrenal gland lies in the retroperitoneal perinephric space, weighing approximately 4 grams and with a thickness of <10 mm (Figure 13.13). The right adrenal is triangular and lies above the upper pole of the right kidney, posterior to the inferior vena cava. The left adrenal is crescent-shaped and lies medial to the kidney above the left renal vein.

13.3.3 Physiology

The adrenal gland has a unique functional and anatomical arrangement. The cortical steroid

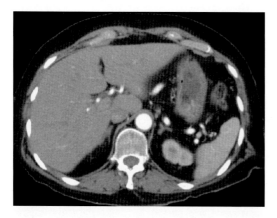

Figure 13.13. Axial contrast-enhanced abdominal CT image demonstrates the normal location and contour of the adrenal glands.

hormones are synthesized from a common precursor, cholesterol, and secreted from the three concentric zones of the adrenal cortex. Aldosterone secretion from the outermost zona glomerulosa is modulated by the renin-angiotensin-aldosterone system whereas cortisol secretion from the zona fasciculata and adrenal androgen secretion from the innermost zona reticularis are under control of the hypothalamic-pituitary-adrenal axis. The adrenal medulla secretion of the principal catecholamine, epinephrine (adrenaline), is under central sympathetic nervous system control.

13.3.4 Adrenal Cortical Scintigraphy

[131]I-6β-Iodomethyl-19-norcholesterol (also known as iodocholesterol or NP-59) is the current radiopharmaceutical of choice for adrenal cortical imaging due to its high avidity for the adrenal cortex. Although iodocholesterol remains investigational in the USA, it is commercially available in Europe and Asia, and ^{131}I-6-iodocholesterol is in clinical trials. The main disadvantage of iodocholesterol scintigraphy is the high radiation dose and it should be used selectively, with other imaging modalities.

The incorporation of these agents into adrenocortical cells is related to the precursor status of cholesterol for adrenal steroid synthesis and to the transport of cholesterol and radiocholesterol by low-density lipoprotein (LDL) [22]. The number of LDL cell surface receptors and their affinity for LDL-cholesterol determine the degree of radiocholesterol uptake by the adrenal cortex. An increase in the serum cholesterol reduces uptake by downregulating LDL receptors. Any increase in circulating ACTH results in increased radiocholesterol uptake. Although radiocholesterol is stored in adrenal cortical cells, it is not esterified and therefore not incorporated into adrenal hormones. Several medications, including glucocorticoids, diuretics, spironolactone, ketoconazole, and cholesterol-lowering agents, may interfere with radiocholesterol uptake [22].

Following injection, the uptake of the radiocholesterols is progressive over several days, and there is prolonged retention within the adrenal cortex, permitting imaging over a period of days to weeks. Although adrenal uptake for all of these agents is ≤0.2% per gland, total body exposure is relatively high (Table 13.5).

Table 13.5. Adrenal imaging

Radiopharmaceutical	[^{131}I]iodocholesterol
Activity administered	35 MBq (1 mCi)
Effective dose equivalent	105 mSv (10 rem)
Patient preparation	Thyroid blocked
Collimator	High-energy, general purpose, parallel-hole
Images acquired	Posterior, lateral, anterior, and obliques of the abdomen. Images taken at about 4 and 7 days post-injection, 20 min exposure per image

The imaging protocol is presented in Table 13.5. Emphasis is given to the posterior view of the abdomen, and lateral views may be required to differentiate gallbladder uptake from activity in the right adrenal gland. Due to problems with soft tissue attenuation and relatively high variability of percentage uptake between normal glands, the quantitation of differential uptake is troublesome. Only when uptakes differ by more than 50% should they be considered abnormal [22].

Although radiotracer uptake reaches its maximum by 48 hours, imaging is usually delayed to day 4 or 5 to allow clearance of background activity. The right adrenal gland frequently appears more intense than the left due to its more posterior location and the superimposition of hepatic activity (Figure 13.14). Visualization of the liver, colon, and gallbladder is physiological. Gastric and bladder activity due to free iodine will usually clear within 48–72 hours post-injection. Bothersome gastrointestinal activity related to enterohepatic circulation of radiocholesterol can usually be cleared by the administration of laxatives.

Cushing's Syndrome

The diagnostic accuracy of iodocholesterol scintigraphy for detecting adrenal hyperplasia, adenoma, or carcinoma as the cause of glucocorticoid excess is approximately 95%. However, it is rarely necessary in the evaluation of Cushing's syndrome. Bilateral symmetrical uptake is seen in ACTH-dependent Cushing's syndrome related to pituitary hypersecretion (Cushing's disease) or ectopic ACTH secretion (Figure 13.15). Adrenal uptake is generally ≥0.3% of the administered dose per gland and will frequently exceed 1% in cases of ectopic ACTH secretion. However, biochemical testing combined with CT and/or MRI is usually successful in localizing the site of ACTH secretion without scintigraphy, except in occasional cases of ectopic ACTH syndrome.

Although non-functioning adrenal adenomas are not ^{18}FDG-avid, functioning cortical adenomas causing Cushing's syndrome may be detected by ^{18}FDG PET [23]. Virtually all adrenocortical carcinomas are detected by ^{18}FDG PET and can be accurately staged by PET as well [24].

In patients with recurrent Cushing's syndrome following prior bilateral adrenalectomy, adrenal scintigraphy may be the most sensitive means of localizing functional adrenal remnants [22]. Despite the use of CT, MRI, venography, arteriography, and selective venous

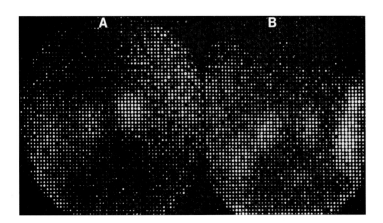

Figure 13.14. Normal ^{131}I iodocholesterol scan demonstrating normal degree of adrenal symmetry. On the posterior abdominal image (A), the right adrenal appears more intense due to its more posterior (and cephalad) location, whereas on the anterior image (B), the left adrenal appears more intense.

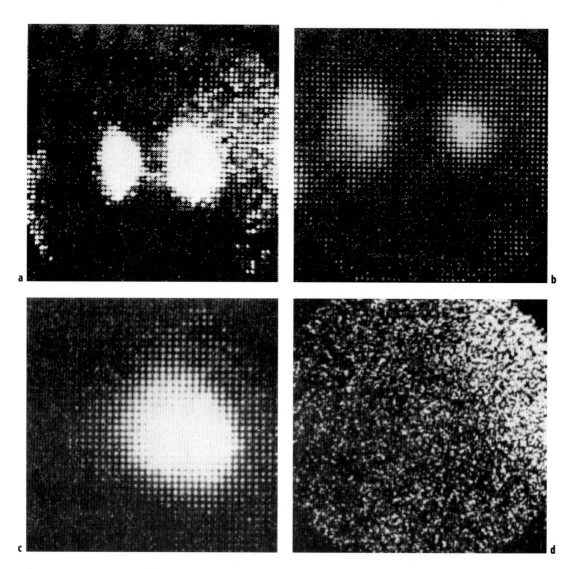

Figure 13.15. The pattern of ^{131}I iodocholesterol imaging in Cushing's syndrome. **a** ACTH-dependent, bilateral hyperplasia. **b** ACTH-independent, bilateral, nodular hyperplasia. **c** Adrenocortical adenoma. **d** Adrenocortical carcinoma. (With permission from Gross MD, Thompson NW, Beierwaltes WH, et al. Scintigraphic approach to the localization of adrenal lesions causing hypertension. Urol Radiol 1981–82; 3(4):242.)

hormone sampling, many of these remnants are difficult to detect without the use of adrenal scintigraphy.

Primary Aldosteronism

Primary aldosteronism presents with hypertension, hypokalemia, and excessive aldosterone secretion with suppression of plasma renin activity and is generally thought to account for <1% of the hypertensive population. However, recent studies

utilizing the plasma aldosterone/plasma renin activity ratio as a screening test suggest that primary aldosteronism has a prevalence as high as 12% [25]. The differentiation of adenoma from bilateral hyperplasia is difficult with biochemical testing without performing bilateral adrenal vein sampling. Aldosteronomas are typically less than 2 cm in diameter and cannot be differentiated from non-functioning adenomas by CT or MRI; hyperplasia is often inferred by absence of a detectable mass.

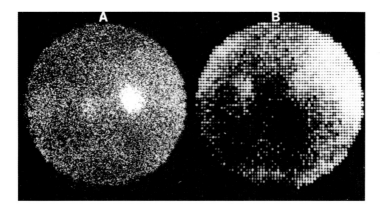

Figure 13.16. Dexamethasone suppression ^{131}I iodocholesterol scintigraphy in primary aldosteronism. A, Day 5 posterior image in a patient with an aldosteronoma; physiological left adrenal activity is faint. B, Day 4 posterior image demonstrates early bilateral symmetric activity in a patient with adrenal hyperplasia. (Reprinted with permission. © American Society of Contemporary Medicine and Surgery. Grekin RJ, Gross MD. Endocrine hypertension. Compr Ther. 1983 Feb;9(2):65–74.)

Aldosterone is not regulated by pituitary ACTH secretion. An adenoma cannot be diagnosed on a baseline scan because both adrenal glands are visualized in all patients with primary aldosteronism, and the degree of asymmetry may be identical in patients with bilateral hyperplasia or adenoma. To increase the specificity, the dexamethasone suppression scan is necessary [22]. Dexamethasone suppression, 4 mg for 7 days before and continued for 5 to 7 days post-injection, results in scans in which the normal cortex is visualized no earlier than the 5th day after iodocholesterol injection. Unilateral adrenal visualization or "break through" before the 5th day post-injection or marked asymmetrical activity thereafter is consistent with adenoma (Figure 13.16). Bilateral adrenal visualization before the 5th day suggests bilateral adrenal cortical hyperplasia. Bilateral uptake after the 5th day may occur in normal subjects. Accuracy of the dexamethasone suppression scan exceeds 90%.

Hyperandrogenism

Dexamethasone suppression radiocholesterol scintigraphy has been used successfully to identify an adrenal source of androgen hypersecretion. Because cholesterol is the precursor for synthesis of gonadal steroids, iodocholesterol imaging has successfully localized both neoplastic and non-neoplastic (e.g. hyperthecosis) ovarian and testicular sources of excess androgen secretion.

13.3.5 Adrenal Medullary Scintigraphy

Pheochromocytomas are catecholamine-secreting neoplasms arising from chromaffin cells. Approximately 10% are malignant, 10% are bilateral, 10% occur in children, and 10–20% are extra-adrenal in origin (paragangliomas), usually in the abdomen or pelvis but occasionally in the neck or mediastinum. Bilaterality, extra-adrenal sites, and malignancy are more common in children. Because anatomical imaging studies are nonspecific and may not be sensitive for the presence of extra-adrenal foci, bilaterality, or metastatic disease, adrenal medullary scintigraphy may play a pivotal role in the management of patients with pheochromocytoma, paraganglioma, or even neuroblastoma (see Section 16.7). This is especially important in view of the several-fold higher perioperative complication rate associated with reoperation.

Radiopharmaceuticals

Metaiodobenzylguanidine (MIBG) is a guanethidine analogue similar to norepinephrine that is taken up by adrenergic tissue via expressed plasma membrane norepinephrine transporters and intracellular vesicular monoamine transporters. Uptake may be inhibited by a variety of pharmaceuticals including sympathomimetics, antidepressants, and some antihypertensives, especially labetalol. These must be withheld for an appropriate length of time before MIBG administration.

Table 13.6. Pheochromocytoma and sympathomedullary imaging

Radiopharmaceutical	^{123}I-MIBG	^{131}I-MIBG
Activity administered	400 MBq (10 mCi)	20 MBq (0.5 mCi)
Effective dose equivalent	6 mSv (600 mrem)	3 mSv (300 mrem)
Patient preparation	Lugol's solution or a saturated solution of potassium iodide (100 mg twice a day) begun the day prior to administration of the radiopharmaceutical and continued for 4 days afterwards	Lugol's solution or a saturated solution of potassium iodide (100 mg twice a day) begun the day prior to administration of the radiopharmaceutical and continued for 7 days afterwards
Collimator	Low-energy, high-resolution, parallel-hole	High-energy, general purpose, parallel-hole
Images acquired	Whole body images, anterior and posterior, 10 minutes per step, at 24 h (and 48 h as needed). SPECT of abdomen	Whole body images, anterior and posterior, 20 minutes per step, at 24 and 48 h (and 72 h as needed)

Although both ^{131}I and ^{123}I have been used to label MIBG, ^{123}I is preferable because of its favorable dosimetry and imaging characteristics. Plasma clearance of MIBG is rapid, with 50–70% of the dose excreted unchanged into the urine within 24 hours. Due to the release of free radioiodine from the radiopharmaceutical, the co-administration of stable iodine to block thyroid uptake is necessary.

Technique

The imaging protocol is presented in Table 13.6. Although posterior images of the abdomen are most important, whole body imaging is recommended for detection of paragangliomas and metastatic disease. When ^{123}I-MIBG is utilized,

the image quality is superior (Figure 13.17), sensitivity is higher, and SPECT can be routinely used to more accurately localize abnormalities; fusion with CT or MR data is promising. Physiological activity is typically seen within the liver, spleen, bladder, and salivary glands. Faint activity is seen in the normal adrenal medulla in 16% of cases using ^{131}I-MIBG and in over 25% of cases using ^{123}I-MIBG. Relatively faint activity is also seen in the myocardium and lungs, especially early. Free radioiodine will localize to the gastric mucosa and later in the colon. The uterus may be visualized during menstruation. Importantly, no skeletal activity is normally present. Anatomical variations in the renal collecting system may lead to false positive imaging results.

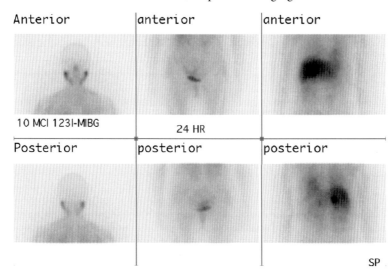

Figure 13.17. Anterior and posterior ^{123}I-MIBG images show a unilateral right pheochromocytoma without additional abnormal foci to suggest metastatic disease. Note the physiological distribution of the MIBG and the improved image quality as compared to ^{131}I-MIBG (Figure 13.18).

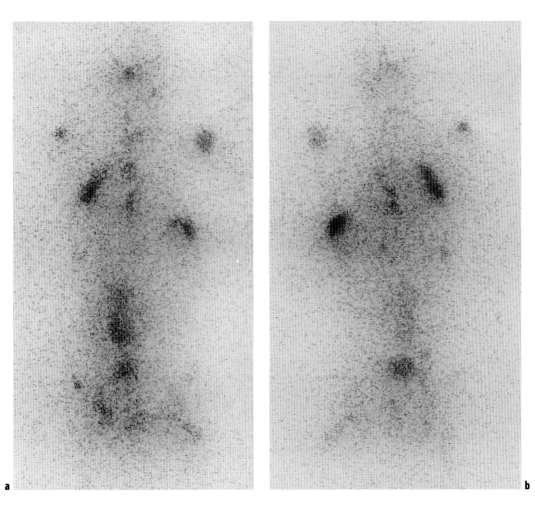

Figure 13.18. Metastatic pheochromocytoma: 48-hour whole body posterior **a** and anterior **b** ^{131}I-MIBG images demonstrate multiple nodal and skeletal metastases.

Clinical Applications

The diagnosis of pheochromocytoma is made by the laboratory demonstration of elevated catecholamines in the plasma and/or urine. Since most adrenal pheochromocytomas are larger than 2 cm in diameter, they are readily identified using CT or MR imaging. Since adrenal masses occur in approximately 3% of the population, functional imaging with MIBG has been recommended to confirm that the mass is a pheochromocytoma and to exclude multiple tumors and metastatic disease preoperatively (Figures 13.17 and 13.18). However, some have not advocated the use of functional imaging in the preoperative assessment of patients with a solitary adrenal mass in the context of proven catecholamine excess due to the low (2%) yield of unsuspected findings [26]. However, in patients with suspected pheochromocytoma who have negative imaging findings with CT and MRI, MIBG scintigraphy can be very useful, especially in view of its high negative predictive value.

Although the sensitivity of CT for the detection of metastatic and extra-adrenal pheochromocytoma is high, CT specificity is relatively poor in the post-surgical patient. The evaluation of suspected recurrent pheochromocytoma requires multiple modalities and should include whole body MIBG imaging (Figure 13.18). False negative MIBG results in such cases may be related to the presence of interfering pharmaceuticals or necrotic tumor. However, malignant pheochromocytoma may dedifferentiate and thus no longer accumulate MIBG. In these instances, [18]FDG PET imaging or ^{111}In octreotide scintigraphy may better demonstrate the extent of metastatic disease (Figure 13.19). Benign pheochromocytoma is also often [18]FDG positive although [18]FDG is more often taken up by malignant pheochromocytoma [27]. Dopamine is a better substrate for the norepinephrine transporter than other amines, and the use of ^{18}F-fluorodopamine (DA) PET is promising for the determination of metastatic disease extent, especially in patients whose tumor is not MIBG-avid [27].

Most neuroendocrine tumors express somatostatin receptors, and somatostatin receptor scintigraphy (SRS) using ^{111}In octreotide has been reported to be highly sensitive (>90%) for the detection of head and neck paragangliomas. However, SRS has been reported to have a sensitivity as low as 25% for the detection of primary adrenal pheochromocytoma [28]. SRS is at least as sensitive as MIBG imaging for detection of metastatic pheochromocytoma (87% versus 57% of lesions) [28]. Therefore, SRS is not recommended as a first-line modality for detection of suspected primary pheochromocytoma.

^{123}I-MIBG imaging may be especially useful in children who more frequently have hereditary syndromes (multiple endocrine neoplasia, von Hippel–Lindau, neurofibromatosis, familial pheochromocytoma, and Carney's triad) and are at higher risk for multifocality, extra-adrenal disease and malignant disease. Bilateral uptake due to medullary hyperplasia may be demonstrated by MIBG scintigraphy, but sensitivity is insufficient to exclude contralateral disease [28]. It must be remembered that MIBG imaging, SRS, and [18]FDG PET may detect other neuroendocrine tumors such as medullary thyroid carcinoma, carcinoid, and islet cell tumors as well as neuroblastoma and small cell lung carcinoma (see Section 16.7). This is especially important in patients with hereditary syndromes. Functional imaging with MIBG is especially useful in differentiating pheochromocytoma from neurofibromas in affected individuals.

13.3.6 Conclusions

In summary, radiocholesterol imaging of the adrenal cortex is most useful in (1) the differentiation of hyperplasia from adenoma in pri-

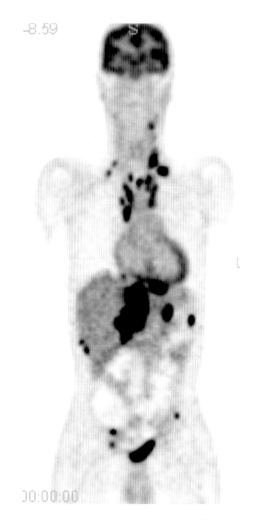

Figure 13.19. Metastatic pheochromocytoma. A [18]FDG PET image demonstrates widespread nodal and parenchymal metastases in this 39-year-old man who presented with labile hypertension. Biopsy of a hypermetabolic cervical node revealed pheochromocytoma. (With permission from Scanga DR, Martin WH, Delbeke D. Value of FDG PET imaging in the management of patients with thyroid, neuroendocrine, and neural crest tumors. Clin Nucl Med 2004; 29(2):86–90.)

mary aldosteronism when CT and MR imaging are equivocal, (2) in the detection of functioning adrenal remnant in the patient with recurrent/persistent Cushing's syndrome despite prior bilateral adrenalectomy, and (3) in the characterization of ACTH-independent adrenal cortical nodular hyperplasia.

Pheochromocytoma and paragangliomas are diagnosed by demonstrating circulating catecholamine excess and are virtually always localized accurately by CT or MR imaging. MIBG imaging is complementary to CT/MR and can be utilized before initial surgery to confirm that the detected mass is a pheochromocytoma and to detect multifocal, extra-adrenal, and metastatic disease. ^{123}I-MIBG is preferable to ^{131}I-MIBG because of better dosimetry, higher quality images, the ability to use SPECT, and probably higher sensitivity. MIBG uptake is higher in sporadic, benign, unilateral, and adrenal pheochromocytoma than in familial, malignant, bilateral, and extra-adrenal pheochromocytoma. In the evaluation of patients with recurrent malignant pheochromocytoma, functional imaging plays a key role. MIBG imaging is useful for detection of MIBG-avid metastatic disease that can subsequently be resected, debulked, or treated with high-dose ^{131}I-MIBG (Chapter 16). For dedifferentiated pheochromocytoma that is not MIBG-avid, SRS using ^{111}In octreotide or PET utilizing ^{18}FDG or ^{18}F-DA is useful.

References

1. Kusic Z, Becker DV, Saenger EL, et al. Comparison of technetium-99m and iodine123 imaging of thyroid nodules: correlation with pathologic findings. J Nucl Med 1990; 31:393–399.
2. Mazzaferri EL. Management of a solitary thyroid nodule. N Engl J Med 1993; 328:553–559.
3. Shakir F, Fitzsimmons TR, Jaques DP, et al. Diagnosis and management of the autonomously functioning thyroid nodule: the Walter Reed Army Medical Center experience, 1975–1996. Thyroid 1998; 8:871–880.
4. Graham GD, Burman KD. Radioiodine treatment of Graves' disease. An assessment of its potential risks. Ann Intern Med 1986; 105:900–905.
5. Hedley AJ, Lazarus JH, McGhee SM, et al. Treatment of hyperthyroidism by radioactive iodine. J R Coll Physicians Lond 1992; 26:348–351.
6. Humphrey ML, Burman KD. Retrosternal and intrathoracic goiter. Endocrinologist 1992; 2:195–201.
7. Sfakianakis GN, Ezuddin SH, Sanchez JE, et al. Pertechnetate scintigraphy in primary congenital hypothyroidism. J Nucl Med 1999; 40:799–804.
8. Grigsby PW, Siegel BA, Bekker S, et al. Preparation of patients with thyroid cancer for ^{131}I scintigraphy or therapy by 1–3 weeks of thyroxine discontinuation. J Nucl Med 2004; 45:567–570.
9. Spies WG, Wojtowizc CH, Spies SM, et al. Value of post-therapy whole-body I-131 imaging in the evaluation of patients with thyroid carcinoma having undergone high-dose I-131 therapy. Clin Nucl Med 1989; 14:793–800.
10. Haugen BR, Pacini F, Reiners C, et al. A comparison of recombinant human thyrotropin and thyroid hormone withdrawal for the detection of thyroid remnant or cancer. J Clin Endocrinol Metab 1999; 84:3877–3885.
11. Lupin E, Mechlis-Frish S, Zatz S. Serum thyroglobulin and iodine-131 whole-body scan in the diagnosis and assessment of treatment for metastatic differentiated thyroid carcinoma. J Nucl Med 1994; 35:257–262.
12. Alzahrani AS, Bakheet S, Mandil MA, et al. ^{123}I isotope as a diagnostic agent in the follow-up of patients with differentiated thyroid cancer: Comparison with post ^{131}I therapy whole body scanning. J Clin Endocrinol Metab 2001; 86:5294–5300.
13. Grunwald F, Kalicke T, Feine U, et al. Fluorine-18 fluorodeoxyglucose positron emission tomography in thyroid cancer: results of a multicentre study. Eur J Nucl Med 1999; 26:1547–1552.
14. Hooft L, Hoekstra OS, Deville W, et al. Diagnostic accuracy of 18F-fluorodeoxyglucose positron emission tomography in the follow-up of papillary or follicular thyroid cancer. J Clin Endocrinol Metab 2001; 86:3779–3786.
15. Wang W, Larson SM, Fazzari M, et al. Prognostic value of [18F]fluorodeoxyglucose positron emission tomographic scanning in patients with thyroid cancer. J Clin Endocrinol Metab 2000; 85:1107–1113.
16. Pacini F, Agate L, Elisei R, et al. Outcome of differentiated thyroid cancer with detectable serum Tg and negative diagnostic ^{131}I whole body scan: comparison of patients treated with high ^{131}I activities versus untreated patients. J Clin Endocrinol Metab 2001; 86:4092–7097.
17. Szakall S Jr, Esik O, Bajzik G, et al. 18F-FDG PET detection of lymph node metastases in medullary thyroid carcinoma. J Nucl Med 2002; 43:66–71.
18. Hauty M, Swartz K, McClung M, et al. Technetium ^{210}Tl scintiscanning for localization of parathyroid adenomas and hyperplasia: a reappraisal. Am J Surg 1987; 153:479–486.
19. Taillefer R. Parathyroid scintigraphy. In: Khalkhali J, Maublant JC, Goldsmith SJ, eds. Nuclear Oncology: Diagnosis and Therapy. Philadelphia: Lippincott; 2001: 221–244.
20. Denham DW, Norman J. Cost-effectiveness of preoperative ^{99m}Tc MIBI scan for primary hyperparathyroidism is dependent solely upon the surgeon's choice of operative procedure. J Am Coll Surg 1998; 186:293–304.
21. Gotway MB, Reddy GP, Webb WR, et al. Comparison between MR imaging and ^{99m}MIBI scintigraphy in the evaluation of recurrent or persistent hyperparathyroidism. Radiology 2001; 218:783–790.
22. Gross MD, Shapiro B, Bui C, et al. Adrenal scintigraphy and metaiodobenzylguanidine therapy of neuroendocrine tumors. In: Sandler MP, Coleman RE, Patton JA, Wackers FJT, Gottschalk A, eds. Diagnostic Nuclear Medicine, 4th edn. Philadelphia: Lippincott Williams & Wilkins; 2003: 6715–6733.
23. Shimizu A, Oriuchi N, Tsushima Y, et al. High [18F] 2-fluoro-2-deoxy-D-glucose (FDG) uptake of adrenocortical adenoma showing subclinical Cushing's syndrome. Ann Nucl Med 2003; 17:403–406.
24. Bechereo A, Vierhapper H, Potzi C, et al. FDG-PET in adrenocortical carcinoma. Cancer Biother Radiopharm 2001; 16:289–295.
25. Mulatero P, Stowasser M, Loh K-C, et al. Increased diagnosis of primary aldosteronism, including surgically correctable forms, in centers from five continents. J Clin Endocrinol Metab 2004; 89:1045–1050.

26. Miskulin J, Shulkin BL, Doherty GM, et al. Is preoperative iodine 123 meta-iodobenzylguanidine scintigraphy routinely necessary before initial adrenalectomy for pheochromocytoma? Surgery 2003; 134:918–923.

27. Ilias I, Yu J, Carrasquillo JA, et al. Superiority of 6-[18F]-fluorodopamine positron emission tomography versus [131I]-metaiodobenzylguanidine scintigraphy in the localization of metastatic pheochromocytoma. J Clin Endocrinol Metab 2003; 88:4083–4087.

28. vander Harst E. de Herder WW, Bruining HA, et al. J Clin Endocrinol Metab 2001; 86:685–693.

Further Reading

Braverman LE, Utiger RD, eds. Werner & Ingbar's The Thyroid: A Fundamental and Clinical Text, 8th edn. Philadelphia: Lippincott Williams & Wilkins; 2000.

Sandler MP, Coleman RE, Patton JA, Wackers FJT, Gottschalk A, eds. Diagnostic Nuclear Medicine, 4th edn. Philadelphia: Lippincott Williams & Wilkins; 2003.

Ilias I, Pacak, K. Current approaches and recommended algorithm for the diagnostic localization of pheochromocytoma. J Clin Endocrinol Metab 2004; 89: 479–491.

14

Gastrointestinal Tract and Liver

Leslie K. Harding and Alp Notghi

14.1 Anatomy and Physiology

The functions of the gastrointestinal tract (GI tract) are digestion and absorption of food, and elimination of waste as feces. After ingestion, food passes down the esophagus and is temporarily stored in the stomach, where it is mixed with digestive juices, and broken down into small particles. It then passes through the duodenum, jejunum, ileum, large intestine, and finally the rectum and anal canal (Figure 14.1). During its passage through the tract it is mixed with saliva, gastric juice, bile and pancreatic juice, and other enzymes which are secreted by the small bowel. The digested food particles are thus absorbed and further metabolized in the liver, which is involved in storage and breakdown of many metabolic products.

In the majority of the gastrointestinal tract the thin outer layer of the bowel is the peritoneum, beneath which is a longitudinal and a circular layer of muscle. In some parts of the bowel, the circular muscle is condensed to form sphincters which regulate the passage of bowel contents through the tract. Between the inner mucosal layer of the bowel and the muscle is a submucosal layer which contains a rich lymphatic, autonomic nerve, and blood supply. Mucus-secreting cells in the mucosa lubricate the bowel contents, and in the submucosal layer are the glands that secrete the digestive enzymes. The liver, pancreas, and GI tract all are intimately involved in digestion, absorption, and metabolism of food and interact with each other via the nervous system and hormonal excretion.

14.1.1 Esophagus

The esophagus is approximately 25 cm long, and unlike the majority of the bowel has an outer covering of elastic fibrous tissue. The circular muscle of the gastric end is thickened to form the cardia (lower esophageal sphincter), which helps prevent gastric contents refluxing into the esophagus. After food is broken down by the teeth and mixed with the salivary juice, a bolus is formed at the back of the tongue. The nasal passages are closed off and the bolus is propelled by a wave of peristaltic activity through the esophagus and into the stomach.

14.1.2 Stomach

The stomach comprises a proximal fundus, a middle body, and a distal antrum and pylorus (Figure 14.2). At the distal end of the stomach the circular muscle forms the pyloric sphincter which controls food passing from the stomach into the duodenum. The main nerve supply is by branches of the vagus nerve, but there is also a sympathetic supply.

Inside the longitudinal and circular fibers of muscle of the stomach is an inner layer of oblique fibers. This additional muscle layer gives the stomach a churning motion which ensures that food is broken down and mixed with gastric juice.

The mucosal layer of the stomach consists predominantly of two forms of cells, the parietal cells which secrete acid and gastric juice, and

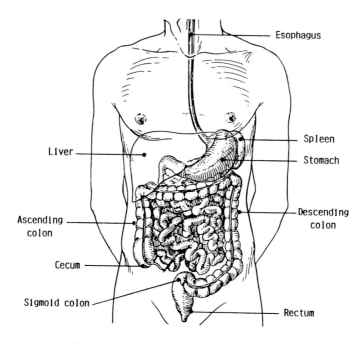

Figure 14.1. General arrangement of abdominal organs.

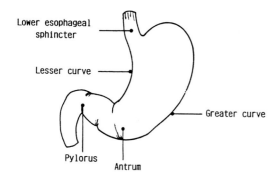

Figure 14.2. The stomach.

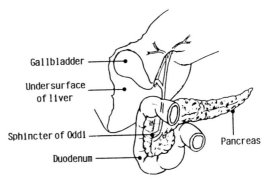

Figure 14.3. The duodenum, pancreas, and gallbladder.

the supporting cells. Gastric juice contains hydrochloric acid, renin which curdles milk, and a protein-digesting enzyme. It also contains intrinsic factor, which is necessary for vitamin B_{12} absorption. Secretion of gastric juice has two main phases. The first or cephalic phase occurs with the sight, smell, or taste of food. This phase is under control of the vagus nerve. Secondly, when food reaches the stomach, the hormone gastrin, which is produced by the stomach, stimulates the glands in the stomach wall to produce more gastric juice.

14.1.3 Small Intestine

The small intestine comprises the duodenum, jejunum, and ileum. The duodenum is C-shaped and curves round the head of the pancreas. It is approximately 25 cm long. The combined pancreatic and bile ducts drain into the medial aspect of the duodenum at the sphincter of Oddi (Figure 14.3). After a meal, both contraction of the gallbladder and relaxation of the sphincter of Oddi are controlled mainly by the hormone cholecystokinin (CCK), which is produced in the walls of the duodenum. Bile contains bile salts, which emulsify fats. Pancreatic juice contains a number of enzymes, particularly important in digestion of proteins.

The jejunum is the middle part of the small intestine and is approximately 2 m long; it blends into the ileum, which is approximately 3 m in length, and both are coiled within the abdomen. The position of the various loops is not fixed, but they are held by the peritoneum to the posterior wall of the abdomen.

The small intestine is the absorptive area of the bowel; microscopically it consists of finger-like projections of mucosa which have a very rich blood and lymphatic supply. Foodstuffs are broken down to monosaccharides, glycerol, fatty acids, and amino acids in the small bowel. These are absorbed and conveyed via the portal vein to the liver.

The ileum terminates at the ileocecal valve, which is in the right lower abdomen. It controls the flow of small-intestinal contents into the large intestine.

14.1.4 Colon and Rectum

The large intestine is approximately 1.5 m long and comprises the cecum, ascending colon, transverse colon, descending colon, sigmoid colon, and rectum (Figure 14.1). The main functions of the large intestine are reabsorption of water and storage of feces. Feces comprise indigestible cellular material, live and dead microorganisms, epithelial cells from the wall of the gastrointestinal tract, and mucus secreted by the epithelium in order to lubricate the feces and allow defecation. The anal sphincters as well as pelvic floor muscles are important for normal evacuation of the rectum.

14.1.5 Liver

The liver is the largest organ in the body, weighing 1200–1500 g. It is situated in the right upper quadrant of the abdomen, protected by the ribcage. It consists of a large right lobe and a smaller thin left lobe.

Circulation

The liver receives about one-fifth of the resting cardiac output; 25% is via the hepatic artery and 75% via the portal vein, which drains the stomach, intestines, and spleen. These vessels enter the liver at the porta hepatis and divide into major right and

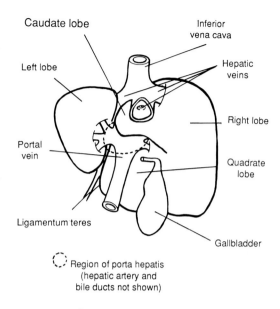

Figure 14.4. Posterior view of liver.

left branches. The division between the territories supplied by the two branches does not correspond to the anatomical right and left lobes.

The blood flowing through the sinusoids drains into a vein at the center of each lobule. The venous drainage ultimately forms three major veins which drain into the inferior vena cava within the upper part of the liver posteriorly (Figure 14.4). Veins from the caudate lobe enter the vena cava directly.

The terminal branches of the hepatic artery and portal vein supply liver lobules, which consist of columns of hepatic cells (hepatocytes) separated by sinusoids through which the blood flows. The sinusoids are lined by Kupffer cells – phagocytic cells that remove particulate matter from the bloodstream.

Biliary Drainage

Small canaliculi between the hepatocytes receive secreted bile and drain into bile ducts which run alongside the branches of the arterial and portal vein at the edge of the lobule. The bile ducts drain into the right and left hepatic ducts, which meet in the porta hepatis to form the common hepatic duct. The cystic duct connects the gallbladder to the common hepatic duct, forming the common bile duct which drains into the second part of the duodenum (Figure 14.3). Bile enters the gallbladder where it is concentrated and then discharged by gallbladder contraction during a meal.

Metabolic Function

The liver makes a major contribution to the body's metabolism. Food substances, absorbed into the portal blood from the gut, are stored or metabolized, and many other compounds are synthesized. A number of hormones, including insulin, glucagon, growth hormone, catecholamines, and thyroxine, regulate the metabolic pathways involved. Enzymes such as alkaline phosphatase and transaminases, present in the hepatocytes, are released in abnormal amounts into the bloodstream after liver damage. Measurement of the circulating levels of such enzymes can be used to detect liver disease, and together with bilirubin and plasma protein concentrations, are referred to as "liver function tests".

Bile

Bile contains salts which are emulsifying agents important for fat digestion. More than 95% of bile salts are reabsorbed in the terminal ileum and re-excreted via the biliary system (enterohepatic circulation). Malabsorption at the terminal ileum results in bile salt loss, reduced bile salt excretion, and thus fat malabsorption. The main waste product excreted is bilirubin, which is derived from the breakdown of hemoglobin. Excess bilirubin circulating in the blood (hyperbilirubinemia) gives rise to jaundice. This may be: "prehepatic", due to excess bilirubin production (hemolytic anemia); "hepatic", due to failure of hepatocytes to secrete bilirubin (e.g. in hepatitis); or "post-hepatic", due to bile duct obstruction (e.g. by gallstone or tumor).

14.2 Esophageal Motility

Once swallowing is initiated, the primary esophageal wave of contraction takes most of the bolus of food down the esophagus and into the stomach, the remainder being rapidly cleared by secondary waves of peristalsis. Problems of esophageal motility occur in a variety of disorders. In achalasia there is both an absence of peristalsis in the lower two-thirds of the esophagus and poor relaxation of the lower esophageal sphincter, due to degeneration of nerve plexuses in this area. Scleroderma is a disease with excess fibrosis, especially evident in the skin, which becomes rigid and shiny, but the disease also affects the

Table 14.1. Esophageal motility

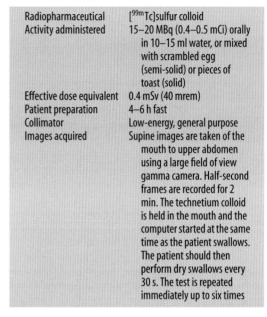

Radiopharmaceutical	[^{99m}Tc]sulfur colloid
Activity administered	15–20 MBq (0.4–0.5 mCi) orally in 10–15 ml water, or mixed with scrambled egg (semi-solid) or pieces of toast (solid)
Effective dose equivalent	0.4 mSv (40 mrem)
Patient preparation	4–6 h fast
Collimator	Low-energy, general purpose
Images acquired	Supine images are taken of the mouth to upper abdomen using a large field of view gamma camera. Half-second frames are recorded for 2 min. The technetium colloid is held in the mouth and the computer started at the same time as the patient swallows. The patient should then perform dry swallows every 30 s. The test is repeated immediately up to six times

gastrointestinal tract, notably the esophagus. This results in difficulty in swallowing, and aspiration of food into the lungs. A third group of patients have diffuse spasm of the esophagus, with uncoordinated motility.

14.2.1 Imaging

The details of the imaging study vary from department to department [1–3]. Technetium colloid has been most commonly used as a non-absorbable marker, although other alternatives are equally appropriate, such as ^{99m}Tc-DTPA. It is usually given in liquid form (with water) or semi-solid form. The imaging protocol is given in Table 14.1.

14.2.2 Appearances

It is conventional to divide the esophagus into upper, middle, and lower portions. Up to 10% of the bolus may remain normally in the lower esophagus. The remainder of the bolus of colloid should traverse the esophagus in under 15 s. Normal transit for upper, middle, and lower moieties of esophagus is 2, 4, and 6 seconds respectively (Figure 14.5). Condensed images maybe used to show the progress of activity through esophagus. The x-axis shows time and the y-axis is the spread of activity from mouth to stomach (Figure 14.6).

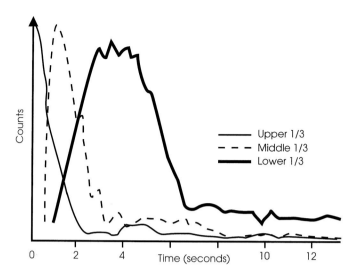

Figure 14.5. Normal esophageal transit showing fast passage of activity through esophagus with no remnant activity. Each curve represents the activity in one third of the esophagus.

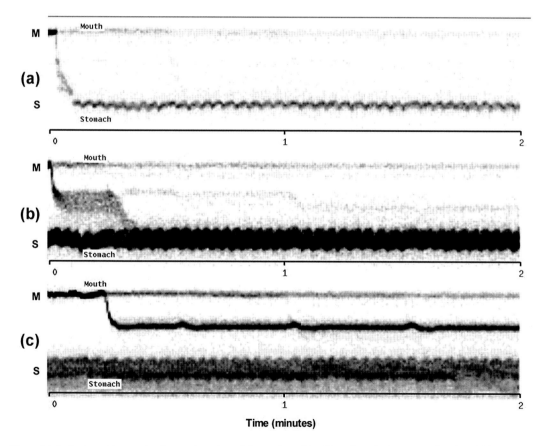

Figure 14.6. Condensed images showing esophageal transit in a patient with mid-esophageal stricture using liquid meal (**a**), semi-solid meal (**b**), solid meal (**c**) (M = mouth, S = stomach).

Table 14.2. Gastroesophageal reflux

Radiopharmaceutical	[^{99m}Tc]colloid
Activity administered	8–12 MBq (0.2–0.3 Ci) in 150 ml 0.1 M HCl and 150 water
Effective dose equivalent	0.2 mSv (20 mrem)
Patient preparation	Fasting
Collimator	Low-energy, general-purpose
Images acquired	An anterior view of the mouth to the upper abdomen is taken. After drinking the radiopharmaceutical, an upright picture is taken at 10–15 min. If there is any residual activity in the esophagus, 15–30 ml of water is taken to clear this activity. The patient is placed supine under the gamma camera and an abdominal binder applied. Pressure in the binder is increased from 0 to 100 mm of mercury by 20 mm increments at intervals of 30 s, with images being taken at each stage. The test is terminated when reflux occurs

14.2.3 Problems

The test is easy to perform, but its reproducibility is low. It is therefore important to perform more than one swallow, and some authors recommend up to six in order to detect an abnormal result [1]. Various methods of looking at transit have been proposed, but the simple transit time is probably the most satisfactory.

14.2.4 Role of Nuclear Medicine in Diagnosis

Apart from the clinical history, disease of the esophagus is normally diagnosed using barium swallow and endoscopy. However, these tests are of little value for examining motility. Pressure measurements in the esophagus are the reference method, but these are difficult to do, inconvenient for the patient, and need experienced personnel who undertake these tests regularly. Some centers now perform nuclear esophageal transit as a simple alternative.

14.3 Gastroesophageal Reflux

Reflux of gastric contents into the esophagus can be demonstrated in a number of subjects who have no symptoms or endoscopic evidence of esophagitis. Other patients, however, complain of heartburn, regurgitation of bitter fluid into the mouth, or difficulty in swallowing. The pain of heartburn may be difficult to distinguish from that of ischemic heart disease when the other symptoms are absent.

14.3.1 Imaging

The best-known nuclear medicine test of esophageal reflux is that which uses an abdominal binder. After swallowing a radiopharmaceutical, the pressure in the binder is gradually increased, and the presence and amount of esophageal reflux is noted [1, 2]. In young children, an alternative test (the milk scan, Section 14.4) is used. The imaging protocol is summarized in Table 14.2.

14.3.2 Appearances

There should normally be no reflux. Should reflux occur, its amount is expressed as a percentage of the counts of the stomach. Four percent is taken as the upper limit of normal and this is evident visually.

14.3.3 Problems

The initial results with this technique suggested that it was both sensitive and specific, but results from elsewhere have been varying. The increase in abdominal pressure produced by the binder is not physiological, and many believe that the test is unsatisfactory.

14.3.4 Role of Nuclear Medicine in Diagnosis

Barium swallow and fiberoptic esophagoscopy are the most commonly used tests. However, as previously explained, barium swallow will show reflux in patients who have no symptoms and which must therefore be considered physiological. Esophagoscopy is positive only if there is esophagitis consequent upon the reflux. The most sensitive test is to monitor the pH of the esophagus, and detect any reflux of acid by the stomach by a fall in pH. However, this test is unpleasant for the patient and requires specialized equipment.

14.4 Milk Scan

The milk scan is used to detect gastroesophageal reflux, which is fairly common in children and usually requires no treatment. It occurs predominantly under the age of 2 years, when the children are on a mainly milk diet. Reflux is generally evident radiologically, and in these children a radionuclide study is not required. If, however, there is doubt as to the diagnosis, and the child has symptoms such as failure to thrive, problems feeding and, especially, episodes of wheezing with chest infection, a radioisotope study should be carried out.

14.4.1 Imaging

The child should be lying on its side and the feeding bottle containing the radiopharmaceutical should be shielded from the gamma camera with lead. The imaging protocol is outlined in Table 14.3.

14.4.2 Appearances

The study is reported by examining the images and time–activity curves over the esophagus. Quantification is not helpful. Reflux into the lower third of the esophagus is common in young children and is of no consequence. Reflux into the upper two-thirds of the esophagus is, however, diagnostic. At one stage, aspiration into the lung was considered an important feature. This aspect of the test has a low sensitivity.

14.4.3 Role of Nuclear Medicine in Diagnosis

All patients should have contrast radiology to exclude disorders of swallowing, hiatus hernia, stricture, gastric volvulus, or gastric malrotation. These structural abnormalities cannot be detected using the milk scan. However, milk scanning is sensitive and specific for detecting gastroesophageal reflux.

14.5 Gastric Emptying

Gastric emptying studies are most often performed on patients with suspected gastroparesis (e.g. diabetic GI neuropathy) or who have an unsatisfactory result from peptic ulcer surgery. Symptoms may be due either to gastric stasis, in which case the patient commonly complains of food vomiting, or too-hasty emptying which results in the symptoms of dumping and diarrhea. Goligher et al [4] showed that the percentage of patients showing dumping 5–8 years after ulcer surgery varied between 1% and 22% depending on the type of operation. Those that involved resection of part of the stomach were associated with a higher incidence of dumping, but proximal gastric vagotomy (PGV) produced dumping in only 1%. Both dumping and stasis may be difficult to evaluate clinically, and it is important to check that there is an abnormality of emptying before a further operation is performed to relieve symptoms.

Gastric emptying measurements are also used to assess the effect of drugs, anesthetics, diabetic neuropathy, or gastric partitioning operations (to treat severe obesity), on gastric emptying. Gastric emptying studies using radionuclides have been used extensively in studying the physiology of the stomach.

The stomach acts as a reservoir for food, and while in the stomach food is mixed with gastric secretions and broken down into small particles before it is emptied via the pylorus. Both the size of particles in the meal and its composition will affect

Table 14.3. Milk scan

Radiopharmaceutical	[^{99m}Tc]sulfur colloid in 100 ml milk or orange juice
Activity administered	15–20 MBq (0.4–0.5 mCi) oral
Effective dose equivalent	0.4 mSv (40 mrem)
Patient preparation	Undertaken at the time of a normal feed
Collimator	Low-energy, general-purpose
Images acquired	Mouth and stomach are included in the field of view. 1 s frames for 4 min. Repeat with the remainder of the feed in a bottle. Images at 4 h

Table 14.4. Gastric emptying

Radiopharmaceutical	[^{99m}Tc]DTPA
Activity administered	15–20 MBq (400–500 μCi) oral
Effective dose equivalent	0.4 mSv (40 mrem)
Patient preparation	Starve for 4–6 h during which time no alcohol or smoking is allowed. Drugs such as metoclopramide, tricyclic antidepressants, or anticholinesterases should be stopped prior to the study
Collimator	Low-energy, general-purpose
Images acquired	Anterior or preferably anterior and posterior images of the sitting or standing patient are acquired. Images should be recorded every minute for 90 min in the case of a solid meal and for 40 min in the case of a liquid meal

the rate of gastric emptying. For example, foods have to be broken down into small particles before emptying through the pylorus will occur, and the higher the calorific value of foods, the slower the rate of emptying. Gravity normally has little effect on solid gastric emptying, but after vagotomy, especially when it is combined with pyloroplasty, gastric emptying becomes gravity-dependent.

14.5.1 Imaging

One factor that has never been standardized in gastric emptying studies is the composition of the meal given to the patient. A wide variety of meals has been used in studies published in the literature, but the important point is that liquid and a solid meals should be distinguished as they behave differently [1–3]. These may be combined into a meal that has liquid and solid phases, but different radioactive labels are required for the two components of the meal. This creates problems in detection of one radionuclide in the presence of the other one, and problems due to differential attenuation because of their different gamma energies. It is also naive to suppose that the radionuclides are distributed totally into a "solid" or "liquid" component. A "solid" meal is a complex mixture of particle sizes, together with emulsions. The simplest meal to use is 10% dextrose containing DTPA, which may be labeled with ^{99m}Tc or ^{111}In. This proves an entirely satisfactory marker for the liquid phase of emptying, and most importantly it is not absorbed in significant amounts, nor does it become attached to gastric mucus or mucosa [1]. As a solid meal we use 70 g of mincemeat (canned) or soy substitute for vegetarian patients, 25 g dried mashed potato, and 15 g of dried peas. The above are cooked in a total of 200 ml of water to which 20 ml of 1% ^{99m}Tc- or ^{111}In-DTPA is added. Finally the meal is made up to a volume of 400 ml. Alternative meals include radiolabeled omelet and

radiolabeled pancake. The problem with all solid meals is that not all the radioactive label remains stuck to the meal throughout the study. An elegant solution to this problem has been devised. It involves injecting a chicken with ^{99m}Tc colloid, killing the chicken and giving the cooked liver as a meal to the patient. This technique is expensive, impractical, and is not necessary for clinical gastric emptying studies. The routine imaging protocol is given in Table 14.4.

14.5.2 Analysis

An area of interest is drawn round the stomach, taking particular care to fit this closely to the border of the stomach at its lower edge in the region of the antrum (Figure 14.7). After background subtraction, counts in the stomach area and the whole field of view of the gamma camera are corrected for radioactive decay. If both anterior and posterior images are acquired geometric mean curves are

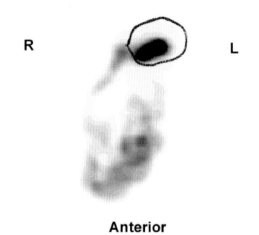

Figure 14.7. Stomach area of interest. Note the close fit to the lower border of the antrum to minimize duodenal overlap.

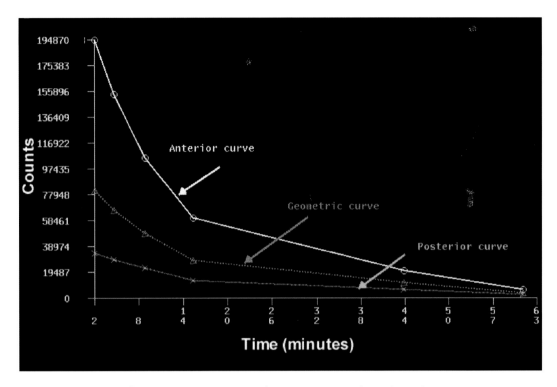

Figure 14.8. Anterior, posterior, and geometric mean curves for gastric emptying.

used (Figure 14.8). The peak counts in the whole field of view correspond to the volume of the meal which has been given to the patient. Counts from the stomach area are expressed as a peak volume, and the half-time ($t_{1/2}$) of the rate of emptying after that peak is calculated. It is important to exclude from this calculation any values representing less than 10% of the volume of the meal, as below this volume errors become large. Not all patients with a low peak volume have symptoms. Our experience is that a volume of less than 240 ml (400 ml meal volume) is associated with symptoms of diarrhea and dumping in about one-third of patients following ulcer surgery. Likewise a solid meal with $t_{1/2}$ over 150 min is associated with symptoms of stasis in only half of the patients. In studies of upper gastrointestinal tract motility, it is not uncommon for some patients who have severe disturbances of motility not to complain. As emphasized earlier, therefore, it is important to ensure that there is an abnormality of emptying before further surgery is offered to symptomatic patients. The normal range for our gastric emptying meal is given in Table 14.5. However, centers using their own meal need to ascertain their own normal range. It is

Table 14.5. Normal range for gastric emptying

Adults	Peak volume Mean (SD)	$t_{1/2}$ volume Median (20–80% range)
5% Dextrose (400 ml)	330 (50)	30 (11–49)
"Solid" meal	–	40 (28–80)
Pediatrics	% administered activity at 60 min Mean	(SEM)
<3 month	65.5	(1.4)
6 month	68	(1.7)
1 year	64	(3.4)
5 years	51	(5.0)

possible to calculate $t_{1/2}$ for antrum and fundus separately to identify function of each segment of the stomach.

14.5.3 Problems

The first problem with this technique is scatter and septal penetration of counts from the stomach region of interest into the rest of the field of view of the gamma camera. This depends on the energy of the radionuclide used, the particular collimator and gamma camera, and its extent should be measured in individual departments using stomach phantoms [1]. The second difficulty that arises is the meal moving forward during emptying, and if only an anterior detector is used, this creates an apparent lag phase in the emptying curve. The error in volume at the end of the study has been quoted as up to 26% in the case of ^{99m}Tc.

A solution to this problem is to take alternate anterior and posterior counts or use a dual-headed gamma camera. The geometric mean of the anterior and posterior counts in the stomach is determined, and this is almost independent of the movement of the meal forwards during emptying.

The last problem is bowel overlap. Some bowel overlap is inherent in the technique, because the distal end of the duodenum tends to loop up behind the stomach. This error is small. Some patients, however, have a very large stomach, and this overlaps loops of bowel to a considerable extent so that the test then becomes invalid. This situation is found to occur particularly in patients with gastric ulcers [1].

14.5.4 Role of Nuclear Medicine in Diagnosis

Nuclear medicine studies are the only satisfactory method of measuring the rate of gastric emptying of solids quantitatively. With liquid meals, naso-gastric aspiration can be used.

14.6 Small Bowel Transit

There is increasing interest in measurement of the small bowel transit as it is now recognized that abnormality of the small bowel transit can account for a number of GI symptoms and problems. In particular, in patients with autonomic neuropathy (diabetic) or with Crohn's disease with segmental involvement of the small bowel, the disease may affect small bowel transit.

14.6.1 Imaging

The same meal as solid gastric emptying is used for small bowel transit measurement. Following standard gastric emptying study, anterior and posterior images of the abdominal region are acquired at half-hourly intervals until the activity is clearly visualized in the cecum.

14.6.2 Analysis

Gastric emptying is measured as described in Section 14.5.2. In the later images the cecum is identified and the percentage of administered activity in the cecum is calculated by drawing a region of interest around it and relating it to decay-corrected geometric mean curves for the whole abdomen and cecum. Ten percent gastric emptying is traditionally considered as the start point and the end point is 10% of the cecal filling. In our experience the normal small bowel transit varies from 4 to 8 hours. However, even with a normal transit, regions where the maximum hold-up occurs in the gut may be identified.

14.6.3 Problems

Due to overlapping and unpredictable position of each segment of the small bowel in the abdominal cavity it is impossible to determine exactly where the activity is during the study. However, the two organs that are fixed and can be identified clearly are the stomach and large bowel. For this reason the main reliable quantitative analysis is the time from start to the end of small bowel transit. Anterior and posterior images are essential so that the geometric mean can be obtained as the depth of activity in the bowel (anterior/posterior) can vary considerably. Decay correction is essential when any ^{99m}Tc radiopharmaceutical is used as the study is prolonged.

14.7 Colonic Transit

Large bowel disorders are common, affecting up to 10% of the population. Despite the large numbers suffering from functional large bowel disorder, the condition has mainly been ignored diagnostically.

There has been increasing use of radionuclide markers for studying large bowel transit. As most patients referred for colonic study are constipated (frequently less than one bowel motion per week), a long-life radionuclide should be used. When studying the large bowel in patients with fast transit, bolus delivery of the radionuclide into the large bowel is preferred. Activity administered orally as a liquid tends to accumulate in the terminal ileum before bolus delivery into the cecum. However this is not consistent and a better approach is the use of a pH-sensitive capsule designed to open in the mid to terminal ileum, thus avoiding the spread of activity due to gastric emptying. Protocols with multiple images up to 10 days have been used, but we find a simplified method of colonic transit measurement satisfactory for most clinical conditions.

14.7.1 Imaging

The patient is asked to refrain from any bowel regulatory medications for at least 48 hours before studying. It may be necessary for the patient to go on a standard diet, but usually the normal diet of patients is used to study the colonic transit. [111]In indium is absorbed onto amberlite resin, which is then encapsulated and coated with a pH-sensitive coating (Eudragit-S BDH Lab. Suppl. Merck Ltd). This coating prevents the activity being released to the acid stomach. The patient is brought to the department at 8.00 a.m. and the capsule administered orally. The first image is then acquired at the end of the first day (8 hours). Both anterior and posterior images are acquired. The patient is then brought back for the following 3 days, for one set of images per day (anterior and posterior). Late images up to 6 days may be required if activity remains in the colon. As the activity administered is small (5 MBq (100 μCi)) it is essential that background activity is measured at least once during the study. The imaging protocol is outlined in Table 14.6.

Table 14.6. Colonic transit

Radiopharmaceutical	[111]In]chloride absorbed on amberlite resin in enteric-coated capsule
Activity administered	5 MBq (100 μCi) oral
Effective dose equivalent	Maximum of 1.3 mSv (130 mrem) in severe constipation Normally <0.5 mSv (50 mrem)
Patient preparation	Overnight fast. No laxatives and bowel regulatory medications for 48 h prior to test and for the duration of the test. Capsule administered in morning
Collimator	Medium-energy
Images acquired	2 minute anterior and posterior images at the end of first day and daily for at least 3 days, if activity persists continue for 6 days

14.7.2 Analysis

Usually on the second or third day the colon is well visualized and its different segments can be identified (Figure 14.9). It is sufficient to divide the colon into four regions: sigmoid and ascending colon; transverse colon; splenic flexure; and descending colon and rectum. The regions of interest are drawn in the anterior and posterior images. The geometric mean for each region at each time point is calculated. After background correction and decay correction the percentage of administered activity in each region at each time point is calculated [5]. The simplest way to display the results is using a schematic diagram with activity shown in different regions with a gray scale and the percentage activity indicated [6].

Colonic transit in general falls into one of the four categories (Figure 14.10). (i) Normal transit, with more than 50% of activity excreted by the end of the third day. Commonly with normal bowel transit all the activity is emptied by the end of the second day. (ii) In generalized delay activity spreads throughout the colon and remains spread out with virtually no activity excreted up to 3 days. (iii) In right-sided delay the activity spreads into the cecum and ascending colon, and remains there with no activity excreted up to 3 days. (iv) In left-sided delay the activity moves normally to

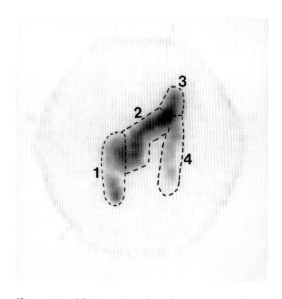

Figure 14.9. Colonic transit study: 24-hour raw image showing activity throughout the colon. 1, Ascending colon and hepatic flexure. 2, Transverse colon. 3, Splenic flexure. 4, Descending colon and rectum.

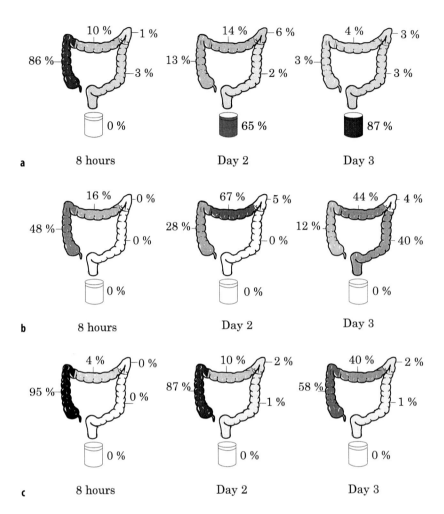

Figure 14.10. Examples of different patterns of colonic transit: **a** normal, **b** generalized delay, **c** right-sided delay.

the left side of the colon (descending colon and rectum) usually within 24 hours, but no activity is excreted to the end of the study. Some patients cannot clearly be identified as belonging to one or the other of these categories, as colonic disorders may represent a spectrum of diseases.

Another method of expressing colonic transit is by using the geometric center. This calculates the progression of the mean mass of activity through the colon using the following formula:

$$\sum_{n=1}^{m} \frac{\%\text{Activity} \times \text{Region}\,(n)}{100}$$

where m is the number of regions. Although a single number to express the whole of transit appears

attractive, the pattern of segmental delay is not available. It is important to perform a colonic transit study before any definitive treatment such as surgery is undertaken as in our experience up to 50% of patients complaining of severe constipation (bowel motion less than once a week) have normal colonic transit. Furthermore, the decision about surgery could be influenced by the type of delay. Left-sided delay seems to be associated more often with pelvic floor disease than colonic abnormalities.

14.7.3 Problems

As with other GI studies the activity moves anteriorly and posteriorly within the abdominal cavity.

Use of a higher energy radionuclide and anterior/posterior view with geometric means overcomes most of this problem. The main difficulty with colonic transit is the mobility of the transverse colon and overlapping of different regions of the colon. Small bowel may overlap with colonic regions but this is usually not a problem as the activity in the small bowel is effectively cleared by the end of 24 hours. Large regions of interest overcome the need for precise delineation of different segments of colon and also reduce the problem with overlapping of segments. In practice the different patterns of colonic transit are so distinct from each other that overlapping is not a major problem.

The most practical way of assessing fecal loss is by calculating the total remaining administered activity in the colon rather than measurement of fecal collections. This overcomes the problem of patients who claim to have had no fecal loss despite a sudden percentage drop in activity remaining in the colon, indicating the collections were not complete or that they did not report bowel motion. Due to radiation scatter, anteroposterior movement and distribution of activity at different times, the calculated percentage activity in the colon is subject to error. Thus the total colon activity (from which the fecal loss is calculated) may vary up to 15% even when there is no fecal loss, and this should be considered when reporting fecal losses less than 20%.

14.7.4 Role of Nuclear Medicine in Diagnosis

Until recently, to determine transit, radio-opaque pellets have been followed through the small and large bowel, using abdominal X-rays. However, the transit of pellets varies depending on their size, shape, and consistency and may not represent the true transit. In general X-ray methods although useful have limited value in studying large bowel transit. Some units measure colonic activity using barometric devices, but this is invasive, uncomfortable for the patient, and requires specialized equipment, which is not readily available. It measures pressure changes and not transit.

In the absence of any other accurate method of measuring colonic transit nuclear medicine has an important role in defining and thus contributing to the treatment of chronic constipation. This is the only method where objective quantitative measurements of colonic transit can be made. The method is relatively new and is complementary to the established methods of manometric and electrical activity measurements of the colon.

14.8 Defecography

Pelvic floor disorders are common, leading to constipation, difficulty in defecation or fecal incontinence. There are several established methods of assessing patients with pelvic floor disorders and the most widely used is a proctogram with defecography using contrast agents and X-rays. The test gives anatomical detail, but is not quantitative, and due to radiation exposure the number of films obtained has to be limited. Manometric measurements of rectal sphincters is also used to assess rectal function. Manometry is complementary to the investigation and helps establish a diagnosis in certain cases. More recently there has been great interest in quantitative physiological measurement of rectal function. Radionuclide investigation enables quantification of the rectal function and allows continuous monitoring during defecation.

14.8.1 Imaging

The patient is asked not to take any bowel regulatory medication for 24 hours before the test. A mixture of ^{99m}Tc-DTPA and porridge is prepared to the required consistency. It is then placed in 50 ml catheter-tipped syringes [7], and a total volume of 150 ml inserted into the rectum. Three markers are used: at the lumbosacral junction, at the tip of the coccyx, and anteriorly at the symphysis pubis. A marker with higher activity is used in the anterior symphysis pubis than the posterior locations as during image acquisition the soft tissue of the leg will be between the camera and this marker. The radioactive porridge is then administered via a catheter placed 5–10 cm inside the rectum. The catheter is then removed and the patient is asked to sit on a commode in front of a large field of view camera with the camera preferably placed on the left of the patient. The field of view should include the rectum and exclude the container for collection of the feces. The image acquisition is then started and the patient is asked to strain and defecate about 1 minute after the start of acquisition. The study is continued until the patient has either evacuated completely or is

Table 14.7. Defecography

Radiopharmaceutical	[99mTc]DTPA in 150 ml porridge
Activity administered	100 MBq (2.5 mCi) rectal
Effective dose equivalent	Maximum of 4 mSv (400 mrem) in complete retention; normally <0.3 mSv (30 mrem)
Patient preparation	No laxative or bowel regulatory medications
Collimator	Low-energy, general-purpose
Images	Radioactive porridge administered rectally. 99mTc marker placed in pubic symphysis, lumbar spine and tip of coccyx. Patient positioned with left side to the camera and patient evacuates while 5 s frame acquisition is in progress

unable to evacuate any further. If the patient has been unable to evacuate a rectal stimulant, such as sodium picosulfate, is administered to facilitate the early evacuation of the activity in order to reduce radiation dose to the patient. The imaging protocol is given in Table 14.7.

14.8.2 Analysis

The anal canal is identified and anorectal angle is calculated. The amount of pelvic floor descent is calculated using the pubo-coccygeal markers. A region of interest is drawn around the rectal activity as well as any rectocele which may be identified. The size of rectocele, percentage of activity in it, and remaining activity in it at the end of the defecation are measured. The rectal evacuation rate, time, and percentage are calculated (Figures 14.11 and 14.12).

14.8.3 Problems

The major problem is the tissue attenuation as the activity descends down into the rectum. Due to increasing thickness of the tissue the total activity

appears to be increased just prior to defecation. However, this is a consistent finding and should be taken into account in interpretation of the results. It is difficult to estimate the exact size of rectocele using radionuclide techniques although its functional significance is evident. If the patient is unable to defecate, the anal canal cannot be identified to measure the anorectal angle. This is, however, rare.

14.8.4 The Role of Nuclear Medicine in Diagnosis

The test is simple and is preferred by the patient to the alternative tests (proctogram and manometric measurements). It gives quantitative measurements of total evacuation, time of evacuation, and percentage of activity remaining in the rectocele, all of which can be assessed on several occasions following treatment and compared objectively. It is more sensitive in identifying rectoceles and also probably the clinical consequences of non-emptying rectocele are more important than a rectocele which empties satisfactorily with defecation. This is a fairly recent test and the full clinical

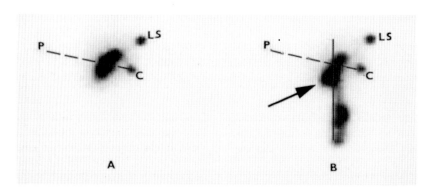

Figure 14.11. Image showing rectocele (arrow) and pelvic floor descent, markers at pubis (P), coccyx (C), and lumbosacral (LS). At rest (A) and straining (B).

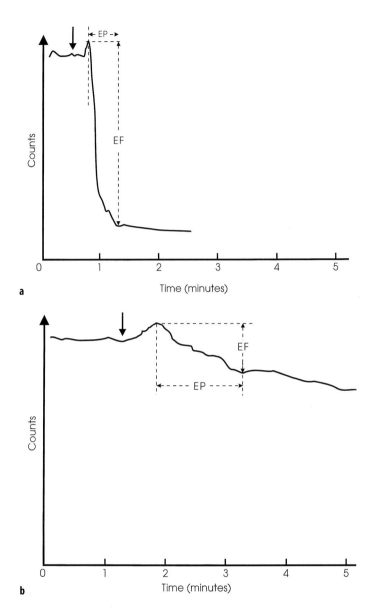

Figure 14.12. Curve of rectal activity normal (**a**) and impaired evacuation (**b**) showing reduced ejection fraction (EF) and prolonged ejection period (EP). The arrow designates the time when patient is asked to evacuate bowel.

impact of the test has not been assessed yet. X-ray proctography gives superior anatomical detail.

14.9 Colloid Liver Scan

A colloid scan is used to examine the liver, spleen, and bone marrow. Colloids are trapped and then taken up by the reticuloendothelial cells (Kupffer cells in liver); 70–80% of tin colloid is taken up by liver, 10–20% by spleen, and 5–10% by bone marrow. The distribution of colloid depends on its size, and the smaller colloid preparations (nanocolloid) have higher bone marrow and spleen uptake than larger tin colloids. Nanocolloid is thus used for bone marrow imaging.

Table 14.8. The colloid liver scan

Radiopharmaceutical	[^{99m}Tc]colloid
Activity administered	75 MBq (2 mCi) IV
Effective dose equivalent	1 mSv (100 mrem)
Patient preparation	None
Collimator used	Low-energy, general-purpose
Images acquired	Anterior (500 kcounts), posterior, right and left laterals (matched for time)

14.9.1 Imaging

Colloid should be administered into a vein. Care must be taken to avoid formation of blood clot in the syringe due to repeated attempts at venepuncture as this may clump the colloid and result in lung extraction. Images are acquired 15 minutes after injection. Costal margin markers are helpful to assess the position of the liver and also a 10 cm marker may be used for liver size measurement. If an abnormal mass is being evaluated it is advisable to use markers to delineate the mass. The standard images are anterior and posterior images with right and left laterals. Occasionally oblique views may be acquired. The patient is usually imaged supine (Table 14.8).

14.9.2 Analysis and Interpretation

The shape and amount of uptake in the liver is noted. The size of the liver is measured. The liver is examined for any photon-deficient areas. With cirrhosis there is reduced liver uptake, increased bone marrow uptake and with portal hypertension excessive splenic uptake.

The liver disease detectable may be focal, which includes metastases, hepatoma, cyst, and abscess, or the abnormality may be reduced diffuse uptake, which is encountered in generalized liver disease such as cirrhosis. However, if the reticuloendothelial system is not affected, such as in viral hepatitis, the uptake may be normal. As caudate lobe venous drainage is separate from the rest of the liver, in Budd–Chiari syndrome there is reduced uptake in the whole liver except the caudate lobe, which is enlarged.

14.9.3 Clinical Interpretation and Problems

Normal liver appearances vary considerably between individuals. In addition, rib impression, breast, the gallbladder, and ligaments may cause varying amounts of apparently reduced uptake in the liver, as does the junction of the left and right lobes.

14.9.4 The Role of Nuclear Medicine in Diagnosis

A colloid liver scan is now rarely performed on its own. It is mainly used with other nuclear medicine investigations. One such use is delineation of tumors when other tumor-specific agents are used, such as octreotide or antibodies (see Chapter 16). It is also used to clarify subphrenic abscess following white cell scan. Ultrasound, which is readily available in most centers and can also be used for guided biopsies and aspirations, is the first line of investigation for focal lesions in the liver. However, in difficult cases where liver cannot be properly visualized with ultrasound, a colloid scan may help. Spleen scanning is useful in looking for a splenunculus in patients after splenectomy.

14.10 Scintigraphic Liver Angiography

As with other methods for measuring blood flow into organs a good bolus injection is of paramount importance.

14.10.1 Imaging

Following bolus injection of the activity, rapid sequence images are acquired 2–3 second intervals. At the same time data should be recorded on a computer for curve quantitative analysis (Table 14.9).

14.10.2 Analysis

There are two methods of analyzing blood flow to the liver, both looking at the differential arrival of the portal venous drainage and the arterial supply to the liver.

Flow Index

A region of interest (ROI) is drawn within the liver, avoiding other organs, and a second one within a kidney. Time–activity curves are then generated (Figure 14.13). The liver curve continues to rise

Table 14.9. The dynamic colloid liver scan

Radiopharmaceutical	[^{99m}Tc]colloid
Activity administered	150 MBq (4 mCi) IV
Effective dose equivalent	2 mSv (200 mrem)
Patient preparation	Fasting
Collimator used	High sensitivity
Images acquired	Bolus injection while patient lying supine. Camera positioned to include liver. 0.5 s frame for 1 min followed by 5 s frames for 1 min. Delayed static images. Anterior and posterior right and left lateral views

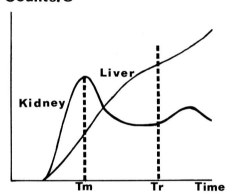

Figure 14.13. Activity–time curves over the liver and a kidney during the first minute after injection.

after the time of the peak on the kidney curve (Tm) due to the portal bolus. An index of arterial to portal flow can be derived either by comparing the height of the liver curve at Tm with its height at Tr (when recirculation begins) [8] or by measuring the slope of the liver curve before and after Tm. A correction must be applied for the fact that the spleen has already removed some colloid from portal blood before it reaches the liver. The total accumulated activity in the liver (Lt) and spleen (St) is found from the geometric mean of total counts in these organs on delayed anterior and posterior views, and measured fractional arterial flow is reduced by a factor of Lt/(Lt + St). With these methods it is assumed that all the activity in the arterial bolus has reached the liver before the portal bolus arrives. This is not correct in practice, and probably introduces an error of 15–20% in most cases. However, such an index can be

useful in detecting conditions in which arterial flow is increased or portal flow decreased.

14.10.3 Role of Nuclear Medicine in Diagnosis

Metastatic deposits derive their blood supply from hepatic arterial branches, and the proportion of liver arterial flow increases in metastatic disease. Measurement of the arterial-portal ratio may indicate the presence of multiple metastases before they are large enough to be seen on plain images. Portal flow is reduced in portal hypertension, which also increases the arterial-portal ratio, and thus can be used to assess cirrhosis. Flow studies are also helpful in assessing vascular patency after hepatic trauma, major liver resection, or liver transplantation.

14.11 Splenic Imaging

The spleen will usually be imaged as part of a liver scan and this often provides sufficient information for clinical purposes (see Table 14.9). A more specific way of showing the spleen is to use heat-denatured erythrocytes, which give excellent splenic visualization and are particularly useful if the splenic uptake is suspected to be poor. This is the investigation of choice when looking for splenic remnants after splenectomy (splenunculi). Red cells are first labeled with technetium as described (see Section 14.14), then they are heated to 39.5°C (for 30 minutes). This distorts the red cell structure and the damaged cells are taken up by the functioning splenic tissue.

14.11.1 Imaging

Imaging is performed using a general purpose collimator, about 30 minutes after the injection of the autologous denatured labeled red cells. Anterior, posterior, and left lateral views are required, although some people prefer left anterior and posterior oblique images.

14.11.2 Analysis and Interpretation

The size of the spleen or splenunculus can be measured using 10 cm markers on one of the images. The normal spleen is kidney-shaped, although the size, shape, and orientation may vary. The normal length of spleen is 12 cm in the long axis. As the left lobe of the liver superimposes on a spleen anteriorly, oblique views are useful to avoid confusion.

14.11.3 Problems

The interpretation of spleen images is usually straightforward. However, the variation in the shape may make interpretation of defects difficult, in particular in the upper pole. An enlarged liver may overlap the spleen and oblique views are required in this circumstance. If the spleen is absent in a colloid scan, a repeat study using denatured red cells may be needed to confirm the absence of a spleen.

14.11.4 The Role of Spleen Scanning in Diagnosis

While radionuclide imaging can be helpful in diagnosing a left upper quadrant mass, ultrasound, CT, or MRI are generally preferred for this purpose. However, it is a useful method to demonstrate splenic remnants after splenectomy, for trauma or hematological conditions.

14.12 Hepatobiliary Scintigraphy

Several amino-diacetic acid compounds labeled with ^{99m}Tc have been used to investigate biliary excretion and the pathway from liver to small intestine. Tribromomethyl-HIDA (mebrofenin) is generally available. It is cleared from the circulation by the hepatic cells and secreted into the bile by carrier mechanisms identical to bilirubin. When liver function is poor there is proportionally increased kidney excretion. HIDA compounds accumulate into the gallbladder and are excreted into the small bowel. Once in the bowel it is possible to investigate and measure bile reflux from duodenum into the stomach. Hepatobiliary scintigraphy is also used to assess the hepatic uptake, bile duct patency, cystic duct patency, gallbladder function (chronic and acute infections), gallstones, common bile duct patency, and sphincter of Oddi dysfunction.

Bile reflux studies are usually undertaken in patients after ulcer surgery. Symptoms of bile vomiting, epigastric pain, and heartburn may occur, especially in those who have had gastric resections, and it is important to establish the presence of reflux before corrective surgery is undertaken. Esophageal reflux of bile tends to cause severe symptoms and is rare in those without gastric resection.

Some authors have attributed the flatulent dyspepsia associated with gallstones to increased bile reflux into the stomach. Patients with this syndrome complain of epigastric discomfort and a feeling of fullness after meals, belching, nausea, vomiting, and heartburn. However, we have found no difference in the incidence of reflux in those with and without symptoms, either in the fasting state or after giving a fatty meal to stimulate gallbladder contraction.

14.12.1 Imaging

Hepatic uptake and clearance can be measured. The patient is positioned prone on a bed with the camera anteriorly so that heart, liver, and spleen are included in the field of view. The patient is then injected with ^{99m}Tc-labeled HIDA and acquisition started immediately. However, if only gallbladder function and reflux is being assessed then the injection can be given first and the patient brought in for imaging 20 minutes later. When gallbladder stimulation is required, either a liquid fatty meal or cholecystokinin (CCK) or its analogue may be given at 40 minutes after HIDA injection to provoke emptying of the bile ducts and gallbladder. It also may provoke reflux into the stomach and esophagus when sincalide is given. It is important to be consistent with the rate of infusion as the rate may affect the response of the gallbladder. Imaging is usually continued for a further 30 minutes but if no gallbladder is visualized then further static images may be required at 2, 3, and 4 hours to assess appearance of activity in the gallbladder. Late images are used to assess common bile duct obstruction, and bile leakage (Figure 14.14). Twenty-four hour images may be required to differentiate large duct biliary obstruction from severe diffuse cholestasis or when investigating for biliary atresia. No activity in the small bowel should be detected even after 24 hours in biliary atresia. The imaging protocol is presented in Table 14.10. If gastric reflux is being investigated and there is any doubt about the presence of activity in the stomach, 100 ml water can be given at $1_{1/2}$ hours. This dilutes activity if it is in the stomach. However, if the situation is still not clear, a small amount

Table 14.10. Hepatobiliary scintigraphy

Radiopharmaceutical	[^{99m}Tc]tribromomethyl-HIDA
Activity administered	60–80 MBq (1.5–2.0 mCi) IV
Effective dose equivalent	1.5 mSv (150 mrem)
Patient preparation	Overnight fast
Collimator	Low-energy, general-purpose
Images acquired	HIDA scan using sincalide: 20 min after injection of the HIDA the patient is positioned supine under the camera and ^{57}Co markers are placed on the iliac crests. 30 min after injection, 2-min images are begun and at 40 min 9 mg/kg in 100 ml IV saline. Sincalide is given over 15 min by intravenous infusion. The image continued and test is stopped at 80 min
	HIDA scan using fatty meal: 20 min after injection of the HIDA the patient is positioned supine under the camera with markers placed on the iliac crest. 5 minutes of 2 minute images are acquired. Patient is then asked to get off the imaging bed and asked to drink 240 ml of Calshake preparation with full fat milk. After 10 minutes (to allow for gastric emptying) the patient is positioned supine under the camera with markers in place for 2 min acquisitions started for a further 30 minutes
	If biliary leak is suspected right lateral and oblique views are acquired and if bile reflux into stomach is suspected then at 80 min 200 ml of water is given to diffuse any activity in the stomach. At 86 min, 6–8 MBq of oral HIDA is given to outline the stomach

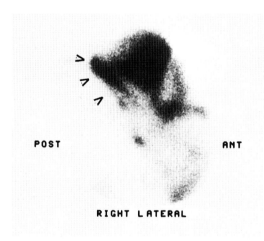

POST   ANT

RIGHT LATERAL

Figure 14.14. HIDA study showing the leakage behind the right lobe of the liver (arrows).

of ^{99m}Tc (10 MBq (200 µCi)) dissolved in 100 ml water can be given to delineate the stomach for comparison (Figures 14.15 and 14.16).

14.12.2 Analysis

The gallbladder is identified in the images and the region of interest is drawn around it. The ejection fraction, ejection period, and rate of ejection are calculated for the gallbladder using the time–activity curves (Figure 14.17). Normal values for CCK and fatty meal are shown in Table 14.11. The sincalide should be infused at a slow rate over 15–30 minutes. A fast injection may result in a low gall-

bladder ejection fraction. The images are checked for the time of appearance of activity in the small bowel and for evidence of reflux into the stomach/esophagus. It is important to note the time of appearance of the gallbladder. In chronic cholecystitis the gallbladder may be visualized later, but more commonly the rate and period of gallbladder ejection is prolonged while the ejection fraction is reduced (Figure 14.18).

14.12.3 Interpretation and Problems

In the presence of right upper quadrant pain, failure to visualize the gallbladder by 4 hours with normal passage of activity to the bowel is diagnostic of gallbladder disease (acute cholecystitis), and indicates cystic duct obstruction. While delayed visualization of the gallbladder usually indicates chronic cholecystitis, a more specific test would be to look at the response of gallbladder to CCK or fatty meal which will be compromised in this condition. Non-visualization of gallbladder, bile ducts, or small bowel may be due to acute biliary obstruction. However, other conditions such as severe hepatic disease may also cause this appearance. In children with cystic fibrosis there is no activity in the small bowel; however, the bile ducts may be visualized in the late images. If bile leakage is suspected then extra views (lateral and oblique views) may help to identify the site of leakage (Figure 14.14).

Other causes of non-visualization of gallbladder are previous cholecystectomy, and non-fasting patients.

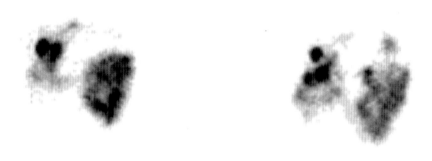

a   b

Figure 14.15. **a** Images 34 minutes after HIDA injection. **b** Reflux has occurred into the stomach in the 38 minute image.

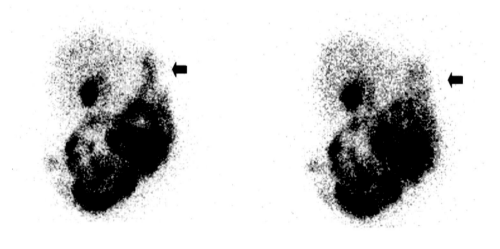

a   b

Figure 14.16. Activity in the stomach **a** is diffused **b** by the water drink.

Table 14.11. Normal range for gallbladder function

	CCK Mean (SEM)	Fatty meal Mean (SEM)
Latent period	2.8 (0.7) min	16 (6) min
Ejection period	9.8 (1.3) min	24 (5) min
Ejection fraction	45 (9.9) %	55 (9) %
Ejection rest	3.5 (2) % per min	2.8 (0.6) % per min

When looking for bile reflux into the stomach, either a liquid fatty meal or cholecystokinin (CCK) may be given to provoke emptying of the bile ducts and gallbladder, so that radioactive bile is available in the duodenum. The incidence of reflux is higher when CCK is used compared with a meal and this may be regarded as a provocative stimulus which is useful, for example, to assess the efficacy of a bile diversion operations.

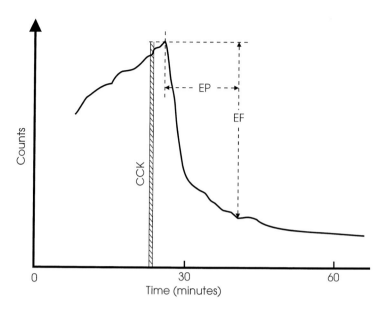

Figure 14.17. Gallbladder activity curve showing normal gallbladder response to CCK infusion (EP = injection period and EF = ejection fraction).

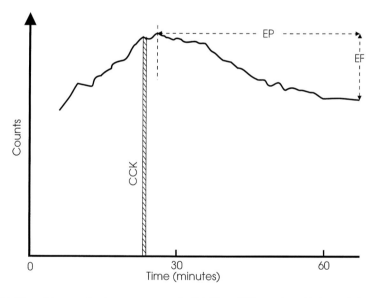

Figure 14.18. Gallbladder activity curve showing poor response of gallbladder to CCK in a patient with chronic cholecystitis (EP = injection period and EF = ejection fraction).

14.12.4 Role of Nuclear Medicine in Diagnosis

The most important application of cholecystography is in the investigation of acute cholecystitis in patients with right upper quadrant pain, for which it has a higher sensitivity and specificity than ultrasound. Occasionally the early hepatic phase of the study may reveal unsuspected focal liver disease, such as abscess or metastases.

In chronic cholecystitis ultrasound is the preferred initial investigation, in particular in the presence of obstructive jaundice and in biliary

Table 14.12. Clinical conditions encountered in cholescintigraphy

Acute cholecystitis (cystic duct obstruction)
Chronic cholecystitis

Postoperative:
   biliary leak
   fistula
   obstruction
Trauma:
   bile leak
   traumatic cyst
Congenital:
   biliary atresia
   choledochal cyst
Obstructive jaundice
Focal liver disease may be detected during the hepatic phase
   of a study
Cholescintigraphy is also used to study enterogastric reflux
   and problems after gastric surgery

colic. However, when ultrasound is not conclusive it is advisable to evaluate gallbladder function with biliary scintigraphy using CCK, which is a more sensitive test for revealing gallbladder dysfunction.

Biliary scintigraphy is helpful to differentiate the different causes of neonatal jaundice (neonatal hepatitis and biliary atresia), in which case 24-hour images are necessary. Some centers calculate liver to heart ratio between $2\frac{1}{2}$ and 10 minutes post-injection (<5 is compatible with biliary atresia), although the reliability of this parameter has been questioned.

Other uses of biliary scintigraphy are to evaluate bile leakage, in particular following surgery and also in evaluating the biliary system following liver transplant (Table 14.12).

Scintigraphy in the only clinically satisfactory test for bile reflux. Various other tests using duodenal intubation have been proposed, but they are unpleasant for the patient. Reflux may be evident at gastroscopy, but the circumstances of the test cannot be described as physiological. HIDA reflux studies are sensitive to 1% of the amount injected refluxing into the stomach. However, we have shown that the reproducibility is only 75%, and this appears to be due to day-to-day variation in the incidence of reflux. Reflux is significantly more common after CCK than the liquid fatty meal; after CCK stimulation reflux occurred in 45% of control patients. The presence of bile reflux does not of itself require treatment, but if a patient has symptoms which suggest bile reflux and reflux is not induced by

CCK, another cause for the symptoms should be sought.

14.13 Meckel's diverticulum

Meckel's diverticulum is the commonest congenital anomaly of the GI tract and occurs in 1–3% of the population. It is rather more common in men than in women (3:2) and is often a coincidental finding. However, 5–7% may contain ectopic gastric mucosa, and this mucosa is prone to all the problems that occur within the stomach, particularly bleeding. Those diverticula that bleed usually present in the first 10 years of life with rectal hemorrhage, but they may cause obstruction of the bowel or become inflamed. The latter two groups are not usually referred to nuclear medicine departments. Imaging depends on the uptake of pertechnetate by the gastric mucosal cells, probably the mucus-secreting cells and not the parietal cells as was first envisaged. Diverticula are variable in position: on gamma camera pictures, they most commonly appear in the lower abdomen; anatomically, they are usually in the ileum within 1 m of the ileocecal valve.

14.13.1 Imaging

It is preferable that the patient is fasting, although in emergency situations this may not prove possible. There is much discussion regarding pretreating the patient with drugs prior to imaging. In our department we use no such treatment. Some departments give oral cimetidine 200 mg three times daily on the day before the examination, with 400 mg early in the morning of the day of the test. The aim is to prevent the release of pertechnetate into the lumen of the stomach or bowel, but without impairing its uptake. In other departments, a mixture of pentagastrin and glucagon is used for the same purpose [1, 4].

Patients are frequently children, and they should be given the radiopharmaceutical and other drug doses proportional to their body weight. While adults are imaged supine, young children should be lying prone on the camera since they usually move less in this position.

The imaging protocol is given in Table 14.13.

14.13.2 Appearances

A positive scan shows a small localized area of uptake (Figure 14.19) which appears at the same time

Table 14.13. Meckel's diverticulum

Radiopharmaceutical	[^{99m}Tc]pertechnetate
Activity administered	350–400 MBq (9–10 mCi) IV
Effective dose equivalent	4 mSv (400 mrem)
Patient preparation	Fasting – see text regarding drug treatment
Collimator	Low-energy, general-purpose
Images acquired	Anterior abdomen, stomach to pelvis, 10^6 counts per image every 5 min for 30 min, and then at 40, 50, 60 min (the last after emptying bladder). Right lateral film at the end of the study. Depending on the position of any abnormal activity, a left lateral or posterior image may be taken

as the stomach, and as the stomach activity accumulates so does that of the diverticulum. It may change in position during the study. There may be confusion due to gastric emptying, or emptying from the lumen of the Meckel's diverticulum. A lateral view at the end of the study usually allows activity in the kidney and ureters, which is in the posterior part of the abdomen, to be differentiated from the diverticulum, which is usually anterior.

14.13.3 Problems

The sensitivity of this test is variously reported, but if the activity appears with the stomach and increases in intensity in the same way as the stomach

a figure of 80% can be achieved. False positive results may occur from the uterus, ureter, duplication of the stomach, or hemangioma of bowel, although activity in the latter will gradually decrease. Infection or intussusception may also give a false positive picture, but these conditions would in any case generally require surgery. It is important to ensure that the bladder is empty, as a full bladder may obscure the Meckel's diverticulum. A bladder diverticulum may be confused with a Meckel's diverticulum. Sometimes there is ectopic mucosa in the small bowel and this also handles pertechnetate. Great care is required in reporting these images, since a positive report would almost always result in the patient being taken to the operating theater.

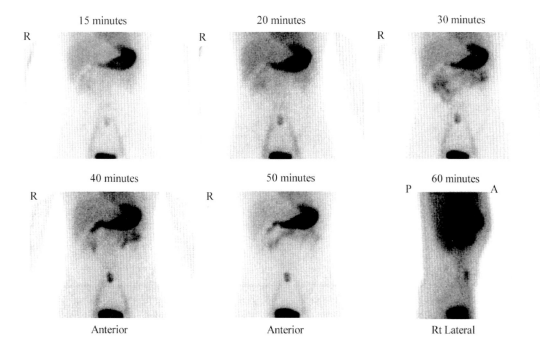

Figure 14.19. A Meckel's diverticulum at the bifurcation of vessels in the abdomen. It appears with stomach and increases in intensity with stomach.

14.13.4 Role of Nuclear Medicine in Diagnosis

Some Meckel's diverticula can be seen on barium follow-through, and by angiography if they are bleeding. Neither of these tests is particularly sensitive. If GI bleeding secondary to Meckel's diverticulum is suspected, colloid or labeled red blood cells (RBC) may be used to detect bleeding (see Section 14.14).

14.14 Gastrointestinal Bleeding

Technetium-labeled RBC or colloid can be used for investigation of suspected GI bleed. Technetium-labeled colloid would enable localization of GI bleed. However, high liver and spleen uptake of the colloid may mask smaller bleed into the gut. Most people prefer technetium-labeled RBC as the images are easier to interpret and delayed images can detect intermittent bleeding.

When using ^{99m}Tc-labeled RBC, in vitro labeling is preferred as labeling efficiency can be checked and free pertechnetate washed. Five milliliters of blood is withdrawn into a syringe, which already contains 100–200 units of heparin to prevent clotting. The sample is carefully labeled with patient identification. Under sterile conditions stannous agent is added to the blood and incubated for 5 minutes. The blood is centrifuged and the supernant discarded. Then 400 MBq of pertechnetate is added and incubated for further 5 minutes. Then 10 ml normal saline is added, mixed and centrifuged. Supernant is separated and activity in it measured to assess the labeling efficiency, then discarded. The ^{99m}Tc-labeled red cells are then resuspended in 10 ml of normal saline ready for injection back into the patient.

14.14.1 Imaging

The patient is positioned supine with the camera positioned to include the whole of the abdominal area. If using ^{99m}Tc colloid then dynamic images are acquired immediately following injection. Then a series of static images are acquired up to 30 minutes. If ^{99m}Tc-labeled RBC is used then either dynamic images or a static image is acquired immediately after the injection of the labeled RBC. Five-minute images are then acquired for one hour; if no bleeding is detected then hourly images are acquired for 4 hours, then at 6 hours and 24 hours to detect intermittent bleeding.

14.14.2 Appearances

The site of active bleeding appears following the visualization of the vessels in the abdominal area. The activity accumulates in the gut. In subsequent images the activity may move. From the shape and movement of the activity one can identifying the bleeding site in small bowel or colon (Figure 14.20). If no site is identified during the early images, a late image may confirm bleeding. However, it may have moved by the time of imaging so the exact site cannot be identified.

14.14.3 Problems

^{99m}Tc colloid imaging for GI bleed only works if the patient is actively bleeding at the time of the injection of the radiopharmaceutical. With this technique, as there is high uptake in liver and spleen, it is not possible to evaluate the upper quadrants adequately.

With ^{99m}Tc-RBC the large vessels in the abdomen are also visualized, as well as angiomas. However, with bleeding the activity increases and moves in the gut in subsequent images while vascular activity remains the same. Although not usually a problem with in vitro labeling, some free pertechnetate can be excreted from the kidneys and accumulate in the bladder and must not be mixed with the site of bleeding.

14.14.4 Role of Nuclear Medicine in Diagnosis

In severe GI bleed endoscopy is usually the first line of investigation. Colonoscopy is used for identifying lower GI bleeding sites as well as the cause for bleeding such as carcinoma or diverticula. Angiography can identify bleeding sites; however, it is invasive and mainly diagnostic in more severe bleeding. ^{99m}Tc-RBC is a relatively non-invasive and sensitive test for detecting GI bleed. It can also detect intermittent bleeding. It is often possible to identify the site of bleeding and determine if it is in the small or large bowel. It is often used if other investigations have failed to identify a site or cause of bleeding.

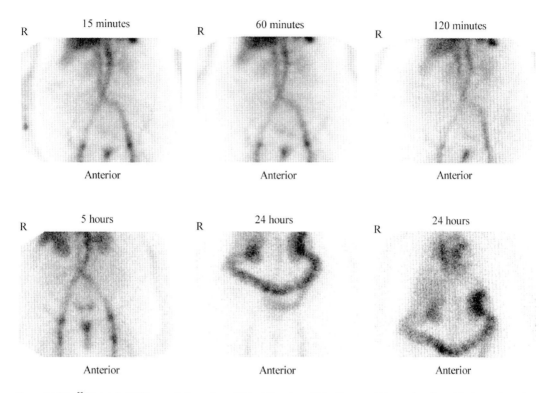

Figure 14.20. ^{99m}Tc-labeled RBC images for intermittent GI bleed. There is no GI bleeding up to 24 hours when the activity is seen throughout the colon indicating bleeding either in cecum or proximal to it the small bowel.

14.15 Tumor Markers

Gastrointestinal tumors are a common cause of death. In the UK they account for 40 000 deaths annually, 7% of all deaths. They initially present with non-specific symptoms such as weight loss, diarrhea, and vomiting, so they may be difficult to diagnose. Colonic and gastric cancers are especially common, and their early diagnosis is important if surgery is to be helpful in treatment. [^{67}Ga]gallium citrate (see Section 16.5) is a non-specific agent which may be taken up by tumors or infected tissue, but its sensitivity in detecting tumors in the gastrointestinal tract is very low. Monoclonal antibodies to tumor proteins have been developed in recent years and offer much promise, but unfortunately their full potential has not been realized. When the antibodies are raised to a given type of protein, they cross-react with other proteins, and are not therefore as specific as might be envisaged.

Carcinoembryonic antigen (CEA) is the best-known antigen, which was originally believed to be present only in fetal gut tissue and adenocarcinomas of the colon. However, the antigen has been found in a number of malignancies including stomach, pancreas, lung and breast tumors, and some non-malignant tissue (see Section 16.8).

Murine B72.3 monoclonal antibody labeled with indium-111 has been used to visualize recurrent or residual colorectal carcinoma. This is an antibody against TAG-72 tumor-associated glycoprotein, which is expressed in 96% of non-small cell lung carcinomas, 100% of epithelial ovarian carcinomas, and 80% of colonic carcinoma and most pancreatic, gastric, and esophageal carcinomas. This is entirely different from CEA antibodies (arcitumomab) and there is no documented cross-reactivity between the two. Both are now commercially available for clinical use (Oncoscint, Eurocetus and CEA scan, Immunomedics). Another commercially available agent for GI tumor imaging is octreotide (Octreoscan, Tyco), which is a peptide labeled by technetium. This agent is widely utilized in different tissues. However, there is many-fold increased uptake in neuroendocrine tumors, in particular in insulinoma and carcinoid tumors. During the last few years ^{18}F-FDG imaging has established itself as the most accurate imaging test when looking for primary, recurrent, or metastatic gut tumors, in particular Ca of the colon. This is discussed elsewhere (see Section 17.5.3).

14.15.1 Imaging

Antibody imaging is difficult, and the count rates are low. B72.3 monoclonal antibody is labeled with 150 MBq (4 mCi) of buffered ^{111}In chloride. Both planar and tomographic views are obtained. After setting the camera on appropriate windows (173 and 247 keV) using a medium energy collimator, planar images are required at 4, 48, and maybe at 72 hours. Tomographic views are required at 48 and possibly at 72 hours. The protocol is outlined in Table 14.14.

Patients with allergy to foreign proteins or atopy should not be given antibodies. The value of an intradermal skin test in detecting those who will react to the antibody is now doubted, and skin tests may cause some inactivation of the antibody in vivo with a reduction in tumor uptake.

14.15.2 Appearances

Liver and spleen show normally and there may be some activity in the urinary bladder. The liver and spleen can be imaged using technetium colloid and then the activity subtracted from the tumor images. This is in particular useful when looking at metastases in the liver when colloid uptake will be reduced while tumor activity will be enhanced using octreotide or other agents. Tomographic views

Table 14.14. Tumor marker study (Oncoscint)

Radiopharmaceutical	Monoclonal [^{111}In]-anti TAGR antigen antibodies
Activity administered	150 MBq (4.2 mCi)
Effective dose equivalent	50 mSv (5000 mrem)
Patient preparation	Intravenous slow injection with pulse and blood pressure monitoring
Collimator	Medium-energy
Images acquired	5 min anterior and posterior abdomen views at 4, 24, and 48 hours and some patients 72 hours. Tomographic views at 48 or 72 hours if available

may be crucial for identifying lesions near to liver and spleen in particular when using octreotide. The uptake is usually intense and focal in insulinoma and other neuroendocrine tumors of the GI tract (epudoma, insulinoma etc.). Octreotide and colloid liver images may be used to identify the extent of carcinoid tumor involvement of liver and other organs (Figure 14.21). When Oncoscint is used there is little or no activity in the bladder and increased activity in the pelvic region usually denotes tumor involvement in the area (anorectal region) (Figure 14.22). Tomographic views enabled a clearer distinction of the tumor activity in the pelvis. As both peptide (octreotide) and antibodies are taken up and broken by the liver the assessment of liver and metastases can be difficult using these agents.

14.15.3 Role of Nuclear Medicine in Diagnosis

Many tumors of the gastrointestinal tract can be identified using contrast radiology, MRI, or endoscopy. Antibody studies have not yet achieved a routine place in initial investigation of such patients. However, they are useful in assessing the extent of the disease, or more importantly recurrence of the disease, in particular when other modalities cannot be used due to previous surgical intervention. There is growing interest in localization of small endocrine tumors using octreotide scans. Positron emission tomography has established itself as a major tool for investigating carcinoma of the colon.

14.16 Protein Loss

Excess protein loss from the gastrointestinal tract may occur in diseases such as protein-losing enteropathy, infiltration of the lymphatics of the colon, some cases of Crohn's disease, and congestive heart failure. The patient has low serum albumin and gamma globulin levels without material loss of protein in the urine.

14.16.1 Method

Chromic chloride can be used for measuring protein loss. The protocol is shown in Table 14.15. An alternative method is to use ^{111}In-labeled transferrin by inoculating patient serum with ^{111}In

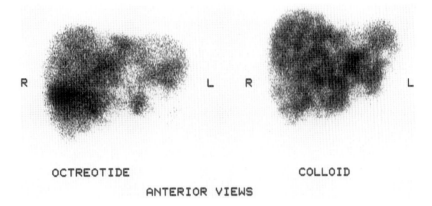

OCTREOTIDE   COLLOID

ANTERIOR VIEWS

Figure 14.21. Octreotide scan of liver showing extensive liver involvement in a patient with carcinoid syndrome (left). A colloid scan shows photon-deficient areas in the involved areas, confirming the metastases (right).

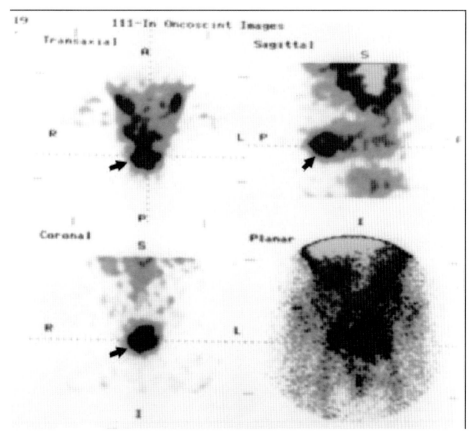

Figure 14.22. Oncoscint scan of colorectal cancer recurrence showing increased activity in the rectal region (arrow). Note the high activity in testes seen in the anterior view.

Table 14.15. GI protein loss

Radiopharmaceutical	[^{51}Cr]chromic chloride or ^{111}In transferrin
Activity administered	3–4 MBq (75–100 μCi) IV
Effective dose equivalent	1.7 mSv (170 mrem)
Specimens	For ^{51}Cr a fecal collection is made over 5 days and the percentage of administered chromium in feces is calculated by comparison with a standard. A large-volume gamma counter is required
Images	For ^{111}In transferrin: anterior and posterior views of abdomen and pelvis at 4 and 24 hours using ME collimator for localization. Whole body uncollimated images at 4 hours and 7 days to assess whole body loss. Loss of more than 10% indicates significant protein loss

chloride in vitro for 15 minutes, then imaging the patient and obtaining whole body counts at 3 hours (baseline) and 5 days. More than 10% labeled protein loss is abnormal. If ^{111}In is used then images acquired at 24 and 48 hours may demonstrate activity in the colon in protein-losing enteropathy and alleviates the need for stool collection [9] (Figure 14.10).

14.16.2 Normal Result

Less than 2% is normally present in the stools over 4 days [1–3]. Chromic chloride binds to transferrin, and if it leaks into the gut there is practically no reabsorption so that the fecal count corresponds to the GI protein loss.

14.16.3 Problems

The main problem with the technique is the urine contamination of feces, especially in the elderly, women and children. Incomplete stool collection will also confound the results, as does gastrointestinal bleeding.

14.16.4 Role of Nuclear Medicine in Diagnosis

There is no other satisfactory method to quantify protein loss from the GI tract.

14.17 Vitamin B$_{12}$ Absorption

An important cause of vitamin B$_{12}$ deficiency is pernicious anemia, which results from lack of intrinsic factor (IF) secretion by the stomach. The patient may be profoundly anemic and have neurological signs (including peripheral neuropathy and subacute combined degeneration of the cord). Pernicious anemia used to be fatal, but is now easily treated with injections of vitamin B$_{12}$. Other causes of vitamin B$_{12}$ deficiency are its destruction by bacteria in blind loops of bowel, damage or resection of the mucosa in the distal ileum where vitamin B$_{12}$ absorption takes place, or a very strict vegetarian (vegan) diet.

Deficiency of vitamin B$_{12}$ in the body is established by measuring its level in the blood. Radioisotope tests are used in differentiating lack of intrinsic factor from the other causes of vitamin B$_{12}$ deficiency. These tests rely on excess vitamin B$_{12}$ being excreted in the urine after absorption from the GI tract. A parenteral injection of 1000 μg of non-radioactive B$_{12}$ (cyanocobalamin or hydroxycobalamin) is given within 2 hours of orally radioactive B$_{12}$ ingestion. Both the excess non-radioactive B$_{12}$ and the absorbed oral radioactive B$_{12}$ preparations are excreted in the urine. Dicopac is a modification of the Schilling test [1–3]. ^{58}Co-B$_{12}$ and ^{57}Co-B$_{12}$ + intrinsic factor is administered on the same day and one 24-hour urine sample is collected; however, this is no longer available. The formal Schilling test is now carried out (Table 14.16).

14.17.1 Normal Result

The normal B$_{12}$ with IF excretion is 14–40%, and that of B$_{12}$ without IF is 14–40%. The ratio of B$_{12}$ with IF to B$_{12}$ without IF is 0.7–1.2 in normal subjects, over 1.7 being indicative of pernicious anemia.

In pernicious anemia B$_{12}$ with IF is absorbed while B$_{12}$ without IF is not absorbed; thus the ratio is much higher, as the percent recovered B$_{12}$ without IF is low. In malabsorption, uptake of B$_{12}$, both with and without IF, will be low.

14.17.2 Problems

The most common problem is an incomplete urine collection. Other difficulties arise due to failure to give the inactive B$_{12}$, renal disease, or

Table 14.16. Schilling test

Radiopharmaceutical	18.5 kBq (0.5 μCi) ^{57}Co-B$_{12}$, orally
Effective dose equivalent	0.05 mSv (5 mrem)
Patient preparation	Patient is injected with 1000 μg non radioactive B$_{12}$ intramuscularly before the test. Patient is then asked to take oral radiolabeled B$_{12}$. 24-hour urine is then collected
	The test is repeated a week later using radiolabeled B$_{12}$ + intrinsic factor
Specimens	The percentage of the recovered radiolabeled B$_{12}$ in 24-urine collection is calculated using a mixed urine sample

gastric stasis. It is not generally appreciated that in untreated pernicious anemia there may be associated malabsorption, which disguises the IF deficiency pattern; however, if the test is requested after treatment then the typical excretion pattern diagnostic of pernicious anemia occurs.

In cases where urine collection may be incomplete, the percentage recovered will of course not be reliable. The other methods of measurement that are independent of urine collection could be used to assess the percentage of activity retained in the body using a whole body counter.

14.17.3 Role of Nuclear Medicine in Diagnosis

No other test measures absorption directly, but the presence of pernicious anemia may be deduced in patients with achlorhydria and parietal cell antibodies.

14.18 SeHCAT

Among the many causes of diarrhea, malabsorption of bile acids is a difficult condition to diagnose clinically. Furthermore, finding an acceptable treatment regime may be problematic, so that proof of the cause of the disease is important. Bile acids are normally absorbed in the bowel by an active transport mechanism and resecreted into the bile. Resection of part of the bowel or Crohn's

disease are the commonest causes of bile acid malabsorption.

SeHCAT, selenohomocholyltaurine, is a taurine conjugate of bile acid with ^{75}Se in the side chain. It is more resistant than taurocholate to bacterial attack, and therefore more specific than breath tests in diagnosis of bile acid malabsorption [1–3]. The protocol is shown in Table 14.17. The SeHCAT study looks at the efficiency of the entero-hepatic cycle, over many cycles; thus a small change in the percentage of reabsorption has a profound effect on total retained SeHCAT over 1 week. This accounts for a wide normal range of 15–90% retained over 1 week.

14.18.1 Normal Findings

Greater than 15% retention at 7 days is a normal result. Results in the 10–15% retention range are equivocal, and figures under 10% undoubtedly abnormal. Those with 1 m or more resection of the terminal part of the ileum generally show less than 2% retention, and patients with spontaneous bile acid malabsorption show less than 6%.

14.18.2 Problems with the Test

Abnormal results may be found in patients already on treatment with aluminum hydroxide or colestyramine. Both of these drugs are used in treatment of bile acid malabsorption.

Table 14.17. Bile acid malabsorption

Radiopharmaceutical	370 kBq (10 μCi) [^{75}Se]HCAT, orally
Effective dose equivalent	0.3 mSv (30 mrem)
Gamma energy	270 keV. All gamma energies up to the photopeak should be recorded – this avoids problems due to change in spatial distribution of the radiopharmaceutical
Detector	Uncollimated gamma camera, as far as possible above the patient, and positioned over the mid-abdomen or if available a whole body scan. Use the mean of the anterior and posterior counts {alternatively, use a whole body counter, when only 37 kBq (1 μCi) [^{75}Se]HCAT is required}
Measure	Distribution at 3 h (100% reference point) and percent retention in the body at 7 days

14.18.3 Role of Nuclear Medicine in Diagnosis

A barium follow-through examination and barium enema are usually performed to assess the extent of disease. However, particularly in Crohn's disease, involvement of the terminal ileum does not necessarily mean functional impairment. The latter is determined using SeHCAT.

14.19 Breath Tests

Breath tests have been in use for 25 years, mostly for testing absorption from the small intestine. More recently there has been growing interest in the use of the ^{14}C-urea breath test for the diagnosis of *Helicobacter pylori* infection. The principle of the breath test is that a substance containing ^{14}C is given by mouth. After ingestion the substance is metabolized with subsequent production of ^{14}C-CO$_2$. This is either produced in the body as an end result of metabolism or in the small or large bowel as a result of bacterial breakdown, in which case it is also taken up by the blood and excreted in the breath [1, 2]. Although the possibilities are many, in practice there are three tests that are performed using this principle. Bile acid absorption is measured using ^{14}C-chologlycine, fat absorption using ^{14}C-triolein, and probably the most commonly performed is to detect the presence of *H. pylori* infection in the stomach using ^{14}C-urea.

14.19.1 Method

After ingesting the substance containing ^{14}C at an appropriate time, the breath is bubbled through a solution containing a known amount of alkaline base (hyamine) solution and a pH indicator (thymolphthalein). The indicator changes color when a known amount of CO$_2$ is trapped in the solution; then by adding liquid scintillant, the amount of ^{14}C-CO$_2$ can be estimated by beta counting. The result is then expressed as a percentage of ^{14}C-CO$_2$ to the known total amount of CO$_2$ (usually 1 mmol) times patient weight in kilograms.

The ^{14}C-urea breath test for *Helicobacter* infection is a sensitive test which relies on the ability of *Helicobacter* to break down urea rapidly. *Helicobacter pylori* may form part of the normal flora

Table 14.18. Urea breath test

Radiopharmaceutical	[^{14}C]urea
Activity administered	100 kBq (3 µCi)
Radiation dose:	
Gonads	<0.008 mGy (<0.8 mrad)
Effective dose equivalent	<0.008 mSv (<0.8 mrem)
Patient preparation	Off antibiotics for 4 weeks and hydrogen pump inhibitors for 3 days. Fasting
Specimens	Breath bubbled through 2 ml M hyamine in a scintillation (thymol-phthalein) changes color from blue to colorless (1 mmol of CO$_2$ collected). Add scintillant, count beta activity

of the mouth, which might give a transient rise in CO$_2$ excretion within the first 10 minutes of ingestion of urea solution. Thus in some centers it is recommended that mouthwash should be performed before initiation of the test. The patient is asked to fast for 2 hours before the test. Activity can be given in liquid or capsule form. There is no need to rinse the mouth if activity is given in capsule form. Then 37–140 kBq (1–4 µCi) of ^{14}C-urea is administered to the patient. Breath samples are obtained at 10 to 20 minute intervals for one hour after ingestion of the urea. The maximum recovered percentage of ^{14}C-CO$_2$ is calculated (Table 14.18).

For bile acid absorption the patient is asked to fast overnight, then a standard meal together with 200–400 kBq (5–10 µCi) ^{14}C-chologlycine is administered and breath samples collected every 30 minutes for 6 hours. The total amount of ^{14}C is then calculated from area under the excretion curve.

For fat absorption test 200 kBq (5 µCi) ^{14}C-triolein is administered orally to a fasting patient with a standard meal (20 g fat). The breath samples are collected half-hourly over an 8-hour period following ingestion. The peak amount excreted is used for calculation. The method is summarized in Table 14.19.

14.19.2 Result

Normally less than 0.2% ^{14}C-CO$_2$ per mmol × patient's weight is recovered in the breath following ^{14}C-urea ingestion (often less than 0.02%).

Table 14.19. Breath test for malabsorption

Radiopharmaceutical	[^{14}C]-labeled compound (chologlycine/trioline)
Activity administered	Typically 200–400 kBq (5–10 µCi)
Radiation dose:	
Gonads	0.1 mGy (10 mrad)
Effective dose equivalent	0.1–3 mSv (10–300 mrem)
Patient preparation	Fasting
Specimens	Breath bubbled through 4 ml M hyamine in scintillation vial till indicator (thymolphthalein) changes from blue to colorless (2 mmol of CO_2 collected). Add scintillant, count beta activity

Results of more than 1% are diagnostic of *H. pylori* infection, while results between 0.2 and 1% ^{14}C-$CO_2 \times$ body weight are neither diagnostic nor exclusive of *H. pylori* infection. They may represent suppressed infection.

In bile acid absorption usually less than 2% of the administered activity is excreted in the breath over a 2-hour period. A higher proportion indicates either fast intestinal transit, when bile acid is delivered to the large bowel before absorption and breakdown of chologlycine, or it may be due to bacterial overgrowth in the small bowel, where the bile acid is deconjugated in the small bowel and thus not absorbed with consequent breakdown in the large bowel.

The normal range for fat absorption is 3.4–6.3% of the administered ^{14}C-triolein. In fat malabsorption the values are below 3.4% of the administered dose over 8-hour period. In diarrhea of other causes the value should be within the normal range.

14.19.3 Problems

One of the problems with this test is the assumption that endogenous CO_2 production is constant. There are several ways of trying to correct for this. In general, production would vary with the metabolic rate. However, the variation in endogenous CO_2 production results in low sensitivity and specificity of the test, except in the diagnosing *H. pylori* with the ^{14}C-urea breath test, where there is more than a ten-fold difference between normal and abnormal result. The breath test requires a beta counter. The carbon-14 test using 200–400 kBq (5–10 µCi) of tracer has an effective dose equivalent in the range of 0.1–2 mSv (10–200 mrem) for tests using bile acid or fat absorption measurement. However, when using the ^{14}C-urea breath test the dose is much smaller, probably less than 0.01 mSv (1 mrem) for

a 100 kBq (2 µCi) test as urea is rapidly broken down either by bacteria or by the body, and CO_2 is quickly excreted in the breath.

14.19.4 Other Investigations

Endoscopy with biopsy and direct culture is the gold standard for diagnosis of *H. pylori* infection. This is usually the test performed in patients with peptic ulcer syndromes for both diagnosing *H. pylori* as well as excluding other important disease such as carcinoma of the stomach. However, treatment of *H. pylori* is not always successful. It is hardly justified to re-endoscope just to establish the success of the treatment and thus the alternative test – ^{14}C-urea breath test or ^{13}C-urea breath test – is performed in follow-up of these cases. This is both convenient for the patient and a reliable test. The ^{13}C-urea breath test uses a spectroscopic analysis for detection of the percentage of ^{13}C in proportion to ^{12}C. For population screening neither of these test is practical and the presence of antibodies against *H. pylori* is probably the correct approach. However, the drawback with the antibody test is that it indicates infection with *H. pylori* in the past and it does not necessarily indicate the presence of infection at the time of the test.

References

1. Robinson PJA. Nuclear Gastroenterology. Edinburgh: Churchill Livingstone; 1986.
2. Freeman LM, Blaufox MD. Gastrointestinal Disease Update 11. New York: Grune & Stratton; 1982.
3. Kircher PT. Nuclear Medicine Review Syllabus. New York: The Society of Nuclear Medicine; 1980.
4. Goligher JC, Hill GL, Kenny TE, Nutter E. Proximal gastric vagotomy without drainage for duodenal ulcer: results after 5–8 years. Br J Surg 1978; 65:145–151.
5. Notghi A, Hutchinson R, Kumar P, Smith NB, Harding LK. Simplified method for the measurement of segmental colonic transit time. Gut 1994; 35:976–981.

6. Notghi A, Mills A, Hutchinson R, Kumar D, Harding LK. Reporting simplified colonic transit studies using radionuclides: clinician friendly reports. Gut 1995; 36:274–275.

7. Mostafa AB, Hutchinson R, Grant EA, et al. Scintigraphic defaecography: how we use it. Nucl Med Commun 1993; 14:274.

8. Fleming JS, Ackery DM, Walmsley BH, Karran SJ. Scintigraphic estimation of arterial and portal blood supplies to the liver. J Nucl Med 1983; 24:1108–1113.

9. De Kaski MC, Peters AM, Bradley D, Hodgson HJ. Detection and quantification of protein-losing enteropathy with indium-111 transferrin. Eur J Nucl Med 1996; 23:530–533.

15

Infection and Inflammation

A. Michael Peters and Heok K. Cheow

15.1 Introduction

Imaging infection and inflammation remains an important activity within clinical nuclear medicine. There are currently no imaging agents that are proven to be specific for infection. The approach to imaging infection is therefore no different to inflammation and the two should be considered together. The main agents for imaging inflammation are radiolabeled white cells and ^{67}Ga. Radiolabeled white cells target inflammatory processes in which the neutrophil is the predominating infiltrating cell. ^{67}Ga is non-specific, since in addition to inflammatory pathology, it also targets several neoplasms. There are many other agents that have been explored for imaging inflammation but they are largely experimental or not widely available.

Leukocytes can be labeled with either ^{111}In or ^{99m}Tc. Since the cell labeling complexes of ^{111}In and ^{99m}Tc label cells indiscriminately, leukocytes have to be separated from other blood cell types prior to labeling. ^{67}Ga citrate, however, is used to label white cells in vivo and does not require prior separation of the cells.

This chapter describes the clinical applications of labeled leukocytes and ^{67}Ga and then briefly touches on some of the more novel agents.

15.2 Physiology of Inflammation

The physiology of inflammation involves essentially three components: endothelial activation, leukocyte migration, and resolution. Endothelium may be activated and leukocyte migration initiated by several proinflammatory mediators, either in association with or without infection. In several non-infective processes, such as inflammatory bowel disease (IBD), the cause of the inflammation is unknown.

15.2.1 Endothelial Physiology

In general, activation of the endothelium is the first stage in the inflammatory process. Endothelium is not a passive barrier separating the interstitial space from blood but a highly specialized tissue responsible for orchestrating cell migration in response to proinflammatory mediators [1]. It achieves this by synthesizing several so-called adhesion molecules, antigenic substances that are expressed on the endothelial luminal surface and display functional selectivity for cognate receptors on circulating leukocytes. They are activated in response to a variety of mediators liberated at the site of inflammation. Some adhesion molecules are constitutively expressed (i.e. expressed all the time) while others are expressed only in response to a specific stimulus. In the case of the latter, the time course of expression may vary according to the stimulus. Adhesion molecules are shed into the circulation, where they can be detected as soluble proteins, but they vary in their tendency to do this. Because adhesion molecules are antigenic, they potentially provide a means for imaging inflammation by binding to specific radiolabeled monoclonal antibodies. It is clear that the adhesion molecules best suited to this approach should not be constitutively expressed or shed into the circulation in appreciable amounts before or after binding to antibodies.

15.2.2 Granulocyte Physiology

Mature granulocytes are highly specialized, short-lived, non-dividing cells with a multi-lobulated nucleus, numerous cytoplasmic granules and a diameter of 12–15 μm. The maturation time of granulocytes in hematopoietic bone marrow is about 15 days. The mean residence time in the circulation is about 10 h (see Section 15.2.3), and survival time in tissues (if they migrate into them) up to about 4 days. The factors controlling granulocyte maturation in, and their release from, bone marrow are poorly understood. The leukocytosis caused by epinephrine (adrenaline) is largely a result of the release of granulocytes from the marginating granulocyte pool; hydrocortisone and endotoxin, however, probably cause leukocytosis by multiple mechanisms including accelerated release of young granulocytes from bone marrow.

In response to an acute infection, as an example of an inflammatory process, the following sequence of events occurs. Firstly, leukocytes arriving at the site of infection marginate on the endothelial surface of small blood vessels, mostly postcapillary venules. They do so by interacting with E-selectin, an endothelial adhesion molecule that is synthesized by the endothelial cell in response to proinflammatory mediators, originating from both host and organism, released at the site of inflammation. Following margination, the granulocytes adhere to the endothelium by binding to endothelial adhesion molecules called integrins. Following adhesion, cells then undergo transmigration by negotiating the interendothelial junctions, which widen in response to the inflammatory stimulus. The separation of endothelial cells from each other is the basis for the accumulation of macromolecules at sites of inflammation and explains why successful imaging of inflammation has been recorded for so many different radionuclide agents.

The next stage in the inflammatory response is recognition and phagocytosis of the invading microorganisms. Various factors, collectively called opsonins, bind to foreign material including damaged autologous cells (opsonization), thereby identifying them for phagocytosis by granulocytes. The principal opsonins are serum immunoglobulins and activated components of the complement system. The latter include components of the classical pathway, activated by specific antibody binding to the foreign cell surface, and components of the alternative pathway which can be activated in the absence of specific antibody. Both pathways go through C3, which is therefore of crucial importance.

Granulocytes express Fc receptors which bind the Fc region of antibody, while the Fab region, the end conferring the antibody's specificity, binds to the foreign cell (the antigen). They also express C3b receptors and, with the Fc receptor, promote adherence of foreign particles to the granulocyte surface. This immune adherence then activates the granulocyte and leads to phagocytosis, which commences as the "throwing out" of pseudopodia surrounding the opsonized particle. After ingestion a phagocytic vacuole, termed the phagosome, containing the particle is formed.

The next stage involves the killing and/or digestion of the foreign particle by the liberation into the phagosome of a variety of enzymes. These enzymes are initially present in cytoplasmic granules which migrate towards and fuse with the phagosome. Upon degranulation and their release into the phagosome, some of these enzymes are also released extracellularly prior to closure of the phagosome, and these may contribute to the tissue injury sustained during the inflammatory process.

Granulocytes are metabolically stimulated during phagocytosis. The first step in the process is granulocyte priming, during which the cell changes its shape, as a result of rearrangements in its cytoskeleton, from broadly spherical to a highly irregular shape. Priming is important in the context of imaging because recent evidence suggests that it is the process most closely linked to the uptake of fluorodeoxyglucose [2] (see Section 15.9). Because primed cells are less deformable, they display a prolonged transit through the pulmonary vasculature and this is the basis for the sustained high lung uptake seen in labeled leukocyte studies in patients with severe systemic inflammation. The main metabolic consequence of priming is a greatly amplified secretion of hydrogen peroxide and other highly reactive oxygen species (such as the hydroxyl radical and superoxide) in response to appropriate "secretagogues". This, the "respiratory burst", results in an increase in oxygen uptake by the granulocyte and is associated with the generation and release of a range of enzymes. In addition to these oxygen-independent mechanisms, other, oxygen-dependent, mechanisms contribute to bacterial killing. These include acids, which decrease the intraphagosomal pH to 4–6, lactoferrin, which binds the essential bacterial nutrient iron, and various other enzymes and proteins of granule origin whose action is not dependent on oxygen.

The termination of the inflammatory response is as important as its initiation, as uncontrolled ongoing inflammation leads to considerable tissue destruction. The physiology of the resolution of inflammation is poorly understood although one important event is granulocyte apoptosis (programmed cell death). Granulocytes harvested from the blood of normal volunteers undergo apoptosis after about 24 h of incubation. Although it has not been demonstrated directly in vivo, it is believed that granulocytes become apoptotic several hours after migration into tissue, after which they are specifically recognized and engulfed by macrophages [3].

The same fundamental process occurs when the inflammation is initiated by non-infective causes, although the adhesion molecules that become activated, the migrating cells, and the time course of the process may all be different.

15.2.3 Granulocyte Kinetics

Granulocyte kinetics can be subdivided into granulocyte distribution, lifespan in blood, and disposal sites.

Distribution

Granulocytes in blood are in dynamic equilibrium between two pools: the marginating (MGP) and circulating (CGP) granulocyte pools [4]. This is based on the finding that within about 20 min of intravenous administration, 50% of labeled granulocytes have apparently left the circulation, and that this figure can be increased substantially, up to 80%, by administration of epinephrine (adrenaline) or by strenuous exercise. It is now recognized that granulocyte migration in the form of endothelial rolling is the prelude to migration, is induced by the activation of E-selectin, and is therefore pathological. Most of the so-called MGP is accounted for by granulocyte pooling within discrete organs throughout the body and its distribution has been quantified with ^{111}In-labeled "pure" granulocytes.

A serious technical problem encountered in such quantitative studies is the susceptibility of

granulocytes to poorly understood, subtle injury, associated with loss of cell deformability, sustained during their in vitro separation [5]. Even if ^{111}In-labeled granulocytes are able to localize infection, they may be inadequate for physiological studies because of immediate sequestration in the lungs (Figure 15.1) followed by uptake in the liver. This problem can be largely solved by careful manipulation of cells in a plasma environment throughout the labeling procedure. This results in rapid cell transit through the lungs with early physiological redistribution to the marginating pools. The susceptibility to this form of activation, which is quite different to the physiological activation described above, seems to be related to the presence of lipopolysaccharide present in trace amounts in saline but apparently inhibited by plasma constituents [6].

Studies with ^{111}In-labeled pure granulocytes have demonstrated that the spleen is the principal organ for pooling granulocytes [7] (as it is for platelet pooling) (Figure 15.2) with important contributions from the lung, liver, and bone marrow. The importance of establishing the normal biodistribution of granulocytes, apart from physiological interest, relates to the evaluation of their integrity for the localization of inflammation and to the interpretation of clinical white cell scans.

Lifespan in the Circulation

Granulocytes have a mean residence time in blood of about 10 h (corresponding to a half-life of 7 h). Their clearance from blood is essentially exponential, i.e. their removal is random rather than age-dependent. This seems inconsistent with programmed cell death and it may be that granulocyte apoptosis is relevant only to the resolution of inflammation. Since labeled granulocytes are cleared from the blood within 24 h of injection, uptake of activity into an inflammatory focus is essentially complete by this time. It is possible that there is a proportion of granulocytes that is longer-lived than 10 h, as suggested by the presence of a slower exponential in radiolabeled granulocyte clearance studies, particularly those based on ^{111}In (Figure 15.3).

Granulocyte Destruction

It was previously thought that granulocytes leave the blood to enter the interstitial space, where they maintain a sterile environment by scavenging

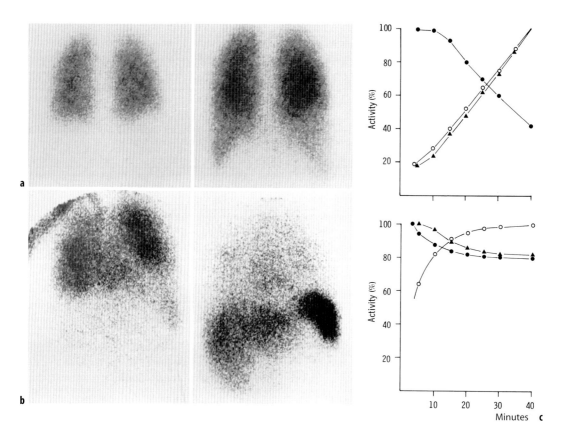

Figure 15.1. Gamma camera images showing transit of ^{111}In-labeled granulocytes through the lungs following intravenous injection. **a** Granulocyes isolated on a Percoll saline gradient and labeled in saline with ^{111}In acetylacetonate. **b** Granulocytes isolated on a metrizamide-plasma gradient and labeled in plasma with ^{111}In tropolonate. The left panels are immediately following injection (note the bolus still in the subclavian vein in **b**) and the right panels at about 10 min after injection. **c** Corresponding time–activity curves recorded in regions of interest placed over the lung (closed circles), liver (triangles), and spleen (open circles). Upper panel, granulocytes in part **a**; lower panel, granulocytes in part **b**. Ordinate, percent of maximum (over 40 min); abscissa, time from injection.

bacteria, and then are ultimately removed by tissue macrophages or excreted in body fluids. Studies with ^{111}In-labeled granulocytes instead suggest that, in normal subjects, the vast majority (greater than 95%) are destroyed in the reticuloendothelial system, as are platelets and red cells. Thus at 24 h after injection of radiolabeled granulocytes, the distribution of activity corresponds to the reticuloendothelial system, particularly the spleen and bone marrow (Figure 15.4).

Because the spleen both pools and destroys granulocytes, its activity level following ^{111}In-labeled granulocyte administration remains constant or falls slightly as the activity from pooled cells is gradually replaced by activity from destroyed cells (Figure 15.4b). In patients with sepsis,

the splenic activity shows a more pronounced fall as granulocytes that initially marginate in the spleen are redirected towards the inflammatory focus and utilized for migration (Figure 15.2).

15.3 Imaging Inflammation

A convenient classification of inflammation-targeting agents is as follows:

1. labeled granulocytes or leukocytes (and monoclonal antibodies directed against them);

2. agents that specifically target activated endothelium;

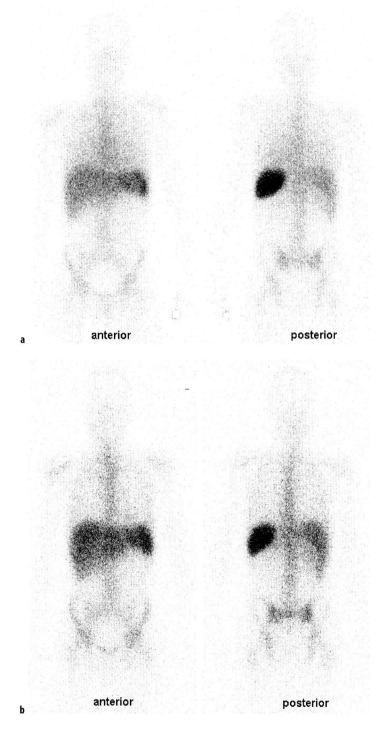

Figure 15.2. Anterior and posterior images showing a normal distribution of labeled cells 4 h **a** and 24 h **b** after injection of ^{111}In-labeled leukocytes. On the 4 h images, there is transient accumulation of labeled cells seen in the lungs **a**, which become clear on the delayed images **b**.

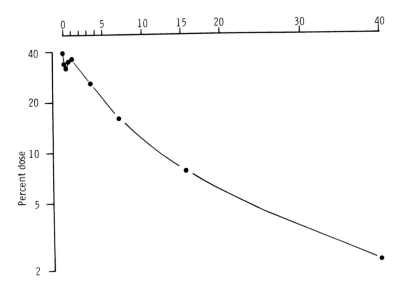

Figure 15.3. Time-course of circulating granulocyte-bound ^{111}In following injection of pure granulocytes isolated on metrizamide-plasma and labeled in plasma with ^{111}In tropolonate. Ordinate, percent of injected dose; abscissa, time for injection (h). Note the early "reappearance" of cells (from about 30 min); this "blip" probably represents release of cells retained in the liver and is another indication of cell activation sustained during labeling.

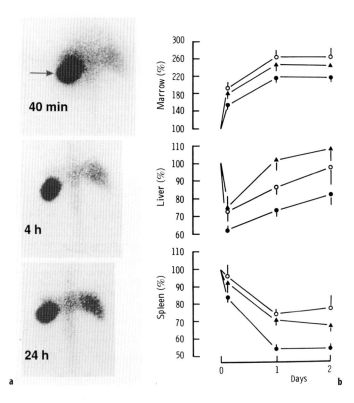

Figure 15.4. a Posterior gamma camera images showing distribution of ^{111}In-labeled granulocytes from 40 min to 24 h after injection in a patient with no evidence of inflammatory disease. Activity at 40 min predominantly represents the distribution of blood granulocytes, while that at 24 h predominantly represents the sites of granulocyte disposal. Note the relative decrease in the splenic signal (arrowed) and increases in bone marrow and hepatic signals. **b** Corresponding time–activity curves (corrected for physical decay of ^{111}In) in regions of interest drawn over the lumbar spine (bone marrow), liver, and spleen. Ordinate, percent of value at 40 min; open circles, normal subjects; triangles, patients with white cell scans negative for inflammatory disease; closed circles, patients with white cell scans positive for inflammatory disease. The time-course of splenic and marrow activities reflects the time-course of blood granulocyte-associated activity (not shown), while liver activity continues to increase after disappearance of blood granulocyte-associated activity, but in the continued presence of "free" plasma [111]In.

3. macromolecules that diffuse through widened interendothelial gaps; and

4. small diffusible radiotracers that target specific granulocyte receptors in vivo after the cells have migrated into the extravascular space.

15.3.1 Radiolabeled Leukocytes

The radionuclides available for leukocyte labeling for the localization of infection are ^{111}In and ^{99m}Tc. For white cell scanning, there are essentially two cell preparations to choose from – mixed (or crude) leukocytes or pure granulocytes. The former is simpler to prepare and perfectly adequate in most clinical circumstances where the patient is neutrophilic and the mixed cell preparation is therefore rich in granulocytes. Pure granulocyte labeling is time-consuming but necessary in some clinical situations; for example:

1. when the patient does not have a raised neutrophil count;

2. cardiovascular lesions, such as endocarditis, when labeled contaminants, principally red cells and platelets, may give rise to a persistent blood pool signal against which it is difficult to see migrated granulocytes;

3. where quantitative studies are undertaken such as quantitation of fecal ^{111}In excretion in the assessment of disease activity in patients with inflammatory bowel disease or ^{111}In excretion in the sputum of patients with bronchiectasis.

Labeling Mechanisms

Ionic ^{111}In, delivered as the chloride in 0.04 M HCl, is unable to penetrate cells and indeed immediately forms a colloidal suspension at non-acidic pH. If, however, it is first complexed with a lipophilic chelating agent, the complex penetrates the lipid bilayer of cells and the ^{111}In binds firmly to intracellular proteins [8]. The fate of the chelating agent is uncertain, but the majority probably leaves the cell. This is an oversimplification of the true mechanism as can be appreciated from the fact that between 10^2 and 10^6 times more chelating agent than the amount required to complex the available ^{111}In ions is required for labeling.

Although the various ^{111}In-complexes label cells indiscriminately, they show variable selectivity for the different cell types. Thus ^{111}In oxinate and ^{111}In tropolonate are selective for leukocytes and platelets compared with red cells; for instance in a mixture of equal numbers of granulocytes and red cells, 90% of ^{111}In tropolonate will label the granulocytes.

A number of other factors influence the efficiency with which a particular complex labels cells. These include temperature (very slow at $4°C$), pH (efficiency falls markedly at pH values less than 6.5), and plasma concentration (reduces efficiency but less critical for ^{111}In tropolonate than ^{111}In oxinate).

^{99m}Tc-HMPAO, like the above ^{111}In-complexes, is highly lipophilic, which is why it was developed for imaging cerebral perfusion (Chapter 12), and also why it readily penetrates blood cells. Its labeling efficiency is relatively independent of plasma concentration. In addition to selectivity for leukocytes, it also displays some selectivity for eosinophils [9] but is not as stable as ^{111}In and elutes from cells at a rate of about 5% per hour.

Labeling Mixed Cells with ^{111}In

1. Intravenous blood is drawn into a syringe containing the appropriate volume of acid citrate dextrose (ACD) (NIH, formula A; 7.5 vols to 42.5 vols of blood). In neutrophilic patients, 50 ml of anticoagulated blood is adequate. Heparin should not be used for anticoagulation because it promotes granulocyte microaggregation in the isolation procedure.

2. A red-cell sedimenting agent, such as hespan or plasmasteril, is added (1 to 10 vols of blood). This promotes the formation of red-cell rouleaux, which, because of their size, then sediment to the bottom of the tube leaving a supernatant rich in leukocytes and platelets with residual individual red cells.

3. The supernatant is removed and centrifuged gently at 150g for 5 min to sediment the leukocytes and red cells; significant numbers of platelets also contribute to the cell pellet. The platelet-rich plasma (PRP) is removed and centrifuged at 1000g for 15 min to obtain platelet-poor plasma (PPP). Alternatively, PPP can be obtained by centrifugation (1000g for

15 min) of a separate aliquot of 20 ml of whole blood withdrawn into a separate syringe (containing ACD) at the initial venepuncture. This is preferable because (a) the PPP is also free of sedimenting agent, and (b) fast centrifugation of PRP may result in some undesirable platelet activation (as a result of platelet pelleting).

4. Depending on the chelate to be used, the cell pellet is resuspended either in 2–5 ml saline, or preferably buffer such as Hepes (for labeling with ^{111}In oxinate) or 1 ml of PPP (for labeling with ^{111}In tropolonate).

5. The chosen ^{111}In-complex is added.

   (a) *^{111}In oxine.* This complex is available commercially in a ready-to-use form. The required amount of ^{111}In is added to the cell suspension; because this will depend on the time since delivery, it is not possible to control the oxine concentration unless the volume of saline within which the cells are suspended is varied to take this into account.

   (b) *^{111}In tropolonate.* This chelate is prepared simply by adding ^{111}In indium chloride directly to a solution of tropolonate in a test-tube. The stock solution of tropolonate, at 4.4×10^{-3} M in 20 mM Hepes saline buffer, pH 7.6, should be stored in small aliquots at $4°$C and protected from light. It is possible to label cells in plasma with this complex, provided the cell concentration is high, and this limits the volume of plasma, in which the cells are suspended for labeling, to 1 ml. This in turn limits the volume of tropolonate solution and ^{111}In indium chloride that can be added; thus about 15 MBq (500 μCi) of ^{111}In in a volume of not more than 50 μl is added to 100 μl of tropolonate solution and this mixture then added to the cell suspension to give a final tropolonate concentration of 4×10^{-4} M, which is the optimal concentration for labeling cells in plasma. (The optimal concentration for labeling in saline is considerably lower.) The limitation in the volume of ^{111}In indium chloride that can be added necessitates the use of material which is at a high specific activity (at least 200 MBq (5 mCi) ml^{-1}).

6. The cells are incubated at room temperature for 5 min. "Excess" PPP (5–10 ml) is then added, which terminates labeling.

7. The suspension is centrifuged again at 150g for 5 min and the supernatant discarded. If larger volumes of PPP are added at step 6, then centrifugation may need to be longer to get the cells down. The pellet is resuspended in 50 ml of PPP and reinjected into the patient.

Labeling Pure Granulocytes with ^{111}In

The procedure is the same as for mixed leukocytes up to step 3 above, whereupon the cell pellet, following removal of all but 2 ml of the supernatant, is carefully layered on to a multiple density gradient column, which may be prepared from Percoll (Pharmacia) or metrizamide (Nyegaard).

Percoll

Percoll is a liquid that contains silica particles coated with PVP. To prepare iso-osmotic stock Percoll solution, 1 vol of 1.5 M NaCl is added to 9 vols of Percoll. This represents 100% Percoll gradient solution. Although Percoll gradients can be made by addition of appropriate volumes of normal saline or buffer, it is preferable to make them by adding autologous plasma because of the deleterious effect on granulocytes of sedimentation through Percoll–saline. Therefore, 100% Percoll is diluted with autologous plasma to give solutions of 65%, 60%, and 50% Percoll in plasma, and 2 ml of each of these are layered onto each other with the most dense at the bottom. Two such gradients are prepared from 1 ml of "crude" cells in plasma (from step 4 above) layered on to each. Following centrifugation at 200g and 5 min, the granulocytes accumulate at the interface between the 50% and 60% gradients, the mononuclear leukocytes localize at the interface between plasma and the 50% gradient and the red cells pellet at the bottom of the tube.

The platelets remain in suspension in the plasma layer. There is usually a clear separation of granulocytes from other cell types although this is slightly variable probably because of slight variability in the density of plasma from patient to patient.

The granulocytes are "harvested", washed in at least 10 ml PPP, and resuspended in 1 ml plasma for labeling with ^{111}In tropolonate as in step 4 for mixed cells. Care is taken to add at least 10 ml PPP at the end of labeling so that any trace of Percoll still remaining at this stage is eliminated.

Metrizamide

Metrizamide, which has been used as a radiological contrast medium, comes as a powder. A stock solution is made by addition of water to give a concentration of 35% w/v, which has a specific gravity of 1.1887 g ml^{-1} (100% metrizamide). The stock solution is then diluted with autologous plasma to give two solutions of 55% and 45% metrizamide:plasma. These are layered, as in the Percoll gradients, and the mixed leukocyte suspension (from step 4 above) added to the top. Cell separation is achieved by centrifugation at 200g for 5 min. Granulocytes localize in the column with more variability than with Percoll, either at the interface between the two metrizamide densities or diffusely in the 45% band. Red cell localization is also rather unpredictable, although this is of less importance because red cells are relatively unselective for ^{111}In oxine and ^{111}In tropolonate. Granulocytes are more difficult to separate on metrizamide-plasma than on Percoll-plasma. Centers setting up granulocyte labeling are strongly advised to carry out pilot experiments to confirm these gradient concentrations under their own laboratory conditions.

Labeling Leukocytes with ^{99m}Tc-HMPAO

Labeling leukocytes with ^{99m}Tc-HMPAO is very similar to labeling mixed leukocytes with ^{111}In tropolonate, being identical up to step 4 above.

The HMPAO (500 mg) is reconstituted by addition of 5 ml pertechnetate to the vial, and 4 ml of this is then added to the l ml of mixed leukocyte suspension to give a total volume of 5 ml, containing 20% plasma and HMPAO at 80 mg ml^{-1}. The l ml of ^{99m}Tc-HMPAO remaining in the vial can be subjected to chromatographic quality control aimed at quantifying the fraction present on the primary, lipophilic, complex.

Separation of pure granulocytes for labeling with ^{99m}Tc-HMPAO is seldom necessary, or appropriate, for two reasons. Firstly, granulocyte labeling is relatively selective with this complex. Secondly, a common reason for using radiolabeled pure granulocytes is for quantitative studies. These are generally inappropriate with ^{99m}Tc-HMPAO because of an elution rate which, although not a problem for clinical imaging studies, is unacceptably high, not only from circulating cells but also from the reticuloendothelial system following normal labeled granulocyte disposal.

15.4 Evaluation of Labeled Granulocyte Function

A number of in vitro tests are available for evaluating the function of granulocytes following isolation and radiolabeling. These include superoxide production, chemotaxis, bacterial killing, respiratory burst, nephelometric aggregation in response to C5a, and phase-contrast microscopy. These tests of granulocyte function are of rather limited use, since by their very nature they cause activation of the cells and cannot therefore distinguish between cells that have become activated as a result of in-vitro manipulation, and quiescent (functionally intact) cells. Activated cells are sequestered in the lung vasculature immediately following injection (Figure 15.1) and display a limited capacity for migration following their release from the lungs. An exception to these tests is phase-contrast microscopy, in which activated cells can be seen to have thrown out pseudopodia, whereas quiescent cells are spherical.

When setting up a leukocyte scanning service (or changing personnel), detailed in-vitro studies of granulocyte function would be appropriate and desirable in order to establish the optimal technique, but they should not be performed without kinetic studies aimed at demonstrating optimal functional integrity in vivo. This is achieved simply by performing dynamic gamma camera scintigraphy immediately following injection. Dynamic data indicating optimal conditions are shown in Figure 15.1. Thus the cells (whether pure granulocytes or mixed leukocytes) should transit the lungs rapidly (such that the lungs are essentially clear by about 20 min) and the radioactivity should appear rapidly in the spleen. The liver should not show prominent activity at any stage. Based on these criteria it should be possible to confirm an adequate technique initially suggested by favorable in-vitro tests.

15.5 Mechanisms of ^{67}Ga Uptake in Inflammatory Foci

The mechanism of ^{67}Ga uptake into inflammatory foci is complex and probably involves at least four steps. Following intravenous injection ^{67}Ga binds to transferrin and circulates as a radiometal–protein complex. Capillaries in inflamed tissue are abnormally "leaky", and the macromolecular complex enters the tissue non-specifically.

Secondly, because of its chemical similarity to ferric iron, ^{67}Ga is trapped in inflamed tissue by cross-chelating to lactoferrin, a protein liberated from degranulating neutrophils that binds ^{67}Ga and ferric iron with greater avidity than does transferrin. The lactoferrin–^{67}Ga complex is then taken up by macrophages, which may explain why ^{67}Ga is able to localize sites of chronic inflammation. Thirdly, the circulating ^{67}Ga–transferrin complex also binds intact to transferrin receptors. Such receptors are expressed in cancers, which may explain why ^{67}Ga localizes malignancies. Fourthly, ferric iron and ^{67}Ga bind siderophores, low-molecular-weight products of bacteria whose role is connected with bacterial ferric iron utilization. This explains why ^{67}Ga may still localize sites of infection in patients with neutropenia.

Although it is clear that ^{67}Ga localization in inflammation is not mediated entirely by leukocytic activity, an additional explanation for the relatively improved performance of ^{67}Ga, compared with radiolabeled leukocytes, in the detection of chronic inflammation is related to the rate of leukocyte turnover in chronic inflammation, and the respective residence times in blood of ^{67}Ga and radiolabeled leukocytes. Thus the residence time in blood of radiolabeled leukocytes is too short, relative to the slow leukocyte turnover in chronic inflammation, for significant accumulation of radioactivity. ^{67}Ga, however, with its longer residence time in blood, has the potential to be accumulated in larger amounts.

15.6 Normal Distribution and Imaging Protocol

15.6.1 Leukocytes

^{111}In

At about 45 min after injection, the normal distribution of ^{111}In following injection of ^{111}In-labeled leukocytes is the blood pool, spleen, and liver, with minimal activity in lungs and bone marrow (Figure 15.4a). At 24 h, when the ^{111}In-labeled cells have been cleared from the circulation, the normal distribution is the reticuloendothelial system, with prominent signals from spleen and bone marrow. Imaging is normally at 4 and 24 h. The regions imaged are dictated by the clinical history. A fixed number of counts should not be aimed for, since the count rate depends critically on whether the view includes areas normally active (such as the spleen) or areas not normally active (such as distal extremities) or active inflammation. The imaging protocol is given in Table 15.1.

^{99m}Tc-HMPAO

Activity quickly appears in the urine after injection of ^{99m}Tc-HMPAO-labeled cells as the result of elution of hydrophilic ^{99m}Tc complex (the precise chemical nature of which is uncertain). This gives rise not only to urinary activity but also to renal parenchymal activity (Figure 15.5), the intensity of which appears to be highly variable. Biliary activity can be visualized in the gallbladder from about 3 h onwards, although, unlike urinary activity which is consistently seen, gallbladder activity is seen in only about 5–10% of cases. Nonetheless, this biliary activity is almost certainly the basis for bowel activity, which is seen

Table 15.1. Indium-labeled granulocytes or leukocytes

Radiopharmaceutical	^{111}In-labeled granulocytes or leukocytes
Activity administered	12 MBq (300 μCi)
Effective dose equivalent	6 mSv (600 mrem)
Patient preparation	None
Collimator used	Medium energy
Images acquired	3 and 24 h post-injection but 45 min and 48 h images may be helpful. Whole body scans may also be useful

INFECTION AND INFLAMMATION

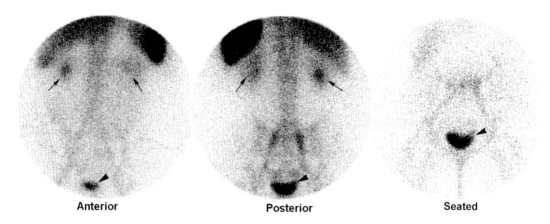

Anterior   **Posterior**   **Seated**

Figure 15.5. Anterior, posterior and seated images showing a normal distribution of activity 2 h after injection of ^{99m}Tc-HMPAO-labeled leukocytes. Normal accumulation of cells is seen in the spleen, liver, and bone marrow. ^{99m}Tc, in the form of labeled hydrophilic complexes that have eluted from the labeled leukocytes, is seen in the kidneys (arrows) and bladder (arrowheads).

Table 15.2. ^{99m}Tc-labeled leukocytes

Radiopharmaceutical	^{99m}Tc-HMPAO-labeled leukocytes
Activity administered	200 MBq (5 mCi)
Effective dose equivalent	4 mSv (400 mrem)
Patient preparation	None
Collimator used	Low-energy, high-resolution
Images acquired	2 and 4 h post-injection but 45 min and 24 h images may be helpful. Whole body scans may also be useful

consistently from 4 h onwards with this agent (Figure 15.6). In addition to the distribution of reticuloendothelial and blood pool activity, therefore, ^{99m}Tc-HMPAO-labeled leukocytes give normal early images which include renal, urinary, biliary, and bowel activities.

Skeletal activity is often prominent with ^{99m}Tc-HMPAO-labeled cells. This is the result of bone marrow uptake, which within the first few hours is the result of margination, and there is no evidence that there is any contribution from bone turnover, as with ^{67}Ga (see below). The imaging protocol is outlined in Table 15.2.

15.6.2 ^{67}Ga Gallium Citrate

There is a prominent blood pool signal for 24 h after injection of ^{67}Ga gallium citrate, which is bound to plasma transferrin. During this time 10–25% of the injected dose is excreted in the urine.

On images up to 24 h, therefore, renal activity is a normal finding but, subsequently, anything more than that faint activity is abnormal.

In addition to urinary excretion, ^{67}Ga is excreted in the feces, as a result of biliary and direct colonic excretion. Bowel activity is prominent up to 72 h and is one of the main drawbacks of ^{67}Ga imaging for abdominal inflammation. Use of laxatives and delayed imaging are ways of circumventing this problem, although laxatives are not very effective and not appropriate in the context of most clinical situations in which patients present for ^{67}Ga scanning for the detection of abdominal sepsis. Moreover, delayed imaging is often not feasible in view of the need for an early diagnosis.

Reticuloendothelial activity becomes progressively more prominent after injection. Initially, liver activity is prominent and it remains so, although after about 72 h it becomes relatively less active while splenic activity increases. Skeletal uptake of ^{67}Ga is related to both reticuloendothelial activity and to bone turnover. Prominent uptake in the growth plates, which is part of the normal distribution, reflects bone turnover. ^{67}Ga is used in osteomyelitis in conjunction with ^{99m}Tc-MDP scanning, active inflammation producing discordance between the two agents. Other sites of normal uptake are the lacrimal glands, nasal mucosa, testes, female perineum and breasts, particularly during lactation when breast-feeding should be avoided. In young children, the thymus may be seen.

ant-hips 3hrs

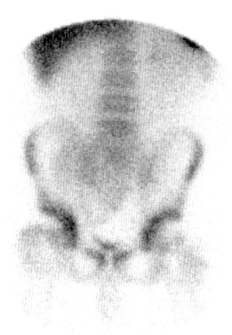

a

anterior 20.5hrs

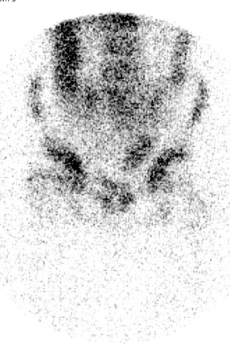

b

Figure 15.6. Non-specific bowel activity seen with ^{99m}Tc-HMPAO-labeled leukocytes. These anterior images show **a** normal distribution of activity at 3 h, with a hint of small bowel activity, but **b** marked activity in the colon at 20.5 h. The patient did not have inflammatory bowel disease.

Table 15.3. ^{67}Ga gallium citrate

Radiopharmaceutical	^{67}Ga gallium citrate
Activity administered	100 MBq (3 mCi)
Effective dose equivalent	11 mSv (1.1 rem)
Patient preparation	None
Collimator used	Medium- or high-energy
Images acquired	48 and 72 h post-injection. Anterior and posterior views of the relevant region. 400 kcounts per image using dual or triple photopeaks

The imaging protocol is given in Table 15.3. The timing of imaging is determined to a large extent by the clinical circumstances. Thus the sick infant with a normal radiograph, an equivocal bone scan and a strong clinical suspicion of acute osteomyelitis will need to be imaged from 12 h or even 6 h after injection. On the other hand, the patient with a history of pyrexia of unknown origin (PUO) of a number of weeks may be imaged from 72 h. Extremities can generally be imaged early, since urinary and colonic activities present no problems and blood pool activity is less of a problem than, for example, in the chest.

15.7 Clinical Applications

15.7.1 Labeled Leukocytes

Abdominal Abscess

Abdominal abscess may present as PUO, as a post-surgical complication, as a complication of some other pathology, such as Crohn's disease, or without an apparent underlying cause.

The accuracy of labeled leukocytes in abdominal abscess is greater than 85%, a figure comparable with computed tomography (CT) and ultrasound. Whole body imaging 4 and 24 h after injection of ^{111}In-leukocytes or 1 and 4 h after ^{99m}Tc-leukocytes are the recommended procedures. An abscess is recognized as a focal accumulation of activity, with an intensity greater than that of the liver, outside the normal distribution (Figure 15.7).

Suspected hepatic abscess should be approached with ^{111}In-leukocytes because of the normal biliary excretion of ^{99m}Tc-HMPAO. It is usually identifiable against the relatively high background of normal hepatic activity (Figure 15.8), especially if 1 h images are obtained in addition to 4 and 24 h images. This is because

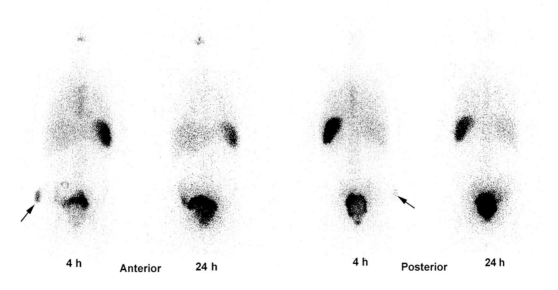

Figure 15.7. The posterior 4 h and 24 h ^{111}In-labeled leukocyte images show intensive activity seen in the pelvis consistent with a large pelvic abscess. The unusual focus of activity seen at the right side of the pelvis seen on the earlier image is an artifact from contamination of the patient's handkerchief after blowing his nose (arrow).

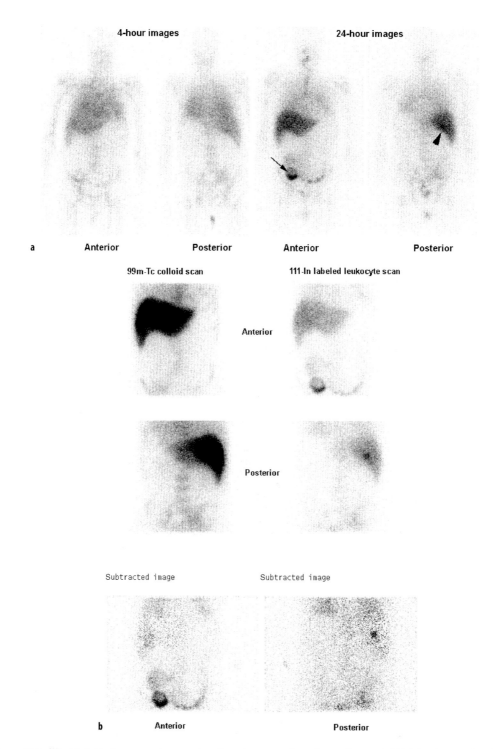

Figure 15.8. ^{111}In-labeled leukocyte scan in a pyrexia patient who was on chemotherapy for non-Hodgkin's lymphoma; 4 h and 24 h post-injection anterior and posterior whole body images are shown **a**. Note that the activity in the lungs has cleared on the 24 h images. An abscess is identified in the right iliac fossa (arrow). A lesion in the liver is just visible on the posterior 24 h image (arrowhead). This lesion was easily identifiable when the leukocyte scan was compared with a contemporaneous ^{99m}Tc sulfur colloid **b**.

INFECTION AND INFLAMMATION

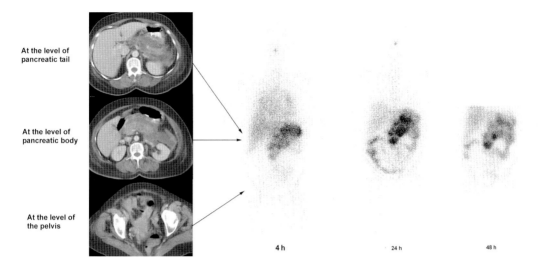

At the level of
pancreatic tail

At the level of
pancreatic body

At the level of
the pelvis

4 h   24 h   48 h

Figure 15.9. Multiple infected collections seen in the pancreatic bed in a patient with acute necrotizing pancreatitis. The activity in the pancreatic bed increases in intensity from 4 h to 24 h before the intensity diminishes. The presence of activity in the bowel at 24 h and 48 h suggests communication between infected collections in the pancreatic bed and the adjacent bowel. The fluid seen in the pelvis is not infected. Computed tomography (CT) was performed 2 days before the ^{111}In-labeled leukocyte study.

normal liver activity falls, often quite markedly, between 1 and 4 h, whereas activity in an abscess increases. The intensity of activity in pus is comparable to that in the spleen but, when an abscess is in close anatomical relationship to the spleen, confusion may be avoided by sequential imaging. Confusion may also arise if the patient is asplenic and this is not known. Whenever doubt exists ultrasound and/or a radiocolloid liver/spleen scan should be performed.

The findings with ^{99m}Tc-HMPAO-leukocytes in abdominal abscess are similar to those with ^{111}In-leukocytes (Figure 15.9). Imaging must be performed before 4 h, and preferably at 1 h in addition, in order to avoid confusion with later normal bowel activity (Figure 15.6). Normal gallbladder activity or renal/urinary activity should be clearly identified as such, and not confused with an abdominal abscess. The pelvic outlet view (with the patient sitting on the face of the gamma camera) is especially useful with ^{99m}Tc-HMPAO-labeled leukocytes in order to clearly delineate bladder activity (Figure 15.10).

A relatively common situation is the communication of an abdominal abscess with bowel (Figure 15.11). Because of the normal gut excretion of ^{99m}Tc-HMPAO, they are more easily diagnosed with ^{111}In-leukocytes. Since communication may be an unexpected finding, ^{111}In-leukocytes should in general be used in preference to ^{99m}Tc-HMPAO-leukocytes in suspected abdominal sepsis. Enteric communication is an important complication which must not be missed as it carries a worse prognosis than uncomplicated abdominal abscess. This is probably due to a degree of silence resulting from spontaneous decompression which leads to a delay in diagnosis based on anatomical modalities such as CT and ultrasound [10]. The appearances on ^{111}In-leukocyte imaging are characteristic, with early views showing appearances typical for abscess, but later views showing evidence of enteric activity with simultaneous drainage of activity from the abscess. The enteric activity moves distally as it does in inflammatory bowel disease. If early imaging is not done, then inflammatory bowel disease may be misdiagnosed; hence the importance of sequential imaging in any case of suspected abdominal abscess.

Because of logistical considerations, ultrasonography should be the first investigation and if an abscess is visualized it may be possible to drain it under sonographic guidance. If the findings are negative or equivocal the next investigation should be either CT or a white cell scan. An advantage of the latter is that the entire body may be examined; on the other hand, if positive on CT, an abscess may then be drained under CT guidance. If CT is negative and the clinical suspicion of abscess is high, a white cell scan should be performed.

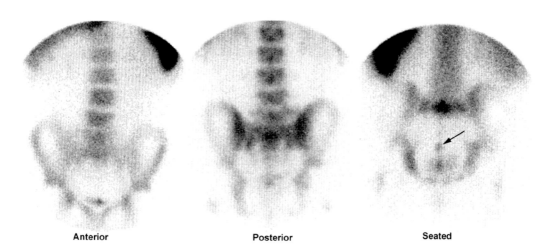

Anterior   Posterior   Seated

Figure 15.10. Anterior, posterior, and seated images of a ^{99m}Tc-HMPAO-labeled leukocyte study showing minor abnormal activity that is most easily detected just behind the bladder on the seated view (arrow). This finding was consistent with a known perianal abscess.

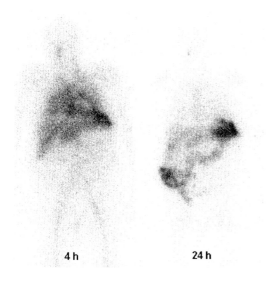

4 h   24 h

Figure 15.11. Abdominal abscess in communication with bowel lumen. The ^{111}In-labeled leukocyte image at 4 h shows a subsplenic collection which can be seen to be spontaneously discharging into the bowel lumen on the image obtained at 24 h.

Other causes of intra-abdominal infection that can be diagnosed with radiolabeled white cells include renal abscesses, abdominal wall abscesses, pelvic inflammatory disease, and hepatobiliary infection. The first and last of these may be difficult to diagnose with ^{99m}Tc-HMPAO-labeled white cells because of normal tracer excretion routes.

Pancreatic sepsis should be investigated with ^{111}In-labeled white cells, since there is a high incidence of spontaneous gut communication. In general the aims of imaging are to detect complications (Figure 15.9) as uncomplicated acute pancreatitis is associated with a negative white cell scan. Patients who develop abscess, fat necrosis, or pseudocyst have positive scans. However, since white cell scanning cannot distinguish between abscess and fat necrosis, a positive scan is of limited value.

Catheter tunnel infection in patients on ambulatory peritoneal dialysis is a major problem. ^{111}In-labeled white cells may be useful in the differentiation of simple peritonitis (Figure 15.12) or exit site infection, which responds to conservative management, from catheter tunnel infection, which usually requires removal of the catheter and termination of peritoneal dialysis.

Inflammatory Bowel Disease (IBD)

^{99m}Tc-HMPAO-labeled leukocytes have replaced ^{111}In-labeled leukocytes for imaging inflammatory bowel disease. Inflammation of the bowel of almost any cause generally shows a prominent accumulation of labeled leukocytes with an intensity that may equal or surpass that of the spleen (Figure 15.13). IBD can be distinguished from abdominal abscess by the distribution of abnormal activity. Imaging is useful in patients with chronic diarrhea in order to separate an organic from a nonorganic cause, and in patients with known IBD

INFECTION AND INFLAMMATION

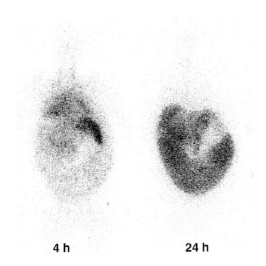

4 h   **24 h**

Figure 15.12. Peritonitis in a patient having continuous ambulatory peritoneal dialysis. Note the early intense lung activity (at 4 h), often seen in patients with extensive inflammatory disease as a result of granulocyte priming. Note the striking reduction in splenic activity on the delayed image that arises from the massive leukocyte accumulation in the abdomen and resulting diversion of labeled cells pooling in the spleen at the early time point towards migration in the inflammatory lesion. Note also the striking absence of bone marrow activity, a feature often seen in very sick patients.

in order to define distribution of disease activity or to distinguish a relapse from mechanical obstruction, abdominal abscess or some non-specific cause of acute illness. Imaging is also useful in very ill patients, especially those with suspected megacolon, in whom radiological studies may be dangerous. The use ^{111}In-labeled granulocytes for disease quantitation by fecal ^{111}In excretion or whole body ^{111}In loss is now confined to clinical research.

In IBD, imaging must be early after cell injection because, having migrated into bowel, granulocytes gain access to the lumen and move distally with its contents (Figure 15.14). The rate of this movement is highly variable and depends on the site of migration (ileum or colon) and on the patient's clinical condition (frequent bowel actions or constipation). The activity may move so rapidly that it is significant with respect to imaging time and "blurs" the image, as in ileitis, or so slowly as not to change between 3 and 24 h. Thus images at 48 h, by showing distal movement, may be necessary to confirm that intra-abdominal activity is present in bowel and not due to an abscess.

^{99m}Tc-HMPAO-labeled leukocytes present a problem in IBD because of non-specific fe-

cal excretion of ^{99m}Tc-labeled secondary complexes (Figure 15.6). This virtually rules out any meaningful imaging after about 4 h, although in the great majority of cases the early views supply the required clinical information. Imaging at 24 h may occasionally be useful to define bowel anatomy and thereby facilitate interpretation of equivocal early images.

Causes of false positive white cell scans in IBD include hematoma, tumor, non-rejecting renal allograft, and uncomplicated bowel anastomosis.

Lung Infection

Lung abscess is readily detected with white cells labeled with [111]In (Figure 15.15) or ^{99m}Tc-HMPAO. Such abscesses frequently complicate bronchogenic carcinoma and may be quite dramatic in size and intensity.

Lobar pneumonia is interesting in that it is usually negative on white cell scanning [11]. It is likely that granulocyte migration terminates early in lobar pneumonia, which can therefore only be imaged if the cells are administered early in the disease. The mechanism of termination, presumably in the face of a continuing chemotactic stimulus, is of great interest in view of the fact that normal anatomy is preserved in the involved lobe following the resolution of pneumonia.

Patients with septic shock, who have clear and sometimes dramatic evidence of sepsis on the white cell scan, may present with the adult respiratory distress syndrome (ARDS). This is associated with increased granulocyte margination in the lungs, which should not be misinterpreted as evidence of damage to the cells resulting from in vitro manipulation during labeling. Such damage produces marked initial pulmonary activity that clears fairly rapidly, usually by about 1–2 h (Figures 15.1 and 15.4). Increased margination of granulocytes, however, as in ARDS, is associated with increased lung activity which remains in parallel with blood pool activity, and therefore persists for longer, usually several hours.

Diffusely increased accumulation of leukocytes in the lung is also seen in association with several other conditions, notably inflammatory bowel disease, systemic vasculitis, and graft-versus-host disease of the gut without pulmonary involvement. Although appearances are similar to those seen in ARDS, there is usually a conspicuous absence of clinical evidence of lung injury in these conditions, questioning the exact role of

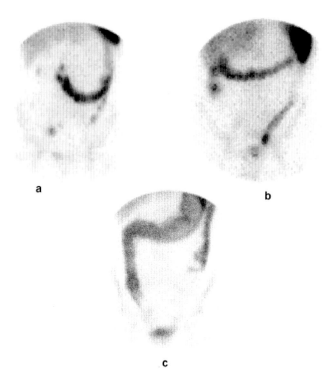

Figure 15.13. ^{99m}Tc-HMPAO-labeled leukocyte imaging in inflammatory bowel disease. **a** Crohn's disease, showing typical skip regions of increased bowel activity involving the large and small bowels. **b** Ulcerative colitis, showing extensive abnormal bowel activity from rectum to ascending colon. **c** Ulcerative colitis, showing increased activity in a dilated colon, consistent with toxic megacolon.

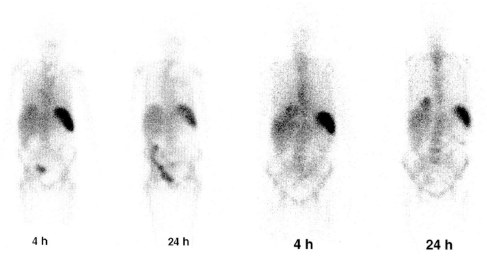

Figure 15.14. Ileocecal tuberculosis. The 4 h image of the ^{111}In-labeled leukocyte scan shows a focal activity in the right iliac fossa. On the 24 h image, the activity has moved up the ascending colon, indicating communication with bowel lumen.

Figure 15.15. Empyema. ^{111}In-labeled leukocyte scan showing increasing intensity of activity at the right lung base from 4 to 24 h. Bowel activity (probably jejunal) is also present probably as a result of swallowed expectorated ^{111}In-labeled sputum.

granulocytes in acute lung injury. Since the increased pulmonary signal persists in ARDS beyond the residence time of granulocytes in the circulation, but not in the other diseases mentioned, it seems likely that granulocyte migration into the pulmonary extravascular space, in addition to increased pulmonary vascular granulocyte pooling, is required for lung damage to occur.

Bronchiectasis is a condition complicated by lung infection in which the affected lobes can be readily imaged with labeled leukocytes. [111]In studies have shown that about one-third of involved lobes are abnormal on CT but negative on white cell scanning, presumably reflecting detection of inactive disease on CT [12]. Furthermore, most patients with this discordance have other lobes that are positive with both modalities, underlying the importance of local factors in determining whether or not disease is active.

As in IBD, ^{111}In-granulocytes may be used to quantify disease activity in bronchiectasis. Thus, granulocytes that have migrated into dilated air passages are ultimately coughed up and expectorated, and the scans, even when intensively positive at 4 h, become completely negative by 5–7 days. Whole body counting over 5–7 days using an uncollimated gamma camera or dedicated whole body counter may demonstrate a loss of up to 50% of the injected activity of [111]In. The rate of loss in normal individuals is about 1% per day. This approach, as in IBD, is largely reserved for clinical research.

Bones and Joints

Imaging the musculoskeletal system with radiolabeled leukocytes is complicated by two problems: firstly, a relatively high incidence of chronic infection, and secondly, the simultaneous uptake of labeled leukocytes by the bone marrow as a result of normal leukocyte destruction in the reticuloendothelial system (Figure 15.4). Opinions are divided of the clinical value of ^{111}In-labeled leukocytes in bone and joint sepsis and this is probably a reflection of these two problems.

Acute osteomyelitis is routinely imaged with ^{99m}Tc-MDP and plain radiography. In chronic osteomyelitis, however, ^{99m}Tc-MDP is not indicated as the initial radionuclide investigation since, in the presence of abnormal plain radiographs the bone scan will inevitably be abnormal. There is usually little difficulty imaging acute exacerbations of chronic osteomyelitis with labeled white cells (Figure 15.16), with uptake intense enough to overcome that due to normal marrow uptake. MDP bone scanning should be reserved for coregistering an abnormal leukocyte image when it is not certain if the increased leukocyte uptake is in bone or soft tissue. This confusion is particularly seen in the diabetic foot or following trauma, where associated soft tissue infection is common and bone architecture is markedly deranged. Alternatively, structural imaging with MRI can be useful in this context.

[67]Ga gallium citrate is often preferred to labeled leukocytes in chronic osteomyelitis, although the latter may be effective. This is a clinical area where optimal leukocyte viability is important for successful imaging.

The accuracy of ^{111}In-radiolabeled leukocytes in the detection of infected joint prostheses appears to be marginally better than their accuracy in other forms of chronic osteomyelitis. However, in one study using pure granulocytes labeled in plasma with ^{111}In tropolonate, infection was correctly diagnosed in all of 18 infected prostheses at a cost of two false positives in 22 other patients who proved to have sterile prostheses [13].

There are few data on the use of radiolabeled white cells in septic arthritis (Figure 15.17), probably because this diagnosis should be excluded on suspicion by joint aspiration.

Other Infections

Leukocyte scanning is occasionally performed for infected cardiac valves, endocarditis, (Figure 15.18) and related conditions of the cardiovascular system. The positivity rate, however, is extremely low, probably because of the small size of the lesions and their tendency to be chronic. Whole body scanning may be important to detect possible metastatic infection.

Cardiovascular lesions more readily detected by white cell scanning are infected prosthetic vascular grafts. Whether the infection starts at the intraluminal or extraluminal side of the graft, it tends to penetrate the graft material as a result of the latter's porous structure. Intraluminal activity in a sterile graft may result from granulocyte adherence, analogous to platelet uptake on a thrombogenic surface, and may be confused with infection. Using ^{111}In-labeled platelets, it has been shown that platelet adhesion on such grafts is maximal at the sites of the anastomosis, and this may also be true for granulocytes.

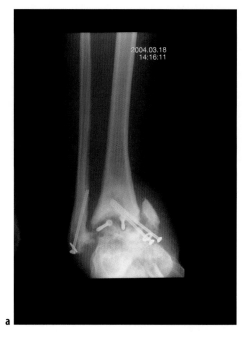

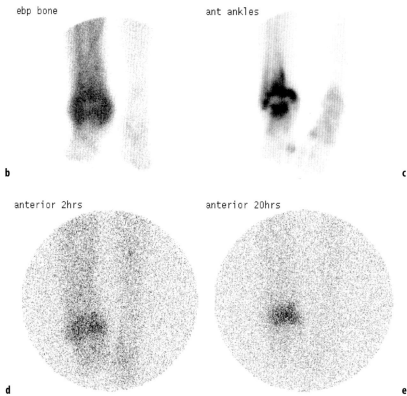

Figure 15.16. Infected fixation screws involving the distal right tibia and fibula (osteomyelitis). The plain radiograph shows fixation screws with an aggressive periosteal reaction around the distal right tibia and fibula **a**. Early blood pool **b** and delay bone scan **c** images (^{99m}Tc-MDP) show marked inflammation around the right ankle. Infection is confirmed on the ^{111}In-labeled leukocyte scan **d**, **e**.

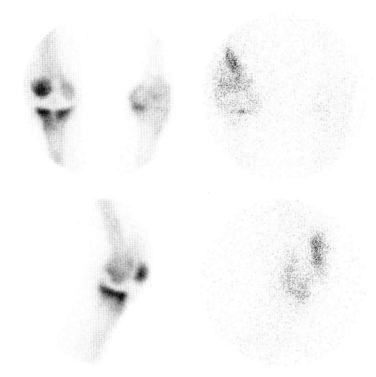

Figure 15.17. Synovitis in a total knee replacement. The combination of ^{99m}Tc-MDP bone and ^{111}In-labeled leukocyte scans established that the labeled cells were localizing around the synovium rather than in the prosthesis. Misinterpretation of sterile synovitis as infection is a common problem in total knee replacements, as the synovium is usually left intact at surgery.

^{111}In-labeled leukocytes have been used to detect cerebral abscesses and distinguish these from cerebral tumors. False positives can, however, occur with infarction. Uptake of ^{111}In-labeled leukocytes in hyperostosis frontalis may be mistaken for intracranial sepsis.

15.7.2 ^{67}Ga Gallium citrate

In the detection of infection, ^{67}Ga is probably most often used in osteomyelitis, particularly chronic osteomyelitis and infected joint prosthesis. As an inflammatory process becomes more chronic its rate of neutrophil turnover declines, and it consequently recruits a smaller fraction of an injected dose of labeled white cells. ^{67}Ga then becomes a preferable alternative to labeled leukocytes.

Intra-abdominal Infection

The main drawbacks in the use of ^{67}Ga for the detection of intra-abdominal inflammation (Figure 15.19) are non-specific bowel activity

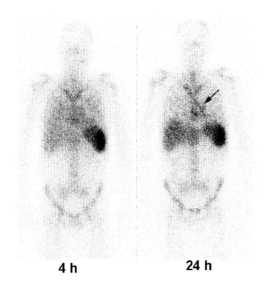

4 h   **24 h**

Figure 15.18. Probable endocarditis. The anterior 4 h and 24 h images of an ^{111}In-labeled leukocyte scan show abnormal activity in the cardiac region (arrow) that changes in distribution between the two time points.

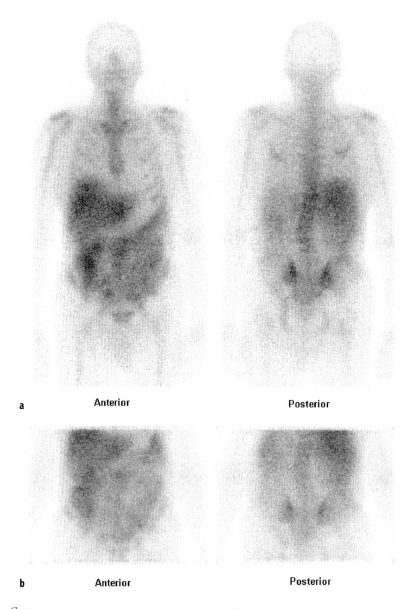

a Anterior Posterior

b Anterior Posterior

Figure 15.19. ^{67}Gallium scintigraphy in a 66-year-old male with pyrexia of unknown origin. Anterior and posterior views obtained at 48 h **a** and 96 h **b** show normal bowel activity.

and, in early images, renal activity. Nonetheless the literature indicates an overall accuracy of up to 90%, comparable with labeled white cells. ^{67}Ga is particularly indicated in the absence of localizing signs. Otherwise ultrasound and/or CT should be the first investigations.

^{67}Ga may be useful in the detection of renal infection and perirenal collections. Faint diffuse renal activity may be seen beyond 24 h and, al-though said to be more prominent in patients with reduced renal function, should not be interpreted as indicating inflammation. Abnormal renal activity is usually prominent, asymmetrical and, with particular regard to inflammatory conditions, distinctly focal.

As with radiolabeled white cells, hepatic abscess is more likely to be detected with ^{67}Ga if sequential imaging is performed, although the decrease in

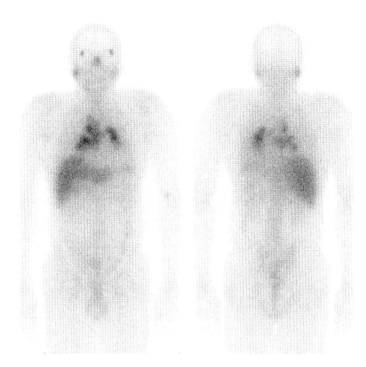

Figure 15.20. Sarcoidosis. ^{67}Ga scan at 72 h in a woman presenting with low-grade fever. The images show abnormal tracer uptake in hilar and mediastinal lymph nodes, and asymmetrically in the parotid glands, consistent with sarcoidosis. Lacrimal gland uptake is also often seen in this condition but is within the normal range in this patient.

normal hepatic activity over time is not as marked as with white cells. Furthermore, the difference between uptake in normal hepatic parenchyma and a hepatic abscess is not as great as with labeled white cells, necessitating a greater readiness to use simultaneous ^{99m}Tc sulfur colloid scintigraphy. ^{67}Ga gives much less splenic activity than radiolabeled white cells, and so left-sided subphrenic abscess should, at least in theory, be easier to detect with ^{67}Ga.

Abscesses with enteric communication are not readily detected with ^{67}Ga because of non-specific bowel activity. This important diagnosis can usually be made with ^{111}In-labeled leukocytes. Similarly, radiolabeled leukocytes are also preferable to ^{67}Ga for the diagnosis of abscess complicating Crohn's disease.

^{67}Ga in the Chest

Accumulation of ^{67}Ga in the lungs is seen in a wide variety of causes of active pulmonary inflammation, including bacterial, fungal, mycobacterial and viral infections, sarcoidosis, pneumoconiosis, and idiopathic pulmonary fibrosis.

Several abnormal patterns may be seen in sarcoidosis, including mediastinal and hilar lymph node uptake, focal pulmonary uptake and diffuse symmetrical pulmonary uptake (Figure 15.20). Abnormal uptake in the chest may or may not be associated with increased uptake involving the salivary glands, nasal region, and lacrimal glands in a constellation giving rise to the so-called "panda" sign. ^{67}Ga scanning may be useful in the confirmation of a diagnosis of sarcoidosis or in monitoring disease activity.

The Immunocompromised Patient

Imaging the complications of the acquired immunodeficiency syndrome (AIDS) has become important over the last few years. Intrathoracic complications of AIDS, as with most other forms of intrathoracic inflammation, are, in general, more effectively imaged with ^{67}Ga than with labeled leukocytes [14]. The reverse is probably true for extrathoracic infections. It is especially important to view the ^{67}Ga scan alongside the chest radiograph. A normal ^{67}Ga scan with a normal chest X-ray excludes infection with a high degree of certainty. On the other hand, a normal ^{67}Ga scan in the presence of obvious respiratory deterioration carries a very poor prognosis, implying an inability to mount an inflammatory response. Focal pulmonary ^{67}Ga uptake usually indicates bacterial pneumonia or *Pneumocystis carinii* pneumonia (PCP). Diffuse pulmonary ^{67}Ga uptake is normally due to PCP but, especially if faint, may be due to other chest infections such as a mycobacterial infection or cytomegalovirus (CMV). A coexisting normal chest X-ray, a heterogeneous distribution of ^{67}Ga activity and intense uptake (greater than liver) all strongly suggest PCP. Lymph node uptake is most often due to mycobacterial infections or lymphoma. Kaposi's sarcoma does not take up ^{67}Ga, so a normal ^{67}Ga scan with an abnormal chest X-ray suggests this diagnosis.

^{67}Ga scans are also often abnormal in AIDS-related enteritides, although the appearances are non-specific and complicated by normal ^{67}Ga excretion in the gut. Outside the chest, leukocyte scintigraphy is generally more useful than ^{67}Ga. Centers with special expertise in cell isolation from HIV-positive blood are able to perform routine white cell scans. An alternative is to use labeled leukocytes isolated from normal donors. These appear to effectively localize inflammation. They may also be useful in hepatitis-B-positive patients.

Cardiac infections that may be visualized on ^{67}Ga scanning include endocarditis, myocarditis (including syphilitic), and pericarditis. ^{67}Ga scanning is seldom clinically indicated in these conditions, although it is occasionally found to be abnormal in them when being used to investigate a patient with undiagnosed fever. Pericardial uptake appears as a circumferential accumulation around the heart, while in myocardial involvement, the area of uptake is wider.

Bones and Joints

Abnormal ^{67}Ga uptake may be intense in acute osteomyelitis. In most cases, the diagnosis can be established on clinical findings, radiography, and ^{99m}Tc-MDP bone scan. Since osteomyelitis commences in the marrow, the ^{67}Ga scan may become abnormal before the MDP bone scan. However, in infants under 6 months of age and particularly in neonates, the bone scan may remain normal.

Two conditions that give abnormal ^{99m}Tc-MDP bone scans, and are not infrequently complicated by acute osteomyelitis, are sickle-cell crises and leukemia. Diagnosing osteomyelitis in these conditions is therefore difficult. Both these conditions present problems for labeling autologous leukocytes; thus sickle cell blood gives a low yield of leukocytes because of difficulties in separating them from sickling red cells, while in the leukemias the white cells themselves are often abnormal. ^{67}Ga has a potential role in such circumstances. Autologous white cell scanning is also difficult in neutropenic patients. Because of its multifactorial uptake mechanism, ^{67}Ga may be preferable.

The role of ^{67}Ga scanning versus radiolabeled leukocytes in chronic osteomyelitis is uncertain. The bone scan is usually abnormal in chronic osteomyelitis, not surprisingly in view of the extended period of increased bone turnover in this condition. The diagnosis of active infection is based on discordant distributions of ^{67}Ga and ^{99m}Tc-MDP.

Various patterns of abnormal uptake of ^{99m}Tc-MDP and ^{67}Ga, including combinations based on both agents, have been suggested to distinguish infection in joint prostheses from loosening, but in general one should be looking for discordance between the two that would help to distinguish between increased bone turnover (which promotes increased MDP uptake) and inflammation (which promotes ^{67}Ga uptake).

^{67}Ga has a limited place in the diagnosis of acute septic arthritis, since joint aspiration is indicated when this is suspected. A role exists for ^{67}Ga, however, in infection of joints such as the disk space and sacroiliac joints, not readily accessible to aspiration.

15.8 Other Agents for Imaging Inflammation

Although it remains the gold standard for imaging inflammation, the main disadvantage of white cell scanning is the need for in vitro manipulation of autologous blood. This has provided the impetus to find agents which can image inflammation as effectively as white cells but which can be given as an off-the-shelf agent by intravenous injection.

Because increased capillary permeability promotes non-specific localization of almost any radiopharmaceutical, it is essential to compare any new agent with an appropriate control agent, for example an irrelevant radiolabeled monoclonal antibody against a specific monoclonal antibody. Indeed, human polyclonal immunoglobulin

G (HIG) was developed for imaging inflammation several years ago and, although at first was thought to localize in inflammation through several specific mechanisms, is now known to target inflammation non-specifically, largely through increased capillary permeability [15]. The indications and findings are broadly in line with [67]Ga. ^{111}In-HIG is somewhat more specific than ^{67}Ga, not showing, for example, abnormal uptake in lymphoma nor physiological uptake in bowel. A marginal advantage over ^{67}Ga is an earlier diagnosis, although this still takes 24 h.

Monoclonal antibodies against granulocytes seemed promising when they were introduced as a means of labeling leukocytes in vivo. However, because the radioactivity in sampled blood is almost exclusively in plasma, it appears that they also work largely as a result of increased capillary permeability, although additional local mechanisms at the site of inflammation may promote their retention [16]. A further fundamental disadvantage is that they label antigenically positive granulocyte precursors in the bone marrow, which far outnumber circulating granulocytes, and therefore give prominent imaging of the bone marrow.

A partly in vivo, partly in vitro technique for labeling granulocytes, which was described very early on in the development of inflammation imaging, is the incubation in vitro of whole blood with ^{99m}Tc-labeled colloid. This, however, unavoidably activates the cells, resulting in a poor intravascular yield. It nevertheless appears to work satisfactorily in IBD, provided the labeling protocol is carefully followed.

In the search for improved specificity in inflammation imaging, labeled antibiotics have been investigated for their ability to specifically target bacteria at sites of infection. They do localize in such inflammation but it is now thought that the mechanisms of uptake are multifactorial and that they are largely non-specific.

Other novel approaches include radiolabeled chemotactic peptides, radiolabeled monoclonal antibodies to endothelium, ^{18}F-fluorodeoxyglucose ([18]FDG), and a range of particles and macromolecules that target inflammation non-specifically and not particularly effectively (e.g. biotin–avidin complexes and liposomes).

A tissue of interest for localizing inflammation is the vascular endothelium, which becomes activated and expresses antigenic proteins during inflammation. Anti-E-selectin labeled with ^{111}In has been successfully used for imaging both acute and chronic inflammation [17], and several other adhesion molecules could be targeted using the same principle. As an alternative to monoclonal antibodies, it should be possible to identify, isolate, and label surface molecules of leukocytes which are responsible for binding endothelial adhesion molecules, thereby reproducing the effectiveness of leukocyte scanning.

Several small radiotracers that rapidly diffuse across the endothelium and target specific leukocyte receptors have been developed for imaging inflammation. These include chemotactic peptides, such as radiolabeled interleukin-8 (IL-8), that target activated granulocytes. They have been shown to work experimentally but are not in clinical use. A variant of this approach is radiolabeled interleukin-2, which targets activated lymphocytes expressing IL-2 receptors. This is an interesting approach which may prove useful in various chronic diseases, associated with a lymphocytic infiltrate [18]. [111]In octreotide, which targets the somatostatin receptor, probably also provides images of inflammation, albeit not very effectively, by binding to activated lymphocytes.

The use of [18]FDG is based on the increased metabolic rate of inflammatory foci (Figure 15.21). Several inflammatory cells accumulate [18]FDG at an accelerated rate when they are activated, especially granulocytes and macrophages. With respect to granulocytes, it appears that priming is the most metabolically active process and largely responsible for [18]FDG uptake. There are several reports of the successful use of [18]FDG PET in chronic osteomyelitis, synovitis, infected joint prostheses, IBD, and granulomatous lesions including sarcoidosis and tuberculosis. However, in none of these studies were comparisons made with labeled leukocytes so the contribution of granulocyte migration to positive images, as opposed to activation of local macrophages and endothelial cells, remains unclear. Moreover, [18]FDG PET has not proved particularly useful for any of the diseases that are common indications for leukocyte scanning, such as IBD and chronic osteomyelitis. It is, however, gaining impetus for the investigation of pyrexia of unknown origin (PUO; see below). The fact that [18]FDG also targets tumors is not necessarily a disadvantage in the clinical setting of PUO, where the aim of the scan is to localize any pathology, inflammatory or otherwise. Atherosclerosis is positive with [18]FDG PET as a result of macrophage infiltration of the arterial wall and it has therefore been suggested that

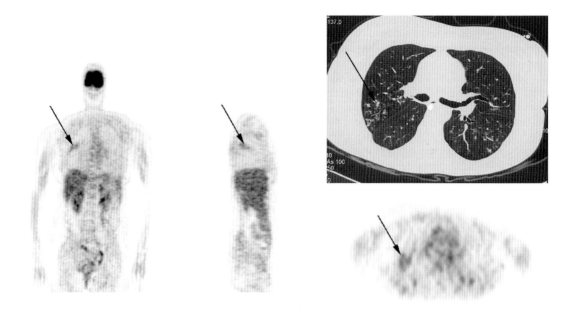

Figure 15.21. Infective consolidation is seen in the upper lobe of the right lung. The computed tomography (top right) identifies focal consolidation in the right lung. This finding is confirmed as a low-grade ^{18}FDG uptake seen in the positron emission tomographic images (arrows).

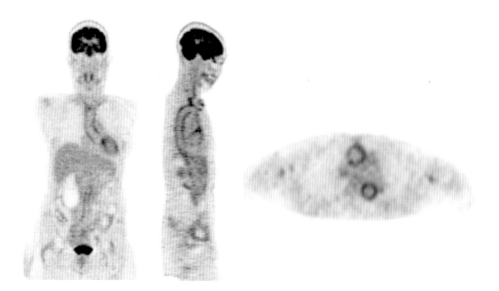

Figure 15.22. An inflammatory process such as vasculitis can be identified using ^{18}FDG positron emission tomography (PET), which in this case shows increased tracer uptake along the ascending aorta in a patient with Takayasu's arteritis. Inflammatory atheromatous plaques may give a similar picture but at a lower level of intensity.

[18]FDG PET may be able to indicate the balance in an atheromatous lesion between inflammatory activity (that predisposes to instability, rupture, and sudden occlusion) and smooth muscle activity (that promotes remodeling and chronic but stable ischemia). [18]FDG PET is also proving useful in the diagnosis of various forms of large vessel arteritis (Figure 15.22).

15.9 Approach to the Patient with an Undiagnosed Fever

Patients with prolonged fever are increasingly referred to nuclear medicine departments with the aim of localizing pathology causing the fever (undiagnosed fever). Indeed, this has become a more frequent reason for requesting an inflammation scan than acute soft tissue sepsis (including abdominal abscess). Since the choice of agent is usually not immediately obvious, this clinical presentation is discussed separately from those described under the specific agents, above.

Patients with undiagnosed fever broadly fall into two groups: firstly, previously well patients with fever of at least 3 weeks duration but no clue as to the cause, the classic description of pyrexia of unknown origin (PUO); and secondly, patients with fever of any duration but associated with features, such as recent surgery, which raise the likelihood of purulent disease (occult fever or occult infection). Several agents have been used to find a cause for undiagnosed fever but there have been several problems in evaluating them, including inconsistencies in clinical presentation, a high proportion of patients in whom no final diagnosis is reached, and proof that any scintigraphic abnormality was in fact the cause of the fever. Since there are several non-infective and non-inflammatory causes of undiagnosed fever, the value of using infection or inflammation as the endpoint in such studies is questionable.

About 10–20% of leukocyte scans yield true positive results in PUO but the yield is higher in occult infection. ^{111}In-HIG also appears to perform well in occult infection, reported series claiming an accuracy at least as good as ^{111}In-leukocytes. ^{111}In-HIG, however, is more likely to be negative than ^{67}Ga when fever is due to neoplasia (Figure 15.20), which accounts for up to 30% of causes of PUO in some series and which has generally been classified as being the cause of "true negatives" in series based on HIG.

A general guideline for choosing an appropriate agent for imaging patients presenting as an undiagnosed fever is to use ^{67}Ga unless there is (1) a history of surgery within the previous 6 months; (2) bacteremia; (3) endocarditis, which may be metastatic, indicating infection elsewhere; (4) a raised C-reactive protein (CRP); and (5) any other feature clearly predisposing the patient to sepsis. Otherwise ^{111}In-leukocytes should be used. In centers with PET facilities, [18]FDG whole body PET is a useful alternative to investigate undiagnosed fever, although evidence for its accuracy is still being gathered [19, 20] and it does not yet have a routine ARSAC (Administration of Radioactive Substances Advisory Committee) serial number.

An attraction of [18]FDG for imaging patients with undiagnosed fever is its potential to be positive not only in the inflammatory causes of undiagnosed fever but also in the neoplastic ones, especially lymphoma (Figure 15.23). As with ^{67}Ga,

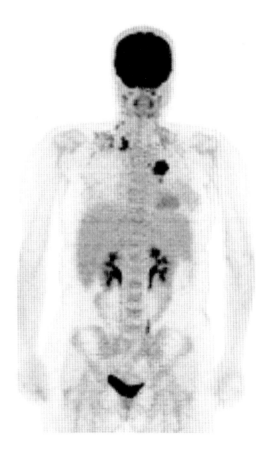

Figure 15.23. Hodgkin's disease. [18]FDG positron emission tomography (PET) showing multiple foci of increased tracer uptake in the right side of the neck, right supraclavicular region, and left hilum.

the endpoint should be a positive image rather than a specific diagnosis. Experience so far indicates that [18]FDG PET is at least as useful as ^{67}Ga in PUO, with the added advantage of a same-day result. Moreover, whilst in patients with cancer there is doubt concerning the accuracy of gamma camera PET compared with dedicated PET, the former may find a greater role in inflammation imaging because, in contrast to staging cancer, image resolution is less critical [20].

References

1. Chapman PT, Haskard DO. Leukocyte adhesion molecules. Br Med Bull 1995; 51:296–311.
2. Jones HA, Cadwallader KA, White JF, et al. Dissociation between respiratory burst activity and deoxyglucose uptake in human neutrophil granulocytes: implications for interpretation of (18)F-FDG PET images. J Nuc Med 2002; 43:652–657.
3. Savill J. Apoptosis in resolution of inflammation. J Leukoc Biol 1997; 61:375–380.
4. Athens JW, Raab SO, Haab OP, et al. Leukokinetic studies. III. The distribution of granulocytes in the blood of normal subjects. J Clin Invest 1961; 40:159–164.
5. Saverymuttu SH, Peters AM, Danpure HJ, et al. Lung transit of [111]Indium-labelled granulocytes. Relationship to labelling techniques. Scand J Haematol 1983; 30:151–160.
6. Haslett C, Guthrie LA, Kopaniak MM, Johnston RB, Henson PM. Modulation of multiple neutrophil functions by preparative methods or trace concentrations of bacterial lipopolysaccharide. Am J Pathol 1985; 119:101–110.
7. Peters AM, Saverymuttu SH, Keshavarzian A, Bell RN, Lavender JP. Splenic pooling of granulocytes. Clin Sci 1985; 68:283–289.
8. Thakur ML, Lavender JP, Arnot RN, Silvester DJ, Segal AW. Indium-111-labeled autologous leukocytes in man. J Nucl Med 1977; 18:1014–1021.
9. Puncher MR, Blower PJ. Autoradiography and density gradient separation of technetium-99m-exametazime (HMPAO) labelled leucocytes reveals selectivity for eosinophils. Eur J Nucl Med 1994; 21:1175–1182.
10. Saverymuttu SH, Peters AM, Lavender JP. Clinical importance of enteric communication with abdominal abscesses. BMJ 1985; 290:23–26.
11. Jones HA, Sriskandan S, Peters AM, et al. Dissociation of neutrophil emigration and metabolic activity in lobar pneumonia and bronchiectasis. Eur Respir J 1997; 10:795–803.
12. Currie DC, Saverymuttu SH, Peters AM, et al. Indium-111-labelled granulocyte accumulation in respiratory tract of patients with bronchiectasis. Lancet 1987; i:1335–1339.
13. Pring DJ, Henderson RG, Rivett AG, et al. Autologous granulocyte scanning of painful prosthetic joints. J Bone Joint Surg 1986; 68B:647–652.
14. Palestro CJ. The current role of gallium imaging in infection. Semin Nucl Med 1994; 24:128–141.
15. Claessens RAMJ, Koenders EB, Boerman OC, et al. Dissociation of indium from indium-111-labelled diethylene triamine penta-acetic acid conjugated non-specific polyclonal human immunoglobulin G in inflammatory foci. Eur J Nucl Med 1995; 22:212–219.
16. Skehan SJ, White JF, Parry-Jones DR, et al. Mechanism of accumulation of ^{99m}Tc-sulesomab in inflammation. J Nucl Med 2003; 44:11–18.
17. Jamar F, Chapman PT, Harrison AA, et al. Inflammatory arthritis: imaging of endothelial cell activation with an indium-111-labeled F(ab′)2 fragment of anti-E-selectin monoclonal antibody. Radiology 1995; 194:843–850.
18. Signore A, Chianelli M, Annovazzi A, et al. ^{123}I-interleukin-2 scintigraphy for in vivo assessment of intestinal mononuclear cell infiltration in Crohn's disease. J Nucl Med 2000; 41:242–249.
19. Blockmans D, Knockaert D, Maes A, et al. Clinical value of (18)F fluoro-deoxyglucose positron emission tomography for patients with fever of unknown origin. Clin Infect Dis 2001; 32:191–196.
20. Meller J, Altenvoerde G, Munzel U, et al. Fever of unknown origin: prospective comparison of ^{18}F FDG imaging with a double-head coincidence camera and gallium-67 citrate SPET. Eur J Nucl Med 2000; 27:1617–1625.

16

Tumor Imaging

Alan C. Perkins

16.1 The Clinical Problem

Figures released from Cancer Research UK show that in 2000 there were over 270 000 new cases of cancer and 155 180 deaths from cancer in the United Kingdom. One in three people will suffer from cancer during their lifetime. Nearly half of all cancer deaths are due to just four types of cancer, those of lung, breast, prostate, and colon. In males and females respectively cancers of the lung and breast are by far the most common, accounting for 25% and 18% of cancers occurring within each sex.

Apart from the action of known carcinogens such as smoking, which is the most important cause of preventable disease in the UK, the causes of cancer are poorly understood. However, factors such as sex, age, race, and internal characteristics such as hormonal imbalance and genetic abnormality have been linked with the etiology of the disease. Environmental factors may also act as a trigger in a person with a preexisting susceptibility to the disease.

The successful management of a patient with cancer requires an accurate knowledge of the extent of the disease. A range of diagnostic investigations is often performed to obtain the necessary diagnostic information. Many of these procedures are invasive and carry inherent risks and morbidity. Imaging techniques such as radiography, ultrasound, magnetic resonance imaging (MRI), and gamma scintigraphy are all capable of demonstrating internal body structures and function with minimal patient trauma.

Because tumor growth occurs at the cellular level, the disease is usually at an advanced stage before the patient becomes aware of its presence. The tumor may have spread to other sites in the body by the time a diagnosis is made, thus presenting additional problems for the complete eradication of the disease. Hence, the earlier the stage at which the diagnosis is made the greater the probability of a permanent cure. Treatment is normally based on the histology and grade of the disease and is usually carried out in the form of surgery, radiotherapy, chemotherapy, or a combination of these.

16.2 Tumor Physiology

Tumors are neoplastic growths which arise from normal body cells that have undergone a fundamental change in structure or function [1]. As a result the cell nuclei lose their ability to control proliferation. Tumors can be of two types: benign and malignant. Benign tumors have a structure similar to their tissue of origin and the cells are normally well differentiated. Their growth is slow and they do not invade into surrounding normal tissues or seed in other sites of the body (metastasize). A benign tumor can threaten the life of the host if it obstructs critical vessels, ducts or tracts within the body, interfering with normal oxygenation, nutrition, or excretion, or if it has a functional activity such as excess hormone production. Surgical removal will usually provide a permanent cure. Malignant tumors or cancers consist of undifferentiated cells having a bizarre atypical structure. They can be found in a diffuse state such as in leukemia where the cells are widely dispersed or in localized cellular associations forming solid tumors. Their growth is rapid and uncontrolled and if not treated they can infiltrate and metastasize to distant sites in the body which serve as new centers of tumor growth.

Malignant cells are characteristically immature and show both morphological and physiological deviations from the normal. Frequently hyperplasia and metaplasia precede the conversion of normal tissue into neoplastic tissue. The structural characteristics of most neoplastic cells resemble in certain ways the immature cells of the embryo and it is often difficult to distinguish the cell type from which the malignancy was originally derived. The cell nuclei are usually large and contain grossly abnormal nucleoli and chromosomes. Cancer cells exhibit a general loss of the capability to synthesize specialized proteins. For example, a differentiated liver cell synthesizes only liver cell enzymes whereas hepatocarcinoma cells may produce few normal enzymes but produce fetal liver enzymes associated with growth. The invasion of tumor cells into other tissues may also be assisted by the production of substances that promote neovascularization.

The progression of the disease generally manifests itself in a set pattern of tumor spread to specific organs of the body depending upon the site of origin. The lymphatic system appears to be the most common pathway for metastatic spread. For example, in general colon carcinoma will initially metastasize to liver whereas carcinoma of the breast will metastasize to bone. Many schemes for tumor staging have been established mainly based on tumor size, lymph node involvement, and the presence or absence of metastases. A typical classification for tumor staging is given in Table 16.1.

Table 16.1. Typical tumor staging

Stage	
1	Tumor limited to the organ of origin
2	Tumor spread to surrounding tissues and lymph nodes
3	Tumor spread extensively into deeper structures and distant lymph nodes
4	Tumor spread throughout the body with distant metastases

Based on Ruben [1].

Knowledge of the pattern of metastatic spread is used as a basis for requesting diagnostic investigations when staging the extent of the disease. Radionuclide bone imaging in the staging of patients with carcinoma of the prostate is a typical example.

16.3 Radiopharmaceuticals

Many substances have been investigated for their ability to localize in tumor tissue. Many imaging radiopharmaceuticals have been developed in an almost ad hoc manner with the prime objective of obtaining a high target-to-non-target (T:NT) ratio of localization. However, there is now a more specific approach to the design of radiopharmaceuticals with the design of ligands targeted to specific tumor receptors. The physiological characteristics exploited for targeting conventional radiopharmaceuticals are largely non-specific. The main characteristics are metabolism, blood supply, and perfusion. The localization of most "tumor seeking" radiopharmaceuticals is probably best considered in terms of altered regional physiology resulting from the presence of the tumor. Such localization would also be expected to occur with other disease states characterized by a similar change in regional physiology. However, the aim of modern radiopharmaceutical design is to target specific tumor characteristics to achieve high diagnostic specificity.

Previously the use of radiopharmaceuticals was based on the differential uptake of a radiopharmaceutical into tumor and normal tissues. Certain radiopharmaceuticals have the ability to localize in some normal functioning tissues and have been termed organ or system specific. These materials simply detect the presence of non-uniformities of perfusion in various inflammations and space-occupying lesions. Examples of these are the uptake of colloids by the reticuloendothelial system or more specifically in the Kupffer cells of the liver, renal imaging with dimercaptosuccinic acid (DMSA), and pulmonary perfusion with macro-aggregated albumin. In each case any disruption in normal function results in an area of reduced radiopharmaceutical concentration commonly termed a "cold spot". Detection of a "cold spot" in a relatively "hot" organ is a non-specific process and may result from many disorders that disrupt normal organ function. This approach cannot provide a specific diagnosis as various space-occupying lesions will produce similar appearances. For example, abscesses or polycystic disease of the liver and kidneys may give similar appearances to tumor deposits when imaged with colloids or DMSA respectively. In such cases additional clinical information is required in order to achieve the correct diagnosis. The relatively poor detection efficiency of the gamma camera for cold spots in a hot background is also a fundamental factor against this approach. In the case of liver imaging, ultrasound and X-ray computed tomography are capable of delineating smaller lesions than colloid scintigraphy.

The more satisfactory functional approach to tumor imaging is to use a particular characteristic of tumor tissue not found in normal tissues. Utilizing such a property involves the concentration of a tracer at the tumor site, resulting in an area of increased activity. This targeting approach offers greater specificity although many radiopharmaceuticals used for tumor diagnosis will also concentrate in some benign lesions. The main factors influencing the concentration of radiopharmaceuticals in tumor tissues are listed in Table 16.2. The mechanisms for targeting radiopharmaceuticals can mainly be divided into three groups: metabolism, extracellular mechanisms, and cell surface receptors. These functional mechanisms have been exploited for a range of radiopharmaceuticals that are used in both diagnosis and therapy [2].

The first process of metabolism utilized is the fundamental physiological uptake of molecules normally occurring in the body. The classical example of this is the use of radioiodine to demonstrate the function of the thyroid gland. Another example can be found in the use of metaiodobenzylguinidine for use in the diagnosis (and therapy) of neuroendocrine tumors. The second mechanism is based on extracellular mechanisms for the uptake of radiopharmaceuticals. The bone-seeking agents fall into this group along with radiolabeled cells. The third grouping includes the

Table 16.2. Principal factors influencing the concentration of radiopharmaceuticals in tumor tissues

1	Increased metabolic activity
2	Increased blood flow
3	Altered microvasculature contributing to EPR effect
4	Extracellular uptake
5	The presence of cell-specific receptors or tumor-associated antigens

cell surface receptors currently being used for the new generation of targeted radiopharmaceuticals which are finding both diagnostic and therapeutic applications. These include radiopharmaceuticals based on hormones, peptides, and antibodies.

One feature of tumor growth is the development of a good blood supply to provide the oxygen and nutrients necessary for cellular replication. The new tumor vessels are inherently leaky compared with normal blood vessels. This is due to wide inter-endothelial junctions, large numbers of fenestrae and transendothelial channels formed by vesicles as well as discontinuous or absent basement membranes. As a result, capillary permeability of the endothelial barrier in newly vascularized tumors is significantly greater than that of normal tissues. This may lead to increased uptake of some agents since this is a function of both local blood flow and microvascular permeability. The amount of tissue accumulation of a conjugate is proportional to plasma clearance. The enhanced permeability and retention (EPR) due to poor lymphatic drainage of the tumor may lead to prolonged accumulation and retention of macromolecules in tumor interstitium.

The influx of a tracer into tissues is mainly a function of tissue perfusion together with increased capillary and endothelial permeability towards the material in microcirculation [3]. The growth of blood vessels around neoplastic tissue results in a local alteration in circulation. The alteration in blood flow results in augmented delivery of tracers to the tumor site. It is a major factor in the localization of bone imaging agents such as ^{85}Sr, ^{18}F, and [^{99m}Tc] phosphates. Local increased blood volume will result in a differential concentration of tracer between a tumor and its surrounding tissues which, in some cases, may be sufficient for non-specific diagnostic purposes. Increased vascular permeability accompanied by prolonged extravascular residence time also provides mechanisms by which tracers may concentrate in tumors. Diffusion across the blood–brain barrier is a well-recognized process for the localization of [^{99m}Tc]sodium pertechnetate in brain tumors. In general neoplastic tissues, areas of inflammation, and certain responses to infarction are characterized by increased permeability of the capillary beds to macromolecules. Often the total perfusion to these areas is increased in comparison to surrounding tissues, due to neovascularization and enlargement of intercapillary pores. Hence, in all three conditions the entry of macromolecules into the interstitial fluid space from the intravascular space is increased. In addition, with neoplasia and inflammation there may be a delay in the growth of new lymphatic vessels adding to the residence time of macromolecules in the interstitial space. In cases of tissue necrosis, increased macrophage activity may result in the ingestion of the labeled macromolecule. Pinocytosis may even result in the ingestion of the macromolecules by other cells within the lesion.

Radiolabeled macromolecules such as albumin, fibrinogen, and gamma globulins exhibit localizing behavior in tumors, inflammatory lesions, and as a response to infarct formation. Same radionuclides such as gallium and indium bind to macromolecules, in these cases mainly transferrin, which has a specific cellular receptor site on some cell surfaces.

It should be appreciated that targeting radiopharmaceuticals to solid tumors is difficult and this is why other strategies have been employed for radionuclide therapy, such as intralesional, intra-arterial and intracavitary administration, for example, as in the treatment of glioma and superficial bladder cancer.

16.4 Radionuclide Bone Imaging

The use of radiopharmaceuticals to trace abnormal physiology precursive to tumor growth can, in some cases, offer diagnostic information unobtainable by any other imaging modality. Nuclear imaging has contributed significantly to the diagnosis, treatment planning, and the evaluation of treatment response in many cancer patients [3]. Bone imaging using [^{99m}Tc]-labeled phosphate compounds is more sensitive than radiography for identifying bone metastases from carcinoma of the prostate and breast [4]. This is because the alteration in osteoblastic action and/or blood supply occurs at an earlier stage than the difference in bone density needed to produce a radiographic change.

Bone scintigraphy can be of use in conjunction with X-rays for the diagnosis and assessment of the extent of primary bone tumors although its main utility is in the detection of bone metastases. The characteristic sign of bone metastases is that of multiple hot lesions scattered over the whole skeleton, commonly in the ribs, spine, and pelvis. Radionuclide bone imaging is especially useful in the staging and follow-up of patients with carci-

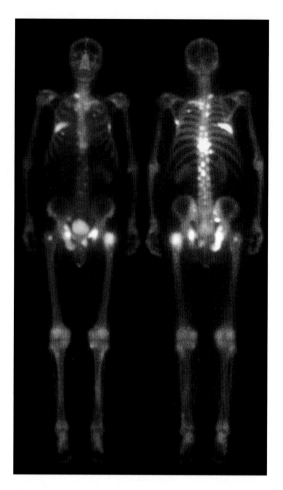

Figure 16.1. Whole body images (left, anterior and right, posterior) of a male patient with multiple metastases from carcinoma of the prostate recorded 3 hours following injection of 600 MBq (15 mCi) ^{99m}Tc-MDP.

nomas of the breast and prostate. An example of widespread metastases in a patient with carcinoma of the prostate is shown in Figure 16.1. Bone imaging is also of value where metastases are clinically suspected in patients with carcinomas of lung, kidney, bladder, and of gastrointestinal and gynecological origins, and in patients with bone pain and malignancy of unknown origin.

Diffuse bone metastases resulting in radionuclide bone images showing uniform uptake of tracer (superscans) are observed in about 10% of patients with bone metastases when presenting with carcinoma of the prostate [5]. Serial imaging following treatment with estrogen showed that in some patients a patchy distribution developed which, in fact, indicates an improvement in the patient's condition. In such instances additional information from radiographs has been found essential for the critical diagnosis but of relatively little value for monitoring changes during treatment.

16.5 [^{67}Ga]Gallium Citrate

The tumor localization of intravenously administered [^{67}Ga]gallium citrate was discovered by Edwards and Hayes [6]. The water-soluble salt [^{67}Ga]gallium citrate, an inorganic cation of group IIIa in the periodic table, has previously had wide clinical use as a tumor-seeking radiopharmaceutical and was at one time considered to be a general tumor localizing agent. Gallium-67 decays by electron capture with a physical half-life of 78 h and emits two major gamma photon energies suitable for imaging, 185 and 300 keV. The usual adult dose is 80–150 MBq (2–3 mCi) administered intravenously 48 to 72 hours prior to imaging (Table 16.3). Preliminary bowel cleansing is often recommended to prevent accumulation of gallium in the gut. On entering the bloodstream approximately 30% of the dose binds strongly with the serum proteins, chiefly transferrin. The remainder of the gallium complex diffuses throughout the extracellular spaces or is excreted by the kidneys. Approximately 12% of the administered dose is excreted by this route during the first 24 hours. At the time of imaging (48–72 hours after injection) high concentrations of activity are usually observed in the liver, spleen, and bone marrow.

Table 16.3. [^{67}Ga]gallium citrate imaging

Radiopharmaceutical	[^{67}Ga]gallium citrate
Activity administered	150 MBq (3 mCi)
Effective dose equivalent	17 mSv (1700 mrem)
Patient preparation	Oral laxatives and bowel cleansing enemas
Collimator	Medium energy, parallel, general purpose
Images acquired	Anterior and posterior thorax, abdomen and pelvis, 48 and 72 h post injection; 400 kcounts per image (dual photopeaks)
SPECT	64 × 20 s increments in 360° rotation. Useful in the thorax

[^{67}Ga]gallium citrate has been advocated for the diagnosis and staging of a wide variety of malignancies such as bronchogenic carcinoma, Hodgkin's disease, and lymphoma. Sensitivities of >90% have been reported for the use of gallium in malignant lymphoma, Hodgkin's and non-Hodgkin's disease, and Burkitt lymphoma. It is considered of value in the staging of disease in patients for whom invasive procedures are contraindicated and in locating metastases in sites not easily examined, such as para-aortic lymph nodes. Gallium imaging has previously been found to be particularly useful as an adjunctive diagnostic aid in assessing patients with radiographic evidence of a lung mass.

However, the interpretation of gallium citrate images needs to be made with caution as this agent is far from tumor specific. Although a review of the literature showed relatively high sensitivities for tumor detection (over 90%), published reports vary in opinion. The main limitation to the use of gallium is the variable bowel uptake and more particularly concentration in abscess and inflammation. Currently its main indication would appear to be in the diagnosis of lymphoma [7]. However, the more widespread availability of PET is expected to limit this.

16.6 Radioiodine and Thyroid Carcinoma

The high specificity of radioiodide for metastatic sites of functioning thyroid tumors occurs because the tumor tissues concentrate iodide while there are only a limited number of other tissues with cell membrane binding sites for iodide (cells of the thyroid, gastric mucosa, and salivary glands). After oral administration iodide is rapidly absorbed from the gastrointestinal tract with some absorption taking place from the stomach but a greater amount occurring from the small intestine. After gastrointestinal absorption or intravenous administration, iodide becomes distributed throughout the extracellular fluid and also diffuses into the red cells, where it accounts for approximately 65% of the iodide in blood. Iodide is removed from the plasma almost entirely by the thyroid and kidneys. Iodide trapped by the thyroid is readily oxidized to iodine which combines with tyrosine to form, first, 3-monoiodotyrosine (MIT) and then 3,5-di-iodotyrosine (DIT). The thyroid hormones

Table 16.4. Imaging thyroid and thyroid metastases

	Thyroid morphology	**Thyroid metastases**
Radiopharmaceutical	[^{123}I]sodium iodide	[^{131}I]sodium iodide
Activity administered	20 MBq (0.5 mCi) (oral or IV)	400 MBq (11 mCi) (oral or IV)
Effective dose equivalent	4 mSv (400 mrem)	24 mSv^a (2400 mrem)
Patient preparation	Withdrawal of any thyroid medication (thyroxine, 3 weeks prior to study, carbimazole and T$_3$, 10 days prior to study)	Withdrawal of any thyroid medication (thyroxine, 3 weeks prior to study, carbimazole and T$_3$, 10 days prior to study)
Collimator	Low-energy, converging-hole, high-resolution	High-energy, parallel-hole, general purpose
Images acquired	Anterior, right anterior oblique, left anterior oblique, 2 h post-administration; 50–100 k counts per view	Anterior and posterior whole body 72 h post-administration; 100 kcounts or 600 s per view

^{a} Figure based on the assumption that the thyroid gland has been removed, hence there is more rapid elimination of the iodide.

thyroxine (T$_4$) and tri-iodothyronine (T$_3$) result from the coupling of two molecules of DIT and one molecule of MIT and one molecule of DIT respectively. The radioisotopes of iodine ^{123}I and ^{131}I are of value in the evaluation of thyroid function, location, size, and morphology as well as the investigation of thyroid nodules and masses (Table 16.4).

Well-differentiated thyroid tumors retain sufficient function to concentrate iodide. These account for about 75% of thyroid cancers. Anaplastic tumors are unable to take up iodide and will therefore appear as photon-deficient areas on the thyroid image. However, similar appearances may be due to thyroid cysts, nodular goiter, and autoimmune thyroiditis. The presence of a solitary cold nodule does raise the question of malignancy and ultrasound is probably the examination of choice to determine morphology. The majority of thyroid tumors may be removed surgically. However, inoperable histologically differentiated cancers may be treated by the administration of serial doses of between 4000 and 74 000 MBq (0.1–2 Ci) ^{131}I.

Follow-up imaging is of value to detect remnant thyroid tissue in cases where surgery has been incomplete (due to tumor adherent to the trachea or in cases where enlarged lymphatic glands extend beyond surgical reach) or to ensure the effectiveness of radioiodine ablation. Whole body imaging for the identification of metastatic lesions is of considerable value and may be repeated for the follow-up of these patients. Imaging may also be performed following therapeutic doses to confirm uptake of radioiodine in metastatic tumor tissue. Caution is necessary in the interpretation of whole body images as radioiodine is frequently visualized in stomach, bowel, urinary bladder, and the salivary glands. The use of surface markers may aid in the localization of sites of radionuclide uptake.

16.7 Metaidobenzylguanidine

The molecular structure of metaiodobenzylguanidine (MIBG) is similar to that of norephinephrine (noradrenaline) and this accounts for the uptake of this radiopharmaceutical in catecholamine storage vesicles. MIBG may be used in the diagnosis and localization of active catecholamine metabolic tumors and their metastases and has been aptly termed a neuroendocrine tumor seeking agent [8]. This group of tumors include adrenal medullary tumors (pheochromocytoma), neuroblastomas, and catecholamine-producing carcinoid tumors.

Radioiodinated MIBG is usually supplied as a sterile isotonic solution of pH 4–7. Since it is a norepinephrine (noradrenaline) analogue there is a possibility of adrenergic side effects, especially if injected rapidly (these include tachycardia, chest pain, transient hypertonia, and abdominal cramp). The simultaneous administration of reserpine and tricyclic antidepressants should be avoided as these drugs decrease the enrichment of MIBG in adrenergic storage vesicles.

Following intravenous injection, the half-life of radioactivity in blood is about 40 hours. The activity is largely excreted in the urine and to a lesser degree via the bowel. Liver and urinary tract are commonly seen on images recorded during the first 24 hours. The normal adrenal medulla may not be visualized using [^{123}I]MIBG. Providing the cost is not a prohibitive factor, the use of ^{123}I in

Table 16.5. MIBG imaging

Radiopharmaceutical	[^{123}I]MIBG	[^{131}I]MIBG
Activity administered	400 MBq^a (2 mCi)	20 MBq^a (0.5 mCi)
Effective dose equivalent	6 mSv^b (600 mrem)	3 mSv^b (300 mrem)
Patient preparation	Withdrawal of tricyclic antidepressants 7 days prior to study; oral sodium iodide, 60 mg for 3 days	Withdrawal of tricyclic antidepressants 7 days prior to study; oral sodium iodide, 60 mg for 3 days
Collimator	Low-energy, parallel-hole, general purpose	High-energy, parallel-hole, general purpose
Images acquired	Anterior and posterior abdomen as required; 4 and 24 h post-injection, 400 kcounts or 600s per view	Anterior and posterior abdomen as required; 24 and 48 h post-injection; 400 kcounts or 600 s per view
SPECT	64 × 20 s increments in 360° rotation; useful in thorax and abdomen	

^{a} The radiopharmaceutical should be administered as a slow intravenous injection over a period of 20–30 seconds.
^{b} With the thyroid blocked.

preference to ^{131}I is recommended, particularly for imaging small lesions and in cases where emission tomography is required. The imaging protocol is outlined in Table 16.5.

16.7.1 Pheochromocytoma

The diagnosis of pheochromocytoma has been made easier by the introduction of sensitive biochemical assays for plasma and urinary catecholamines. However, MIBG scintigraphy is of considerable value in the preoperative localization of tumor sites and in cases of suspected postoperative recurrence. Sensitivities and specificities of well over 90% have been reported. An example of a positive study using [^{123}I]MIBG is shown in Figure 16.2.

16.7.2 Neuroblastoma

This tumor comprises embryonic cells from the sympathetic nerve cells. Twenty-four hour urine collection has shown these tumors to produce high levels of catecholamines. Although neuroblastoma can normally be diagnosed using X-ray CT, the uptake of MIBG can be used to provide a more specific diagnosis and for the evaluation of tumor spread, particularly to bone marrow metastases.

16.8 Radiolabeled Monoclonal Antibodies

Antibodies are produced naturally in the body by plasma cells as a mechanism of defense. This mechanism may be exploited in a suitable animal species following immunization with a suitable antigen or immunogen. In such cases the antisera contain a number of cross-reacting antibodies known as polyclonal antibodies. In vitro cloning techniques have enabled the production of homogeneous cultures of hybrid cells (hybridomas) producing single antibody types (monoclonal antibodies) of definable chemical properties. It is now possible to produce large amounts of monoclonal antibodies and antibody fragments directed against almost any molecular structure and they offer great potential to nuclear medicine. Furthermore, humanization of the antibody molecule minimizes the amount of foreign protein administered to the patient and hence reduces the potential for generation of an immune response. When labeled with an appropriate radionuclide, antibodies represent a range of radiopharmaceuticals with exceptional targeting properties. However, it must be appreciated that the antibody is specific for the antigen and therefore it is the distribution of the antigen in the tissues that is important. It is clearly desirable for the antigen defined by an antibody to be present in tumor tissues in large amounts but absent from normal tissues.

Antibodies are proteins. Most clinical studies to date have been carried out using mouse immunoglobulins (IgG1 and IgG2: molecular weight approximately 150 kDa) although a number of chimeric and human monoclonal antibodies have been investigated clinically. The antibody molecule may be thought of as a Y-shaped molecule with the ends of the two upper arms (variable Fab regions) being the binding sites and the vertical lower portion of the molecule being

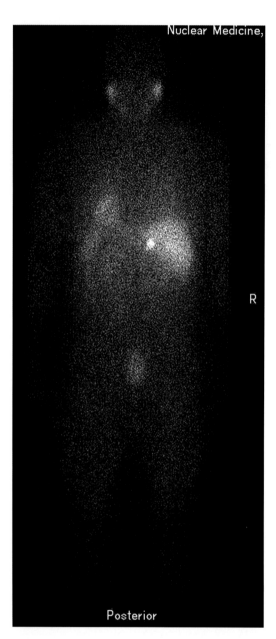

Figure 16.2. Posterior whole body image of a patient recorded 4 hours following injection of 400 MBq (10 mCi) ^{123}I-MIBG. A small focus of uptake can be seen in a pheochromaocytoma of the right adrenal gland.

Table 16.6. Some monoclonal antibodies that have been used for clinical imaging

Tumor type	Antibody description
Gastrointestinal tumors	Anti-CEA (carcinoembryonic antigen, e.g. CEA scan (FAB$_2$)
	B72.3 (IgG1) high molecular weight glycoprotein (TAG 72)
	PR1A3 (IgG1) epithelial cell surface antigen
	NS19.9 (IgG1) carbohydrate antigen associated with gastric and small bowel tumors (antigen CR19.9)
Ovarian and breast tumors	OC125 (IgG1) raised against ovarian adenocarcinoma (antigen CA125)
	B72.3 (IgG1) high molecular weight glycoprotein (TAG 72)
	OVTL-3 (IgG1) raised against OvCa cells
	HMFG1, HMFG2 (IgG1) human milk fat globule antibodies
	H17E2 (IgG1) placental alkaline phosphatase (PLAP) SM3 (IgG1) stripped mucin
Prostate tumors	Anti-PAP (IgG1) prostatic acid phosphatase
	Capromab pendetide (Prostascint, IgG1) directed against PSMA
Thyroid tumors	ID4 (IgG2a) anti-human thyroglobulin
Melanoma	225.28s (IgG2a) 94 kDa high molecular weight melanoma associated antibody (HMW MAA)

molecular weight of fragments promotes more rapid elimination from the body following injection, thus reducing background activity. However, the absolute uptake of fragments within tumors is reduced. As a guide, the uptake of intact antibodies into tumor tissues is generally less than 0.01% of the administered dose per gram of tumor. In studies using ^{111}In or ^{99m}Tc-labeled fragments, high renal uptake dominates the images.

Of the many monoclonal antibodies that have been produced, relatively few have been selected for clinical use [9] (Table 16.6). However, a few monoclonal antibodies are now commercially available as product licensed radiopharmaceuticals and are supplied pre-radiolabeled or as a preparation for a simple one-step labeling with ^{111}In or [99m]Tc. Imaging details are given in Table 16.7.

The choice of radionuclide for antibody labeling has a marked effect on image quality. The most suitable radionuclide is ^{99m}Tc, although

termed the constant region (Fc). Enzymatic treatment of the molecule with papain will cut the molecule to produce two monovalent Fab fragments and one Fc fragment. Enzymatic digestion with pepsin removes part of the constant region to produce a bivalent F(ab′)2 fragment. The lower

Table 16.7. Radiolabeled antibody imaging

Radiopharmaceutical	Approximately 1 mg tumor associated monoclonal antibody	Approximately 1 mg tumor associated monoclonal antibody	Approximately 1 mg tumor associated monoclonal antibody
Radionuclide	[123]I	[111]In	[99m]Tc
Activity administered	80 MBq (2 mCi)	80 MBq (2 mCi)	800 MBq (20 mCi)
Effective dose equivalent	6 mSv (600 mrem)	10 mSv (1000 mrem)	8 mSv (800 mrem)
Patient preparation	Oral sodium iodide for 3 days	Oral laxatives and bowel preparation may be necessary	Oral laxatives and bowel preparation may be necessary
Collimator	Low energy, parallel hole	Medium energy, parallel hole	Low energy, parallel hole
Images acquired	Anterior and posterior whole body images as required, 600 kcounts; 4–24 h	Anterior and posterior whole body images as required, 600 kcounts; 24, 48 and 72 h	Anterior and posterior whole body images as required, 600 kcounts; 4–24 h
SPECT	64 × 20 s increments in 360° rotation. Useful in thorax, abdomen and pelvis	64 × 20 s increments in 360° rotation. Useful in thorax, abdomen and pelvis	64 × 20 s increments in 360° rotation. Useful in thorax, abdomen and pelvis

Approximate figures given. Organ doses will depend upon the antibody and fragments used and may vary with repeat administrations.

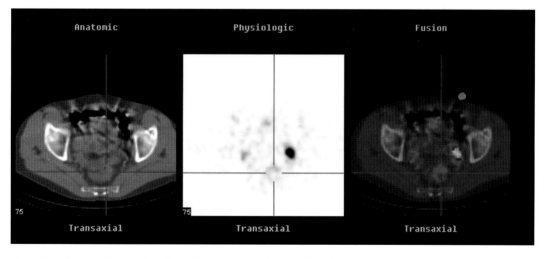

Figure 16.3. Transverse images of a patient with a carcinoma of the descending colon recorded after administration of 750 MBq (20 mCi) ^{99m}Tc-CEA scan. Left, CT image; center, SPECT image; and right, fused image pair.

[123]I and ^{111}In may be used, the latter allowing for delayed imaging 2 or 3 days following administration. One of the main differences between the radionuclides used for antibody labeling is the physiological fate of the radionuclide following antibody catabolism. In the case of radioiodine the radiolabel is rapidly eliminated from the body, predominantly by urinary excretion, whereas radiometals such ^{111}In are retained at sites of antibody catabolism. When imaging with radioiodine-labeled antibodies, concentrations of tracer in the thyroid, stomach, and urinary tract may lead to false positive results despite the administration of oral potassium iodide. However, when imaging with ^{99m}Tc or ^{111}In, high uptake throughout the reticuloendothelial system limits the detection of liver metastases but bone marrow uptake provides useful landmarks for tumor localization in both planar and tomographic views. Recording an early blood pool image followed by images acquired on two or three subsequent occasions will assist in determining tumor uptake from non-specific uptake, e.g. bowel activity. The use of combined SPECT/CT imaging can also aid in the localization of tumor sites (Figure 16.3).

Before administering it to the patient, it is important to know if the antibody is of murine origin. Murine monoclonal antibodies are foreign proteins which are themselves capable of evoking an immune response in the patient. The use of an intradermal or subcutaneous test dose of antibody is not warranted as there is now evidence that this is more likely to sensitize the patient, resulting in problems when repeat doses for further imaging studies or therapy are administered. In vitro assays for human anti-mouse antibody (HAMA) are currently being developed for monitoring patients prior to antibody injection, thereby minimizing this problem. Developments in genetic engineering and biotechnology have resulted in a new generation of chimeric and humanized materials for both diagnostic and therapeutic use.

16.9 Receptor-mediated Imaging

An interesting recent development in radionuclide tumor imaging has been the use of peptides for receptor-mediated imaging. Examples of these include naturally occurring peptide hormones such as somatostatin (SS), vasoactive intestinal peptide (VIP), melanocyte stimulating hormone (MSH), estrogens, and progesterones. Of all these agents, somatostatin has so far proven to be of greatest interest. Somatostatin is a peptide hormone consisting of 14 amino acids and is present in the hypothalamus, brainstem, gastrointestinal tract, and the pancreas. It has an inhibitory effect on growth hormone secretion and many neuroendocrine and non-neuroendocrine tumors contain high numbers of somatostatin receptors. The somatostatin analogue octreotide was produced by Sandoz Pharma Ltd in 1988 under the name of Sandostatin. This has been radiolabeled with ^{123}I and ^{111}In and extensive clinical trials have been undertaken [10]. The most clinically promising agent has been ^{111}In-[DTPA-D-Phe^1]-octreotide (^{111}In-pentetreotide or Octreoscan). This radiopharmaceutical has been used mainly for imaging tumors derived from the neural crest in particular gastro-entero-pancreatic (GEP) tumors such as gastrinoma, insulinoma, VIPoma, glucagonoma, and carcinoid syndrome. It has also been indicated for imaging small cell tumors of the lung, medullary thyroid carcinoma, renal cell carcinoma, breast cancer, melanoma, Hodgkin's disease, and non-Hodgkin's lymphoma.

Imaging details are given in Table 16.8. Following administration approximately 20% of the ad-

Table 16.8. Somatostatin receptor imaging using [^{111}In]pentetreotide

Radiopharmaceutical	[^{111}In-DTPA-D-Phe1]-octreotide
Activity administered	110 MBq (3 mCi)
Effective dose equivalent	9 mSv (900 mrem)
Collimator	Medium energy, parallel, general purpose
Images acquired	Anterior and posterior thorax, abdomen and pelvis, 4 and 24 h post-injection; 400 kcounts per image (dual photopeaks)
SPECT	64 × 20 second increments in 360° rotation. Coronal, axial, and 3-dimensional views are useful in the abdomen

ministered activity locates in the liver and can be excreted via the bile into the gut. Imaging may be carried out for up to 48 hours after dosing. However, intestinal activity may be a problem in images recorded after 4 hours. In many instances positive uptake using pentetreotide indicates a favorable prospect for treatment with cold octreotide.

There has been considerable interest in the use of somatostatin receptor imaging in patients with solitary pulmonary nodules. This may be carried out with ^{99m}Tc-depreotide (Neospect). Imaging of the chest is normally carried out between 2 and 4 hours after injection of approximately 700 MBq (20 mCi) of the radiopharmaceutical. This results in an effective dose of the order of 11 mSv (1100 mrem). An example of a positive study is shown in Figure 16.4.

16.10 Intraoperative Tumor Localization

Imaging techniques are commonly used as part of the diagnostic work-up of patients prior to surgical treatment. The effectiveness of such treatment is invariably dependent upon the complete removal of all tumor tissue. Microscopic disease not immediately visible to the surgeon may remain in situ, resulting in ineffective treatment. Even with state-of-the-art imaging there are many instances where the surgeon may benefit from additional information on the localization and extent of disease [11].

TUMOR IMAGING

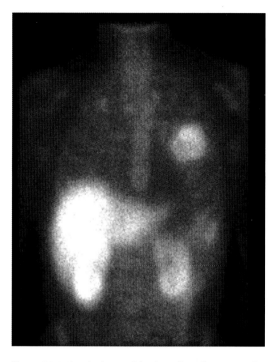

Figure 16.4. Anterior image of the chest of a male patient with a tumor of the left lung recorded 2 hours following injection of 700 MBq (20 mCi) ^{99m}Tc-depreotide. High retention of the tracer is also seen in the liver and kidneys.

The intraoperative technique requires the positive accumulation of an appropriate radiopharmaceutical which should be administered prior to surgery. After a suitable period of time (normally the same as that required for imaging investigations) a well-collimated sterile radiation detector (the surgical probe) is used to scan the operative site during surgery (Figure 16.5). The main established surgical procedure is for the localization of osteoid osteoma, a benign but painful bony tumor which occurs mainly in the long bones of young children. Symptoms of osteoid osteoma may be relieved with analgesics, but orthopedic surgery is the only effective cure. Radionuclide bone imaging is part of the normal diagnostic evaluation of these tumors. Administration of the standard amount of ^{99m}Tc bone agent prior to surgery enables the accurate probe-guided localization of the tumor nidus, thus aiding excision and preserving normal bone. Intraoperative procedures are also proving to be of value in the localization of a large number of different tumors using ^{99m}Tc and ^{125}I-radiolabeled antibodies, [^{123}I]MIBG and [^{111}In]pentetreotide (Table 16.9).

A number of factors need to be considered before undertaking a routine intraoperative study:

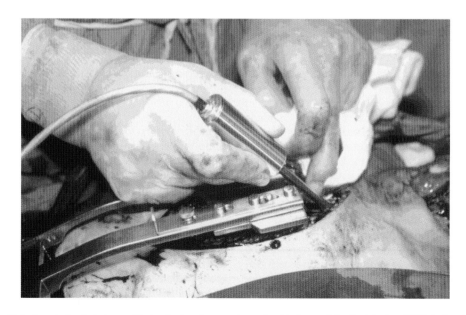

Figure 16.5. A surgical probe being used for localization of an ectopic parathyroid adenoma following injection of ^{201}Tl-thallous chloride.

Table 16.9. Examples of intraoperative probe tumor localization

Radiopharmaceutical	Tumor/Lesion
[^{99m}Tc]Nanocoll	Sentinel node
[^{99m}Tc]HDP	Osteoid osteoma
	Osteoblastoma
	Hamartoma
	Brodie's abscess
[^{99m}Tc]colloid	Probe guided lymph node biopsy for tumor staging (e.g. from melanoma or breast)
[^{123}I]MIBG	Neuroblastoma
	Pheochromocytoma
[^{111}In]pentetreotide	Somatostatin receptor positive tumors, e.g. insulinoma, medullary thyroid carcinoma
[^{99m}Tc]vDMSA	Medullary thyroid carcinoma
[^{99m}Tc] [^{123}I] [^{111}In] antibodies	Colorectal tumors
	Ovarian tumors
	Lymph node mapping from breast tumors and melanoma

1 A radionuclide imaging study should be performed prior to planning the intraoperative procedure.

2 A standard adult or pediatric amount of radioactivity should be adequate for use with most intraoperative probes.

3 The optimum time for surgery after administration is generally the same as that for the equivalent imaging procedure.

4 Non-specific sites of accumulation of activity (e.g. the urinary tract) may interfere with intraoperative measurements.

5 Radiation protection measures must be considered with respect to operating theatres and staff.

16.10.1 Sentinel Node Detection

The subcutaneous injection of small colloidal particles of size between 10 and 1000 nm allows the identification of lymphatic drainage. This procedure is often used to identify forms of edema, especially in the arms and legs. Nominally 40 MBq (1 mCi) ^{99m}Tc-albumin nanocolloid is used to outline lymphonodular reticulocyte function by recording a series of static images up to 3 h following subcutaneous injection in the web spaces between the fingers or toes.

Although the radiopharmaceuticals for lymphoscintigraphy were originally developed for mapping out the lymphatic vessels, more recently they have been used for the identification of the first regional draining node from a metastasizing tumor (the sentinel node). The identification and biopsy of the sentinel node has had a dramatic effect on the management of patients with certain tumors, in particular breast carcinoma and melanoma. Once identified and excised, the node may then be examined histologically for the presence of tumor cells. Positive identification of tumor within the sentinel node will indicate metastatic spread from the primary site. This procedure has become a valuable alternative to complete axillary lymph node dissection in patients with multifocal breast cancer [12].

The technique typically involves injection of between 10 and 50 MBq (300 μCi to 1.5 mCi) ^{99m}Tc-albumin nanocolloid into the tissue parenchyma adjacent to the tumor. The regional drainage of the tracer is then considered to follow that of the tumor itself. The node may be identified by dynamic imaging or by recording a series of static images following injection. Greater than 95% of the injected activity will remain at the site of injection. However, after a period of time a series of draining "hot spots" may be seen. The first site of accumulation is the sentinel node. In some cases a body outline is obtained to aid localization of the node by acquiring a transmission image using a ^{99m}Tc or ^{57}Co flood source or a scanning line source (e.g. ^{153}Gd) placed behind the patient. Once the site of the node has been identified, an indelible mark can be placed on the skin to assist the surgeon in locating the node.

Surgical removal may be aided by use of an intraoperative sterile surgical probe. Characterization, calibration, and testing of these devices is important prior to surgical use. During surgery the surgeon can use the probe to localize the increased count rate from accumulation of the tracer in the node, which will direct him to the site for surgical excision.

16.11 PET Imaging in Oncology

Positron emission tomography is one of the true forms of metabolic imaging that is now firmly established as one of the most sensitive imaging modalities in clinical oncology [13, 14]. The principles of PET imaging are described in Chapters 3 and 17. Although PET was previously widely considered to be an expensive imaging modality there is now evidence to show that it is a cost-effective modality. A wide range of positron emitting radiopharmaceuticals are currently available. However, the current leading clinical agents are based on ^{18}F and ^{11}C. ^{18}F-FDG is the most widely used radiopharmaceutical. This tracer follows the metabolic path of glucose, as far as phosphorylation, but is not further metabolised. It allows a measure of the increased glucose uptake exhibited by tumor cells. Many of the clinical applications of FDG imaging are now mature and the technique is the method of choice for diagnosing and staging a growing number of tumor types, lung and lymphoma being the notable examples.

It is appropriate to consider the fact that FDG is a non-specific tracer and it is to be expected that more specific tracers will enter clinical use. Markers of cellular proliferation such as ^{18}F-FLT (fluorothymidine) and ^{11}C-methionine are examples of the new generation of PET radiopharmaceuticals used in the staging of tumors and in monitoring response to therapy.

It is also important that the development of PET-CT systems for functional anatomical imaging is having a dramatic impact on patient management and has already led to a fusion of nuclear medicine and radiological specialties.

16.12 The Role of Nuclear Medicine in the Diagnostic Process

Many nuclear medicine procedures provide complementary diagnostic information to other imaging modalities, such as X-ray CT, ultrasound, and MRI. In some cases, for example thyroid carcinoma and pheochromocytoma, radionuclide imaging can provide a specific diagnosis. The relatively poor anatomical resolution of radionuclide imaging when compared to other techniques has resulted in a decline in the clinical demand for some investigations, e.g. brain and liver imaging. However, the introduction of the newer functional radiopharmaceuticals outlining tumor physiology, including PET tracers, has rejuvenated the role of nuclear medicine in clinical oncology and techniques are now being extended into the operating theatre.

Tumor targeting studies have a dual role in the management of the cancer patient, both as a method of detection and as a means of delivering a therapeutic dose [2]. High tumor uptake of the tracer relative to the blood background and other surrounding areas is the primary objective. This has a direct bearing on both tumor diagnosis and therapy. High T:NT uptake ratios are equally as important in determining good image contrast as in delivering the maximum therapeutic tumor dose whilst keeping side effects to a minimum. In this context the mechanisms of uptake required in imaging studies may also provide a means for delivering cytotoxic agents. The therapeutic applications of [^{131}I]sodium iodide and [^{131}I]MIBG are good examples.

The clinical role of radionuclide bone imaging remains unchallenged. Bone imaging is the most common radionuclide imaging procedure carried out within the UK.

The use of gallium citrate has declined mainly because of poor sensitivity and clinical attention is turning to monoclonal antibodies and receptor-specific radiopharmaceuticals. Although the initial claims of antibodies are yet to be substantiated, it is now considered that antibodies have a role in the evaluation of patients with melanoma (melanoma-associated antibodies) and gastrointestinal cancer (anti CEA, B72.3). In many instances clinical management of these diseases is difficult. The combined use of assays for determining levels of circulating serum antigen and imaging with the appropriate antibody is now practiced in most centers. The clinical role of immunoscintigraphy would appear to be restricted to the detection of recurrent and metastatic disease. In the case of colorectal carcinoma and ovarian carcinoma, where the abdominopelvic anatomy may be disrupted as a result of previous surgery, the interpretation of X-ray CT images may be difficult, particularly when differentiating between tumor and fibrosis. Radiolabeled antibody imaging is capable of providing valuable diagnostic information in such cases.

An additional range of investigations previously discussed in this chapter involve subcutaneous injections of radiopharmaceutical for the evaluation of lymphokinetics. Lymphoscintigraphy may be performed quickly and cheaply and will accurately outline abnormal lymph node function resulting from malignancy. Radionuclides such as colloidal [^{99m}Tc] injected interstitially around the tumor, into the webs of the feet or subcostally into the posterior rectus sheath, may demonstrate lymph node drainage within 3 hours. It is anticipated that newer materials, such as monoclonal antibodies, may be successfully used in this way.

The interpretation of radionuclide imaging studies should be carried out with full clinical details and due consideration should be given to abnormal radiopharmaceutical biodistribution due to radiotherapy or the simultaneous administration of medications. For example, the administration of cytotoxic drugs such as vinblastin, bleomycin, and cis-platinum may result in increased renal and gastric uptake of tracer.

Lesion detection is dependent upon the radiopharmaceutical T:NT uptake, the energy of the radionuclide used and depth within the body. In many instances radionuclide imaging is not capable of demonstrating tumor masses very much smaller than 10 mm in diameter. This represents cell populations of the order of 10^{13} cells. Clearly there is considerable room for improvement and this will only be achieved by advances in both radiopharmaceutical design and equipment performance.

References

1. Ruben P. Clinical Oncology: A Multidisciplinary Approach for Physicians and Students, 8th edn. Philadelphia: WB Saunders; 2001.

2. Flemming JS, Perkins AC. Targeted Radiotherapy. IPEM Report No. 83. York: Institute of Physics and Engineering in Medicine; 2000.

3. Eary JF. Nuclear medicine in cancer diagnosis. Lancet 1999; 354:853–857.

4. O'Sullivan JM, Cook GJ. A review of the efficacy of bone scanning in prostate and breast cancer. Q J Nucl Med 2002; 46:152–159.

5. Perkins AC, Hardy JG, Wastie ML, Clifford K. Serial radionuclide imaging during treatment of patients with diffuse bone metastases from carcinoma of the prostate. Eur J Nucl Med 1982; 7:322–323.

6. Edwards CL, Hayes RL. Tumour scanning with ^{67}Ga citrate. J Nucl Med 1969; 10:103–105.

7. Biersack HJ, Briele B, Hotze AL, et al. The role of nuclear medicine in oncology. Ann Nucl Med 1992; 6:131–136.

8. Kaltsas GA, Mukherjee JJ, Grossman AB. The value of radiolabelled MIBG and ocreotide in the diagnosis and management of neuroendocrine tumours. Ann Oncol 2001; 12 (Suppl):547–550.

9. Bischof Delaloge A. Radioimmunology and radioimmunotherapy: will these be routine procedures? Semin Nucl Med 2000; 30:186–194.

10. Grotzinger C, Weidenmann B. Somatostatin receptor targeting for tumour imaging and therapy. Ann NY Acad Sci 2004; 1014:258–264.

11. Perkins AC, Hardy JG. Intra-operative nuclear medicine in surgical practice. Nucl Med Commun 1996; 17:1006–1015.

12. Goyal A, Newcombe RG, Mansel RE, et al. ALMANIC Trialists Group. Eur J Surg Oncol 2004; 30:475–479.

13. Ruhlmann J, Oehr P, Biersack HJ. PET in Oncology Basics and Clinical Applications. Berlin: Springer; 1999.

14. Rohren EM, Turkington TG, Coleman RE. Clinical applications of PET in oncology. Radiology 2004; 231:305–332.

17

Clinical PET Imaging

Gary J.R. Cook

17.1 Introduction

The number of clinical applications for PET continues to increase, particularly in the field of oncology. In parallel with this is a growth in the number of centers that are able to provide a clinical PET or PET/CT service. The vast majority of clinical PET applications are oncological in nature but there are also important neurological and cardiological applications.

The advantages of PET over conventional single photon imaging include better spatial resolution, absolute quantitation, and the potential for labeling a large number of biological compounds with positron emitters including ^{11}C-carbon, ^{13}N-nitrogen, ^{15}O-oxygen, and ^{18}F-fluorine. The latter is a particularly important radionuclide for labeling as its half-life of approximately 110 minutes allows the distribution of ^{18}F-fluorine-labeled radiopharmaceuticals to PET scanning facilities that do not have a cyclotron for local radionuclide manufacture. The short half-lives of many other positron emitting radionuclides including ^{11}C-carbon (20 min), ^{13}N-nitrogen (10 min) and ^{15}O-oxygen (2 min) preclude radiochemical labeling and distribution to distant sites.

17.2 Radiopharmaceuticals

In all aspects of clinical PET, ^{18}F-fluorodeoxyglucose (^{18}FDG) is the most commonly used radiopharmaceutical. In oncology, the preferential uptake of this compound by malignant cells compared to most non-malignant tissues and most benign disease processes makes it an ideal tracer to accurately and sensitively identify small volumes of active tumor. This radiopharmaceutical behaves as an analogue of glucose and as many tumors overexpress glucose membrane transporters, especially Glut-1, and have enhanced hexokinase activity, ^{18}FDG is transported and phosphorylated to ^{18}FDG-6-PO$_4$, which being negatively charged remains trapped in the cell. Unlike glucose, this tracer does not undergo further significant enzymatic reactions. Most tumors and normal tissues have relatively low glucose-6-phosphatase activity and so with minimal dephosphorylation of ^{18}FDG, the accumulation of this compound is proportional to glycolytic rate (Figure 17.1). Some tissues such as the liver and some primary liver tumors have higher levels of glucose-6-phosphatase and may therefore show a reduction in ^{18}FDG activity over time.

Although clinical ^{18}FDG PET imaging is conventionally carried out at 1 hour after injection, many tumors continue to accumulate this tracer for a number of hours and it is possible, in some circumstances, that delayed imaging at 3 to 4 hours may enhance tumor to background signal and facilitate differentiation of benign and malignant tissues [1]. An alternative method to improve differentiation of benign and malignant tissue is to acquire scans at dual time points. If scans are acquired at 1 and 2 hours it has been shown that malignant tissue continues to accumulate ^{18}FDG

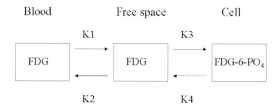

Figure 17.1. A three compartmental model describing the transport, phosphorylation, and trapping of [18]FDG. K1, K2, K3 and K4 are the rate constants describing the exchange of FDG between compartments.

during this time whilst benign tissue does not [2]. Knowledge of the kinetics of tumor [18]FDG accumulation is particularly important when performing serial scans to assess response to treatment. If static scans are performed then these should be acquired at exactly the same time post-injection on each occasion so that any difference in tumor uptake is due to treatment effect rather than simply being due to a shorter or longer accumulation time. An alternative method to minimize timing as a potential source of error in serial scanning is to scan patients at 3 to 4 hours when the uptake of [18]FDG has reached a plateau and where small differences in scan timing make little difference in measured uptake [1].

In clinical routine, the most convenient and simplest quantitative parameter that can be calculated is the standardized uptake value (SUV) (see Section 3.7). This parameter can be regarded as a measure of the concentration of tracer within a volume of interest in relation to the concentration in the rest of the body. There has been much controversy over the use of this parameter and whether it should be corrected for body weight, surface area, glucose levels, and partial volume effect [3]. In an individual patient its use to differentiate benign from malignant lesions is probably limited over subjective interpretation by an experienced observer due to an overlap in values and variation between some benign and malignant processes. However, if performed carefully to ensure minimal precision errors in its application, it may be a simple, relatively robust and clinically practical measure for follow-up of serial scans. More complex quantitative methods can be employed including non-linear regression analysis or the Patlak technique [4] to calculate dynamic parameters of [18]FDG accumulation such as the metabolic rate of [18]FDG (MR_{FDG}). However, these are less prac-

tical in the clinical setting as dynamic scans are required as well as measurement of arterial blood activity over time, either directly or by image analysis of the left ventricle or aorta.

For some tumors [18]FDG lacks sensitivity and specificity and alternative radiopharmaceuticals have been developed to exploit different aspects of abnormal tumor metabolism and biology. There has been interest in the use of labeled amino acids as a measure of tumor amino acid transport and protein metabolism. Unlike [18]FDG, these tracers show little uptake in normal brain cortex and may aid detection of intermediate and low-grade primary recurrent brain tumors and more clearly identify tumor margins. Examples include ^{11}C-methionine and ^{18}F-fluoroethyltyrosine [5, 6]. Other tracers that are involved with membrane synthesis (^{11}C-choline, ^{18}F-choline) [7] are being used in circumstances where [18]FDG is not ideal, including prostate cancer and brain tumors. There is also increasing interest and use of tracers that reflect thymidine kinase activity, and hence DNA turnover and tumor proliferation, such as ^{11}C-thymidine and ^{18}F-fluorothymidine [8]. The use of many of these novel tracers is restricted to centers with a cyclotron and radiochemistry laboratories and have not yet gained the widespread use and availability of [18]FDG.

In cardiac [18]FDG PET scanning, uptake of this tracer is dependent on the availability of various substrates, including glucose and fatty acids. Cardiac activity can be enhanced by oral glucose loading to encourage high insulin levels and a predominance of glucose metabolism. Infarcted myocardium resulting in non-functional scar tissue shows little or no uptake of [18]FDG, whilst ischemic but viable myocardium may show reduced uptake or, in some circumstances, ischemia may lead to uptake that is greater than normal myocardium [5].

When using [18]FDG for brain imaging, high uptake is seen in normal brain cortex, the basal ganglia, and thalami irrespective of substrate conditions. As previously mentioned, other tracers such as amino acids and choline analogues may also be helpful in oncologic brain imaging. A number of other tracers have been used for other neurological disorders of which the most important is probably ^{18}F-fluorodopa for studying dopamine receptors in the movement disorders including Parkinson's disease.

17.3 Patient Preparation

For oncologic imaging it is customary to fast the patient, except for clear fluids, for 4 to 6 hours prior to scanning. This encourages low insulin levels and therefore discourages uptake of [18]FDG into normal muscle and adipose tissue, ensuring a high tumor to background ratio. This approach should also minimize myocardial activity, allowing a clear view of the mediastinum. Cardiac activity can also be reduced by caffeine, which causes increased fatty acid metabolism in the myocardium.

Patients are asked to refrain from vigorous exercise in the 24 hours leading up to their scan to minimize skeletal muscle uptake of [18]FDG and are made as comfortable and relaxed as possible after their injection to minimize uptake in tense muscles. It is known that young patients with low body mass index are prone to showing uptake of [18]FDG into activated brown fat, particularly in cold weather as this is a vestigial organ of thermogenesis . The appearance of intense symmetrical activity in the neck, supraclavicular and paraspinal regions (Figure 17.2) can be minimized by the administration of oral benzodiazepine 30 to 60 minutes prior to injection of [18]FDG.

Unlike glucose, [18]FDG is excreted in the urinary tract and may on occasion mimic foci of malignancy. This can be minimized by keeping the patient well hydrated and/or administering diuretic to reduce urinary stasis and to dilute urinary bladder activity, thereby minimizing reconstruction artifacts and the potential to mistake urinary activity for malignant pelvic lymph nodes. To some extent, some of the potential pitfalls caused by normal variant uptake can be minimized with combined PET/CT scans, where it is easier to correctly differentiate physiological accumulation from disease by having an accurately co-registered anatomical framework to refer to.

While physiological bowel activity can also be misleading when interpreting [18]FDG PET scans, attempts at reducing bowel uptake with various interventions have met with variable results. Most clinical PET departments have no specific preparation protocols to reduce bowel activity as in most circumstances the appearances are typical. This is another area where combined PET/CT can help to avoid incorrectly identifying normal bowel activity as pathology. For PET/CT imaging protocols, bowel contrast is not used

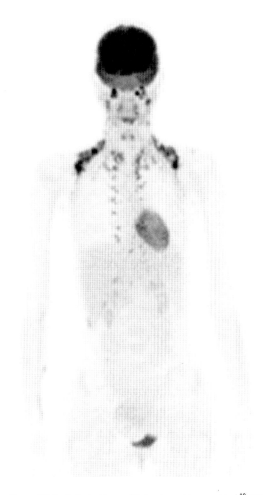

Figure 17.2. Activated brown fat showing avid symmetrical [18]FDG accumulation in the neck, supraclavicular and paraspinal regions.

universally but groups have found success using either water as a negative contrast media or dilute oral barium preparations [9].

17.4 Normal Appearances in [18]FDG PET

The brain's major substrate is glucose and therefore high cortical activity, basal ganglia and thalamic activity is seen with [18]FDG. White matter shows little discernible uptake and cannot be distinguished qualitatively from the ventricles.

Lymphatic tissue in the head and neck region, including Waldeyer's ring, shows moderate uptake of [18]FDG that is symmetrical. Thyroid uptake is not seen in most patients although a mild diffuse activity may be seen in subjects without apparent thyroid disorder.

Little uptake is seen in rested skeletal muscle but myocardial activity can be variable even with dietary preparations described above. Laryngeal muscle activity is seen if the patient talks after administration of [18]FDG and has the potential to interfere with the interpretation of laryngeal malignancy unless the patient is kept silent during the [18]FDG uptake period. The lungs show little [18]FDG activity on attenuation-corrected scans. Bowel activity is variable, the cecum and rectosigmoid regions being the commonest areas to show uptake. The remainder of the colon is often seen and small bowel loops may show activity. It is likely that much of this activity is within the mucosa and bowel contents rather than in smooth muscle [10]. Urinary activity is seen in any part of the urinary tract.

The liver shows moderate homogeneous activity that is usually slightly greater than that of the spleen and bone marrow. Reactive bone marrow following chemotherapy or granulocyte colony stimulating factors can show a homogeneous increase in activity throughout the red marrow.

It is now routine to interpret either CT or external rod source attenuation-corrected images but inspection of the non-corrected data is often useful. Overcorrection can occur at sites of high density when using CT data, e.g. dental fillings, cardiac pacemaker, causing apparent hot spots on the corrected but not on the uncorrected images. When rod sources are used for attenuation correction it is possible to view the resultant transmission scan to obtain rudimentary anatomical information to help localize abnormalities. With PET/CT the CT data can be used for attenuation correction and anatomical localization of [18]FDG abnormalities. Due to differences in breathing patterns between the fast CT acquisition (<1 min) and the subsequent much slower PET emission acquisition (~30 min) some misregistration of data may result, causing photopenic artifacts close to the diaphragm in the corrected images (Figure 17.3). This can be minimized by performing the CT acquisition in relaxed expiration.

A number of potential normal variants, artifacts, and pitfalls have been described that can be minimized with careful patient preparation and recognition by the interpreter [9, 11].

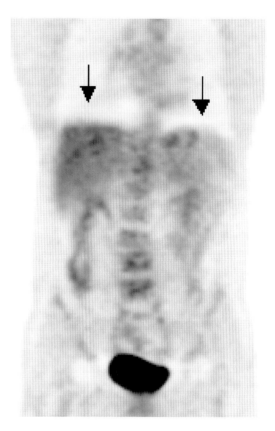

Figure 17.3. Photopenic "banana" artifact at the diaphragmatic surfaces in CT attenuation-corrected PET emission data (arrows) due to differences in breathing patterns between the fast CT and much slower PET emission acquisitions.

17.5 ONCOLOGY

17.5.1 Lung Cancer

Most primary lung malignancies show avid uptake of [18]FDG and as there is relatively low normal activity in the lungs and mediastinum, PET is a very sensitive technique for detection and staging of lung cancer.

[18]FDG PET has proved to be of significant clinical benefit in the evaluation of indeterminate solitary pulmonary nodules. Meta-analyses have shown overall sensitivities of ~95% and specificities of ~80% in cancer detection [12]. High negative predictive values of >95% mean that patients with a negative scan who are not amenable to biopsy can be watched. A lower specificity means that a small number of false positives for

malignancy exist but in general are diseases that will require further investigation and treatment anyway. Examples of false positives include tuberculosis, sarcoidosis, and histoplasmosis but a number of others have also been described. False negatives are rarer but bronchoalveolar carcinoma and some carcinoid tumor may show relatively low uptake of [18]FDG. As a non-invasive tool, it has been suggested that the inclusion of PET in the diagnostic algorithm of indeterminate pulmonary nodules may be cost saving [13].

It is in the preoperative staging of lung cancer where [18]FDG PET shows most value. In a prospective trial 40% of patients were upstaged and 20% downstaged by PET compared to conventional staging procedures [14]. Some patients will therefore have potentially curative surgery enabled and a significant number of patients will have futile surgery cancelled as a result of [18]FDG PET findings (Figure 17.4). It has been estimated that approximately 50% of futile surgery can be avoided by the use of PET [15]. Because of the small chance of false positive uptake leading to inappropriate upstaging of lung cancer, it remains advisable to confirm abnormalities histologically that would deny the chance of curative surgery. It is possible that uptake of [18]FDG, as measured by SUV, could be an independent prognostic factor, even in stage 1 tumors. In one series, patients with an SUV of greater than 20 had a 4.7 times increase in hazard of death by one year compared to those with lower SUVs [16].

With the advent of combined PET/CT it is possible that even more accurate results can be obtained compared to PET alone, or indeed, CT alone or PET and CT reported side by side. In particular, a significant improvement can be made in tumor T staging using this method.

As a functional imaging technique, [18]FDG PET has the potential to distinguish post-treatment effects, fibrosis, and scarring from recurrent tumor in those patients in whom recurrence is suspected but anatomical imaging is unable to differentiate [17].

There are early data to support the use of functional imaging techniques in radiotherapy planning, particularly now that PET/CT is becoming more widely available. It has been shown that including [18]FDG PET data in planning radiotherapy for lung cancer not only improves tumor coverage by detecting additional malignant lymph nodes but that target volumes can also be reduced, minimizing toxicity to normal lung tissue [18].

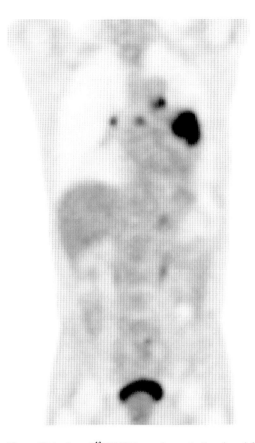

Figure 17.4. Coronal [18]FDG PET image demonstrating a large left-sided non-small cell lung cancer with ipsilateral and contralateral hilar and subcarinal lymphadenopathy. The contralateral hilar and subcarinal adenopathy had not been suspected on CT and upstaged this patient, changing treatment from surgery to chemotherapy.

17.5.2 Lymphoma

The majority of lymphomas, excluding mucosa-associated lymphoid tissue (MALT) tumors and small lymphocytic cell lymphomas, show avid uptake of [18]FDG [19]. Follicular non-Hodgkin's lymphoma often demonstrates lower levels of activity but it has been shown that [18]FDG PET remains a valuable technique in this subtype also [20].

There is a wealth of evidence to show that [18]FDG PET is more accurate than conventional staging procedures in Hodgkin's disease and non-Hodgkin's lymphoma in nodal, extranodal, and bone disease [21–23]. It is most common for patients to be upstaged using PET and a significant proportion will have their management altered as a result [24].

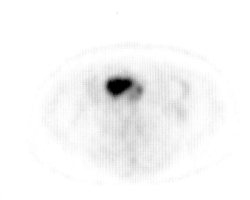
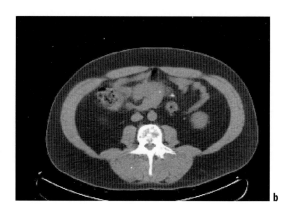

a   b

Figure 17.5. Transaxial [18]FDG **a** and CT **b** images of a patient with non-Hodgkin's lymphoma with a residual mesenteric mass after therapy. This demonstrates abnormal activity in keeping with residual viable tumor. The patient required further therapy.

[18]FDG PET is proving to be a valuable and accurate method to monitor therapy. It is possible to predict which patients are unlikely to eventually relapse after just two or three cycles of chemotherapy by observing significant reductions in metabolic activity at an early stage before anatomical techniques, such as CT, have shown tumor shrinkage [25]. A strategy of scanning patients early in the course of intended therapy may allow an early alteration of treatment in those who are not responding adequately and with the potential to minimize the length of treatment in those who show a good early metabolic response. At the end of treatment of lymphoma it is common for a residual mass to be present. It is almost impossible to tell whether this is simply fibrotic scar tissue or whether active malignant tumor still exists when using CT alone. [18]FDG PET can be used at this stage to accurately assess this issue [26] (Figure 17.5). In those with no abnormal metabolic activity within a residual mass it may be possible to avoid radiotherapy, which has its own long-term side effects and acute toxicity.

17.5.3 Colorectal and Other Gastrointestinal Cancers

At initial diagnosis of colorectal cancer [18]FDG PET is not frequently used as a routine staging procedure although the accuracy for detecting distant metastases is at least as good, if not better than, CT [27] (Figure 17.6). However, it has no role for local tumor and nodal staging within the mesorectum and pelvis, which remains the province of MRI. The main role for PET is in the detection and staging of recurrent tumor that may be amenable to curative resection.

It can be extremely difficult to distinguish recurrent tumor in the pelvis from the effects of surgery and radiotherapy using conventional cross-sectional anatomical techniques, such as CT or MRI. In this situation, [18]FDG PET may be a valuable tool [28, 29], particularly when CT or MRI is equivocal. One potential weakness is in the early months following radiotherapy when an inflammatory reaction may cause uptake of [18]FDG. After 6 months a positive scan is highly suggestive of recurrent disease but before this time a negative scan is still useful.

The accurate staging of recurrent disease in the liver is of the utmost importance as these patients are potentially curable with partial hepatic resection. Although PET is more accurate than conventional CT and CT portography for detecting liver metastases [30], no comparisons have been made to MRI with new liver contrast agents. The sensitivity for the detection of hepatic metastases is reduced for lesions of less than 1 cm. It is likely that the major incremental benefit from PET will mostly be in the detection or exclusion of extrahepatic metastases, which may be previously unsuspected in approximately one-third of patients.

[18]FDG PET is a useful method for detecting small volumes of recurrent disease in patients with rising tumor markers (e.g. carcinoembryonic antigen, CEA) but negative conventional imaging such as CT (Figure 17.7). Approximately two-thirds

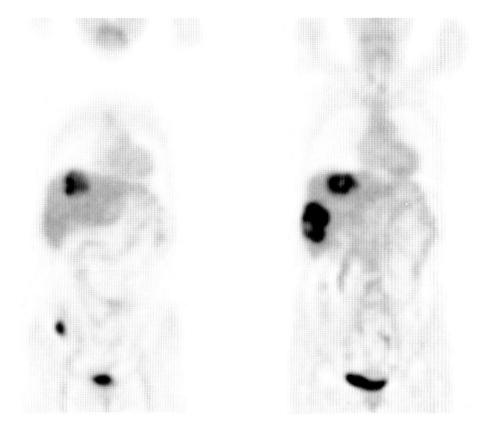

a

b

Figure 17.6. Coronal ^{18}FDG PET slices demonstrating a primary cecal cancer **a** as well as a number of liver metastases **b**.

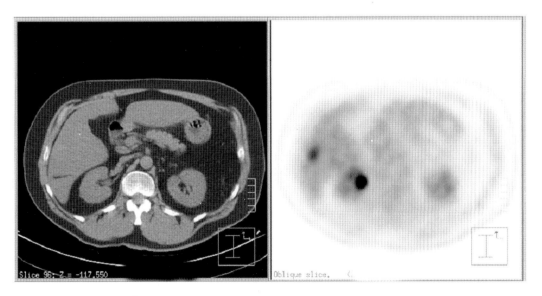

Figure 17.7. Transaxial CT and ^{18}FDG PET images in a patient with a previous history of colon cancer in whom CEA levels were rising but a diagnostic CT scan with contrast had failed to demonstrate recurrence. The PET scan clearly demonstrates a focal metastasis in the right lobe of the liver that was also not seen on this CT acquisition performed as part of a combined PET/CT acquisition.

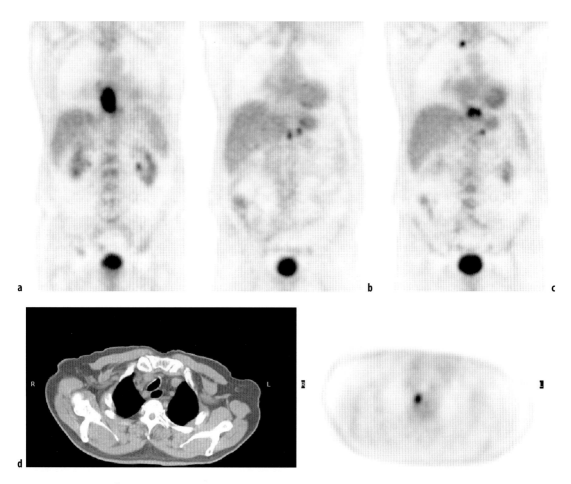

Figure 17.8. Coronal [18]FDG PET images demonstrating a primary esophageal cancer **a**, left gastric lymphadenopathy **b**, and an upper mediastinal lymph node **c**. The latter is also demonstrated on combined transaxial PET/CT images **d**. The 1 cm right paratracheal lymph node was considered to be of borderline significance on CT but was confirmed to be metastatic on the PET scan, upstaging the patient.

of such patients with negative anatomical imaging will have recurrent disease detected by PET [31, 32].

A meta-analysis of 11 studies reporting the use of PET in recurrent colorectal cancer showed an overall sensitivity of 97% and specificity of 76%, with a striking change in management of 29% of patients as a result of PET results [33], making it a cost-effective technique [32].

In staging esophageal cancer, [18]FDG PET has a significant role to play and will save futile surgery in approximately 20% of patients by detecting hitherto unknown distant metastases [34, 35] (Figure 17.8). It is possible to detect nearly all primary tumors with PET but it has a limited role

in T staging and the detection of peri-esophageal lymph nodes, which are the province of CT and endoscopic ultrasound. Optimal presurgical staging requires all three modalities. There are some data to suggest that [18]FDG PET may have a role in assessing response to neoadjuvant chemotherapy. A reduction of 35% or more in SUV at 14 days in patients receiving preoperative chemotherapy has been reported to have a sensitivity of 93% and specificity of 95% in predicting clinical response at 3 months [36]. Response measured by PET also predicts the risk of local recurrence and overall survival [36, 37].

The differentiation of pancreatic cancer from mass-forming pancreatitis can be problematic with anatomical imaging alone. Although it has been shown that carcinoma of the pancreas over-expresses Glut-1 when compared to mass-forming pancreatitis and that the mean SUVs with ^{18}FDG PET are 2.98 ($\pm$1.23) and 1.25 ($\pm$0.51) respectively [38], both false positives and false negatives have been reported for pancreatic cancer [39, 40]. It would appear that hyperglycemic diabetic patients may show poor or absent uptake into malignant tissue whilst those with serological evidence of active inflammation may show high uptake. However, if caution is taken with these two groups of patients, ^{18}FDG PET assessment of pancreatic masses remains a useful non-invasive tool in diagnosis, particularly if other investigations including CT and endoscopic retrograde cholangiopancreatography are equivocal [40].

Lymph node staging of pancreatic cancer with ^{18}FDG PET would seem to be limited, with sensitivities of between 49% and 61% being reported [39, 40]. The detection of hepatic metastases is reasonably good with an overall sensitivity of 70% but metastases of less than 1 cm are frequently missed [40]. ^{18}FDG PET has also been used to assess response to chemotherapy and to detect recurrent pancreatic cancer.

^{18}FDG PET has been shown to have relatively limited sensitivity for the detection of primary liver hepatomas, possibly due to higher background activity in cirrhotic livers and possibly due to higher glucose-6-phosphatase activity leading to dephosphorylation of FDG-6-PO$_4$. Despite a low sensitivity for intrahepatic disease, Trojan et al [41] found that PET contributed to changes in management in 23% of patients in detecting extrahepatic disease. For the detection of metastatic liver disease, ^{18}FDG PET has been shown to have slightly higher sensitivity and specificity (97%, 88%) than CT (93%, 75%) in a series of 64 patients but may be particularly helpful when availability is scarce in those patients with equivocal findings on CT or ultrasound [42].

17.5.4 Head and Neck Cancers

Most squamous cell carcinomas of the head and neck show avid uptake of ^{18}FDG. However, interpretation of head and neck images is one of the more difficult areas of oncologic PET as there are a number of areas of normal uptake seen in the head and neck and precise anatomical localization of le-

sions can be problematic. A thorough knowledge of normal appearances and their variation, including the lymphatic tissues of Waldeyer's ring and a number of muscles, is essential for interpretation. With the availability of PET/CT it is possible to reduce false positive interpretations due to areas of physiological uptake but also to more accurately localize pathological uptake.

For staging head and neck tumors at diagnosis ^{18}FDG PET has a similar or slightly improved accuracy compared to cross-sectional imaging techniques including ultrasound, CT, and MRI [43, 44]. Reactive lymph nodes (a common occurrence in the neck) can show false positive uptake although delayed scanning at 90 minutes has been shown to reduce this and to improve specificity [45]. Sensitivity for lymph nodes of less than 1 cm is approximately 70% but between 83% and 100% when greater than 1 cm [45].

It is not uncommon for squamous cell carcinomas of the head and neck to present as enlarged metastatic lymph nodes with an occult primary. A number of primary lesions will remain occult in spite of conventional imaging and panendoscopy. It is important that primary tumors are localized as treatment options are quite different and it has been shown that locating the primary tumor ensures the most appropriate treatment associated with an improved prognosis [46]. The results for PET have been variable in the detection of occult primary tumors but there is no doubt that in a proportion of patients it is the only method that successfully localizes the primary (Figure 17.9).

Where ^{18}FDG PET would appear to have the greatest value over conventional staging procedures is in the detection and staging of recurrent tumor [47, 48]. Alterations in anatomy and symmetry following surgery and radiotherapy make anatomical image interpretation especially challenging but affect functional imaging to a much lesser extent. Following radiotherapy, results from PET scanning are improved by scanning at 4 months rather than earlier, due to non-specific inflammatory uptake of ^{18}FDG in the early period after radiotherapy. Initial results also suggest that ^{18}FDG PET may be an accurate method to assess response to chemotherapy in patients with head and neck cancer [49].

Because of the complicated anatomy of the head and neck region and the physiological areas of uptake often seen with ^{18}FDG, it is likely that

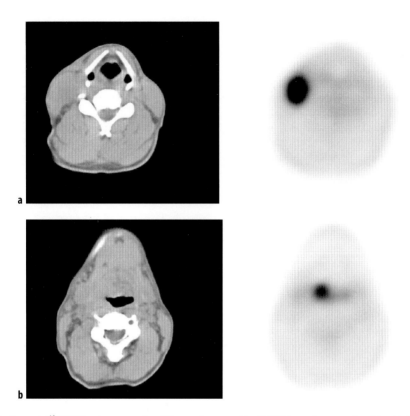

Figure 17.9. Transaxial [18]FDG PET and corresponding CT images from a combined PET/CT scan demonstrating right-sided clinically palpable metastatic nodal activity **a** but also an occult primary lesion at the right tongue base **b**.

combined PET/CT scans will be helpful and there is great interest in using this technique to plan head and neck radiotherapy treatment. The use of this combined modality has the potential to reduce toxicity to normal tissues and to improve coverage of tumor tissue by more accurately defining metabolically active tumor volume [50].

In differentiated thyroid cancer, [18]FDG PET is most valuable in patients with rising tumor markers, e.g. thyroglobulin, in whom radioiodine scintigraphy is negative. It is likely to be less useful in those cancers that remain well differentiated and continue to show accumulation of iodine. In iodine-negative patients [18]FDG PET has been reported to show a sensitivity of 85% for detection of disease [51].

Incidental focal or diffuse thyroid uptake of [18]FDG is not infrequently seen and has been reported to occur in 2.3% of one large series of 4525 patients being scanned for other reasons [52]. Diffuse uptake can be associated with thyroiditis or Graves' disease but focal uptake can be as-

sociated with malignancy. However, it is usually not possible to distinguish malignant from benign incidental thyroid nodules, as the former may also show [18]FDG uptake.

17.5.5 Melanoma

It is generally regarded that the risk of metastases is very low in patients with stage 1 melanoma (Breslow thickness <1.5 mm) and that further staging is not considered cost-effective. In higher-risk patients sentinel node lymphoscintigraphy and biopsy is more sensitive than PET for staging regional lymph nodes for occult metastases [53]. However, a meta-analysis of the use of [18]FDG PET in high-risk melanoma has shown an overall sensitivity and specificity of 90% and 87% respectively [54] and is considered to be cost-effective [55]. It should be noted that the meta-analysis excluded studies for diagnosis of sentinel lymph nodes and microscopic involvement and assessed the role of

PET in detecting distant metastases. Melanoma has an unpredictable pattern of spread in many patients and the whole body capability of PET can be advantageous in this regard.

In suspected recurrent melanoma, the treatment of choice is often surgical and [18]FDG PET is probably the most sensitive method of detecting unsuspected disease but PET may be limited in the detection of brain and skin metastases. From the referring clinician's perspective, [18]FDG PET is considered a helpful investigation with 30% of patients being restaged, 29% undergoing an intermodality and 18% an intramodality change in management [56].

17.5.6 Breast Cancer

The reported accuracy of [18]FDG PET in primary breast cancers varies widely but the larger studies and meta-analyses suggest that the number of false negative and false positive readings preclude its use as a routine diagnostic tool in breast masses and that it is not accurate enough to help reduce the need for biopsies [57, 58]. It is possible that PET may be more helpful in particularly dense breasts where mammography is difficult or when breast implants are present. There is ongoing work to develop PET scanners especially modified for breast imaging and it is possible that accuracy using dedicated equipment designed for breast imaging may improve diagnostic accuracy to some extent.

The accuracy of [18]FDG PET in axillary staging also varies widely in the literature but it would appear that it is not possible to detect small volume disease. A recent prospective multicenter study including 360 patients showed sensitivity, specificity, positive and negative predictive values of 61%, 80%, 62%, 79% respectively and concluded that PET could not be recommended for routine axillary staging at the current time [59].

It is probably in the staging of advanced disease and restaging recurrent disease that [18]FDG PET has most benefit. Detection of locoregional recurrence has been reported with a sensitivity of 89% and specificity of 84% and for distant metastases 100% and 97% respectively, with PET being more sensitive than tumor markers [60] (Figure 17.10). [18]FDG PET detects more bone metastases that conventional bone scintigraphy in the majority of patients but in the subset of patients with predominantly sclerotic disease the sensitivity is less

[61, 62]. Those with predominantly lytic skeletal disease show higher [18]FDG avidity and a poorer prognosis [61]. A lower sensitivity for detection of skeletal metastases has also been noted in prostate cancer patients and it would appear that sclerotic disease is associated with lower levels of [18]FDG uptake [63].

More recently, serial [18]FDG PET has been used in the evaluation of primary tumor response to chemotherapy.

17.5.7 Central Nervous System Tumors

One of the weaknesses of whole body [18]FDG PET imaging is that the detection of cerebral metastases is limited. This is largely because of the difficulty in detecting small lesions that are of similar or slightly lower intensity than normal brain cortex and in view of this some centers do not acquire images of the brain during routine oncological whole body scanning [64].

[18]FDG PET scanning alone may also be suboptimal in patients in whom it is necessary to distinguish recurrent primary brain tumor from gliosis following treatment. There is likely to be some non-specific uptake due to gliosis and the degree of uptake depends on tumor grade. For this reason some groups have used ^{11}C-methionine PET imaging where the tumor to normal brain contrast is much greater and the tumor recurrence can be more precisely determined.

17.5.8 Combined PET/CT Imaging

For clinical oncological imaging there is an increasing preference to purchase combined PET/CT systems rather than PET-only. In addition to the obvious attraction of having an anatomical framework to help interpret the PET images, the CT data can be used for attenuation correction, leading to a significant reduction in scanning time compared to PET systems that use germanium-68 rods as a transmission source for this purpose (Figures 17.5, 17.7, 17.8, and 17.9).

Data are accumulating to show the benefits of combined imaging in oncological diagnosis. As mentioned above, in the staging of non-small cell lung cancer combined PET/CT imaging has shown a significant improvement in diagnostic accuracy, particularly with regard to T staging of primary tumors. Advantages are apparent when

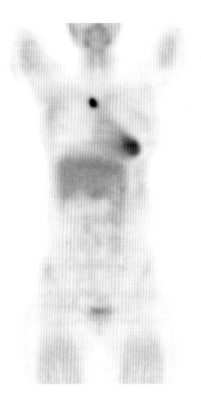

a

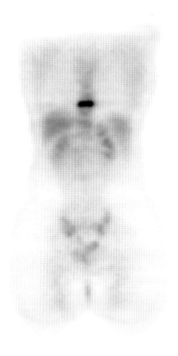

b

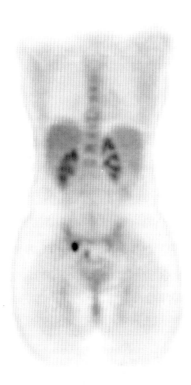

c

Figure 17.10. Coronal ^{18}FDG PET images of a patient with suspected recurrent breast cancer demonstrating skeletal metastases in the sternum **a**, a collapsed lower thoracic vertebra **b**, and the right side of the sacrum **c**.

compared to interpretation of PET data alone, CT alone or even PET and CT interpreted side by side [65]. Other groups have also described advantages to combined image interpretation in a variety of different cancers. Additional value has been claimed in as many as 49% of patients from combined imaging [66] as well as an increased accuracy in staging [67]. Combined PET/CT scanning with ^{18}FDG in oncology would seem to be particularly advantageous in characterizing and localizing lesions, reducing the number of false positives due to benign normal variant uptake and in reducing the number of equivocal results. The CT data can be particularly helpful where ^{18}FDG PET on its own is weak, such as the detection of small sub-centimeter lung metastases, in tumors with limited avidity to ^{18}FDG, and in the detection of incidental, but clinically significant, non-cancer-related pathology.

Clinical PET/CT protocols are evolving but most centers acquire a relatively low current CT scan without intravenous contrast for attenuation correction and for image fusion [67]. Bowel contrast can be given in the form of dilute barium preparations, using water as a negative contrast agent or some units use none at all.

17.5.9 Miscellaneous Oncological Applications

As a whole body technique, ^{18}FDG PET scanning has the potential to identify tumor sites in patients who present with metastases in whom the primary tumor is occult or in patients who present with a paraneoplastic syndrome with an occult primary. PET not only shows reasonable sensitivity and specificity for detection of unknown primary tumors compared to conventional methods such as CT, but also allows accurate staging of the full extent of the disease, affecting subsequent management decisions [68, 69]. Similarly, in patients with paraneoplastic syndromes ^{18}FDG PET can detect primary tumor in a proportion of patients where other non-invasive imaging techniques have failed [70].

A number of other malignancies may benefit from the use of ^{18}FDG PET, including gynecological and testicular cancers, particularly when recurrence is suspected due to rising tumor markers. However, the number of reported studies is less than with the types of cancer mentioned above.

17.6 ^{18}FDG PET in Infection Imaging

Accumulation of ^{18}FDG is known to occur in activated white cells as well as malignant tumor tissue. Although this reduces the specificity of ^{18}FDG PET imaging in oncology imaging, there has been growing interest in the use of this technique to specifically localize infection and inflammation. In a series of patients with fever of unknown origin or suspected focal infection, PET was found to be clinically useful in 37% of the former group and 65% of the latter, often in patients who had had a series of unhelpful alternative investigations [71].

Similarly, whole body ^{18}FDG PET in patients with HIV disease can be clinically useful [72]. Although it may not be possible to distinguish inflammatory/infective uptake from tumor uptake, PET often detects sites of disease that are more amenable to biopsy so that a rapid histological diagnosis can be made. In the brain it is possible to distinguish infectious space-occupying lesions (e.g. toxoplasmosis) from lymphoma, the latter showing higher levels of accumulation.

17.7 Cardiology

The main clinical indications for the use of PET are in assessment and quantification of myocardial perfusion and in the evaluation of myocardial viability. Myocardial perfusion can be assessed by cyclotron-produced tracers such as ^{15}O-water ($H_2^{15}O$) or ^{13}N-ammonia ($^{13}NH_3$) or the generator-produced tracer rubidium-82 (^{82}Rb).

^{13}N-ammonia is the commonest tracer to be utilized in centers with a cyclotron. It freely diffuses across cell membranes and has a near 100% first-pass extraction. Kinetic models can be applied to quantify blood flow and are valid over a range of flow rates [73]. Using this method, regional perfusion can be quantified at rest or after pharmacological stress to detect functionally significant coronary artery disease. ^{15}O-water myocardial perfusion studies are potentially less complicated as water is freely diffusible and does not undergo metabolism, making kinetic modeling simpler. However, the short 2 min half-life of ^{15}O and the high count rates that the PET scanner has to deal with make this tracer less practical. ^{82}Rb is an analogue of thallium and extracted in

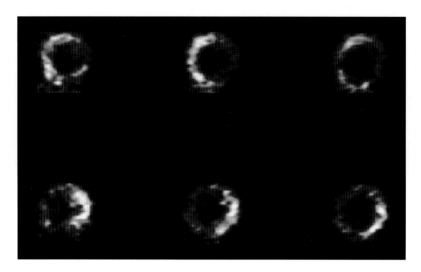

Figure 17.11. Short axis ^{13}N-ammonia blood flow (top row) and ^{18}FDG metabolism scans. These demonstrate reduced blood flow in the lateral wall but this area shows enhanced uptake of ^{18}FDG, demonstrating that it is viable tissue.

proportion to myocardial blood flow, although the relationship between extraction and blood flow becomes non-linear at high flow rates. The major advantage of this tracer is that it is available from a strontium-82 (^{82}Sr)/^{82}Rb generator that has a useful life of over a month. The short 76 second half-life of ^{82}Rb means that rapid image acquisition is required but that repeat studies can be performed at short intervals.

PET methods are reported to be slightly more sensitive and specific than SPECT methods, in part due to improved spatial resolution and count statistics. Nevertheless SPECT remains very valuable and continues to be the most commonly used nuclear medicine method for evaluation of coronary heart disease [74]. The differences in accuracy between PET and SPECT methods are likely to be reduced now that attenuation correction is more commonly used in SPECT. PET methods are more valuable when absolute quantification is required.

The accurate detection of viable myocardium is of extreme importance in patients with left ventricular dysfunction and coronary heart disease. The degree of left ventricular dysfunction correlates with prognosis and both symptoms and prognosis can be improved by revascularization of viable but dysfunctional myocardial segments. The distinction of viable but dysfunctional from infarcted myocardium is challenging and it is currently accepted that ^{18}FDG PET imaging may be the best method. Those with significant areas of

ischemic and dysfunctional but viable (hibernating) myocardium may benefit from revascularization procedures if technically possible but those with infarcted scar tissue are more likely to require medical therapy or cardiac transplantation (Figure 17.11). Cardiac PET imaging techniques are therefore of great importance in influencing subsequent management of patients with severe left ventricular dysfunction. The demonstration of a mismatch between poor blood flow with ^{13}N-ammonia but continued viability with ^{18}FDG has been shown to be predictive of functional recovery after revascularization [75].

Although a mismatch between blood flow and ^{18}FDG uptake can be used to predict functional recovery in dysfunctional myocardium, it is likely that gated acquisitions, allowing measurement of regional wall motion and thickening, will enhance the diagnostic capability of cardiac PET methods.

17.8 Neurology

Although PET techniques have been studied to evaluate and quantify a number of neurological indications, these have been largely research orientated and there are relatively few clinical neurological applications being used in a routine fashion. Areas in which there is some evidence of clinical benefit include dementia, epilepsy, and movement disorders. Dementia is covered in Section 12.3.2 and so will not be discussed further.

17.8.1 Epilepsy

[18]FDG PET has been used in the clinical evaluation of patients with refractory epilepsy in whom surgery is planned. It has been reported to be particularly effective in the lateralization of temporal lobe epilepsy where hypometabolism may be identified in interictal studies. For logistic reasons [18]FDG PET studies are performed interictally, unless a seizure occurs coincidentally after injection of [18]FDG, when hypermetabolism may be identified. It is known that the area of abnormal metabolism overestimates the true epileptogenic focus as defined pathologically and PET is therefore used as a lateralizing method and can be used as one of the many localizing techniques in such patients before surgery. It is common also to perform MRI and EEG studies to confirm the potential site for surgical excision. Although ictal SPECT with cerebral blood flow agents remains the most accurate method for defining epileptogenic foci, this is logistically difficult, requiring hospitalization and the requirement for the ability to inject tracer soon after the start of an ictus. An abnormal [18]FDG PET scan is strongly associated with surgical outcome [76] and asymmetry of temporal lobe metabolism of greater than 15% also predicts successful surgery in temporal lobe surgery [77]. [18]FDG PET is less accurate in localizing extratemporal epileptogenic foci but remains of value in some cases.

17.8.2 Movement Disorders

The main task for functional imaging techniques is to distinguish Parkinson's disease due to nigrostriatal degeneration from Parkinson-like syndromes. The former is characterized by tremor, rigidity, and bradykinesia and can be treated by drugs that increase dopamine levels in nigrostriatal pathways. The latter may be difficult to distinguish from Parkinson's disease on clinical grounds alone but require different treatment. PET can be used to measure dopaminergic activity in the basal ganglia using ^{18}F-dopa. The tracer is taken up into dopaminergic neurons and stored in terminal vesicles. Quantifying uptake in the basal ganglia, either on a static image, or by measuring the rate of uptake on dynamic acquisitions, allows Parkin-

son's disease to be distinguished from other movement disorders, the former showing low levels of accumulation. Some disorders, including progressive supranuclear palsy and multisystem atrophy, that may clinically mimic Parkinson's disease and also show nigrostriatal degeneration may be distinguished by the regional pattern of loss of ^{18}F-dopa uptake in the basal ganglia [78].

17.9 Conclusion

PET has developed rapidly in the last decade to become a clinical imaging tool with many indications in oncology using [18]FDG as a radiopharmaceutical. It has a role in the diagnosis, staging, recurrence detection, and treatment evaluation of many cancers. With the advent of combined PET/CT and the development of new tracers to evaluate other aspects of tumor biology it is likely that its role will become even more firmly established. Similarly, it provides unique information in a number of clinical cardiac and neuropsychiatric applications with established clinical effectiveness.

References

1. Lodge MA, Lucas JD, Marsden PK, et al. A PET study of [18]FDG uptake in soft tissue masses. Eur J Nucl Med 1999; 26:22–30.
2. Hustinx R, Smith RJ, Benard F, et al. Dual time point fluorine-18 fluorodeoxyglucose positron emission tomography: a potential method to differentiate malignancy from inflammation and normal tissue in the head and neck. Eur J Nucl Med 1999; 26:1345–1348.
3. Hallett WA, Marsden PK, Cronin BF, et al. Effect of corrections for blood glucose and body size on ^{18}F]FDG PET standardised uptake values in lung cancer. Eur J Nucl Med 2001; 28:919–922.
4. Hoekstra CJ, Paglianiti I, Hoekstra OS, et al. Monitoring response to therapy in cancer using ^{18}F]-2-fluoro-2-deoxy-D-glucose and positron emission tomography: an overview of different analytical methods. Eur J Nucl Med 2000; 27:731–743.
5. Chung JK, Kim YK, Kim SK, et al. Usefulness of 11C-methionine PET in the evaluation of brain lesions that are hypo- or isometabolic on ^{18}F-FDG PET. Eur J Nucl Med Mol Imaging 2002; 29:176–182.
6. Weber WA, Wester HJ, Grosu AL, et al. O-(2-^{18}F]-fluoroethyl)-L-tyrosine and L-[methyl-11C]methionine uptake in brain tumours: initial results of a comparative study. Eur J Nucl Med 2000; 27:542–549.
7. Picchio M, Messa C, Landoni C, et al. Value of [11C]-choline-positron emission tomography for re-staging prostate cancer: a comparison with ^{18}F]fluorodeoxy-glucose-positron emission tomography. J Urol 2003; 169:1337–1340.

8. Shields AF, Grierson JR, Dohmen BM, et al. Imaging proliferation in vivo with [F-18]FLT and positron emission tomography. Nat Med 1998; 4:1334–1336.

9. Cook GJR, Wegner E, Fogelman I. Pitfalls and artefacts in [18]FDG PET and PET/CT oncologic imaging. Semin Nucl Med 2004; 34:122–133.

10. Qureshy A, Kubota K, Iwata R, et al. Localization and reduction of FDG intestinal uptake: tissue distribution and autoradiography study. Nucl Med Commun 2002; 23:388.

11. Cook GJR, Maisey MN, Fogelman I. Normal variants, artefacts and interpretative pitfalls in PET imaging with 18-fluoro-2-deoxyglucose and carbon-11 methionine. Eur J Nucl Med 1999; 26:1363–1378.

12. Gould MK, Maclean CC, Kuschner WG, et al. Accuracy of positron emission tomography for diagnosis of pulmonary nodules and mass lesions: a meta-analysis. JAMA 2001; 285:914–924.

13. Gambhir SS, Shepherd JE, Shah BD, et al. Analytical decision model for the cost-effective management of solitary pulmonary nodules. J Clin Oncol 1998; 16:2113–2125.

14. Pieterman RM, Putten JW van, Meuzelaar JJ, et al. Preoperative staging of non-small-cell lung cancer with positron emission tomography. N Engl J Med 2000; 343:254–261.

15. Tinteren H Van, Hoekstra OS, Smit EF, et al. Effectiveness of positron emission tomography in the preoperative assessment of patients with suspected non-small-cell lung cancer: the PLUS multicentre randomised trial. Lancet 2002; 359:1388–1393.

16. Dhital K, Saunders CA, Seed PT, et al. ^{18}F-Fluorodeoxyglucose positron emission tomography and its prognostic value in lung cancer. Eur J Cardiothorac Surg 2000; 18:425–428.

17. Patz EF, Lowe VJ, Hoffman JM, et al. Persistent or recurrent bronchogenic carcinoma: detection with PET and 2-[F-18]-2-deoxy-D-glucose. Radiology 1994; 191:379–382.

18. Ciernik IF, Dizendorf E, Baumert BG, et al. Radiation treatment planning with an integrated positron emission and computer tomography (PET/CT): a feasibility study. Int J Radiat Oncol Biol Phys 2003; 57:853–863.

19. Barrington SF, O'Doherty MJ. Limitations of PET for imaging lymphoma. Eur J Nucl Med Mol Imaging 2003; 30 (Suppl):117–127.

20. Blum RH, Seymour JF, Wirth A, et al. Frequent impact of [18F]fluorodeoxyglucose positron emission tomography on the staging and management of patients with indolent non-Hodgkin's lymphoma. Clin Lymphoma 2003; 4:43–49.

21. Moog F, Bangerter M, Diederichs CG, et al. Lymphoma: role of whole-body 2-deoxy-2-[F-18]fluoro-D-glucose (FDG) PET in nodal staging. Radiology 1997; 203: 795–800.

22. Moog F, Bangerter M, Diederichs CG, et al. Extranodal malignant lymphoma: detection with FDG PET versus CT. Radiology 1998; 206:475–481.

23. Moog F, Kotzerke J, Reske SN. FDG PET can replace bone scintigraphy in primary staging of malignant lymphoma. J Nucl Med 1999; 40:1407–1413.

24. Partridge S, Timothy A, O'Doherty MJ, et al. 2-Fluorine-18-fluoro-2-deoxy-D glucose positron emission tomography in the pretreatment staging of Hodgkin's disease: influence on patient management in a single institution. Ann Oncol 2000; 11:1273–1279.

25. Mikhaeel NG, Timothy AR, O'Doherty MJ, et al. 18-FDG-PET as a prognostic indicator in the treatment of aggressive non-Hodgkin's lymphoma – comparison with CT. Leuk Lymphoma 2000; 39:543–553.

26. Wit M De, Bumann D, Beyer W, et al. Whole-body positron emission tomography (PET) for diagnosis of residual mass in patients with lymphoma. Ann Oncol 1997; 8:57–60.

27. Abdel-Nabi H, Doerr RJ, Lamonica DM, et al. Staging of primary colorectal carcinomas with ^{18}F-FDG whole body PET: correlation with histopathologic and CT findings. Radiology 1998; 206:755–760.

28. Moore HG, Akhurst T, Larson SM, et al. A case-controlled study of 18-fluorodeoxyglucose positron emission tomography in the detection of pelvic recurrence in previously irradiated rectal cancer patients. J Am Coll Surg 2003; 197:22–28.

29. Beets G, Penninckx F, Schiepers C, et al. Clinical value of whole-body positron emission tomography with [18F]fluorodeoxyglucose in recurrent colorectal cancer. Br J Surg 1994; 81:1666–1670.

30. Vitola JV, Delbeke D, Sandler MP, et al. Positron emission tomography to stage suspected metastatic colorectal carcinoma to the liver. Am J Surg 1996; 171:21–26.

31. Flanagan FL, Dehdashti F, Ogunbiyi OA, et al. Utility of FDG PET for investigating unexplained plasma CEA elevation in patients with colorectal cancer. Ann Surg 1998; 227:319–323.

32. Valk PE, Abella-Columna E, Haseman MK, et al. Whole body PET imaging with F18-FDG in management of recurrent colorectal cancer. Arch Surg 1999; 134:503–511.

33. Huebner RH, Park KC, Shepherd JE, et al. A meta-analysis of the literature for whole-body FDG PET detection of recurrent colorectal cancer. J Nucl Med 2000; 41:1177–1189.

34. Rankin SC, Taylor H, Cook GJ, et al. Computed tomography and positron emission tomography in the preoperative staging of oesophageal carcinoma. Clin Radiol 1998; 53:659–665.

35. Flamen P, Lerut A, Cutsem E Van, et al. Utility of positron emission tomography for the staging of patients with potentially operable esophageal carcinoma. J Clin Oncol 2000; 18:3202–3210.

36. Weber WA, Ott K, Becker K, et al. Prediction of response to preoperative chemotherapy in adenocarcinomas of the esophagogastric junction by metabolic imaging. J Clin Oncol 2001; 19:3058–3065.

37. Couper GW, McAteer D, Wallis F, et al. Detection of response to chemotherapy using positron emission tomography in patients with oesophageal and gastric cancer. Br J Surg 1998; 85:1403–1406.

38. Reske SN, Grillenberger KG, Glatting G, et al. Overexpression of glucose transporter 1 and increased FDG uptake in pancreatic carcinoma. J Nucl Med 1997; 38:1344–1348.

39. Zimny M, Bares R, Fass J, et al. Fluorine-18 fluorodeoxyglucose positron emission tomography in the differential diagnosis of pancreatic carcinoma: a report of 106 cases. Eur J Nucl Med 1997; 24:678–682.

40. Diederichs CG, Staib L, Vogel J, et al. Values and limitations of 18F-fluorodeoxyglucose-positron-emission tomography with preoperative evaluation of patients with pancreatic masses. Pancreas 2000; 20:109–116.

41. Trojan J, Schroeder O, Raedle J, et al. Fluorine-18 FDG positron emission tomography for imaging of hepatocellular carcinoma. Am J Gastroenterol 1999; 94:3314–3319.

42. Hustinx R, Paulus P, Jacquet N, et al. Clinical evaluation of whole-body ^{18}F-fluorodeoxyglucose positron emission tomography in the detection of liver metastases. Ann Oncol 1998; 9:397–401.

43. Adams S, Baum RP, Stuckensen T, et al. Prospective comparison of ^{18}F-FDG PET with conventional imaging modalities (CT, MRI, US) in lymph node staging of head and neck cancer. Eur J Nucl Med 1998; 25:1255–1260.

44. Kresnik E, Mikosch P, Gallowitsch HJ, et al. Evaluation of head and neck cancer with 18F-FDG PET: a comparison with conventional methods. Eur J Nucl Med 2001; 28:816–821.

45. Brink I, Klenzner T, Krause T, et al. Lymph node staging in extracranial head and neck cancer with FDG PET – appropriate uptake period and size-dependence of the results. Nuklearmedizin 2002; 41:108–113.

46. Haas I, Hoffmann TK, Engers R, et al. Diagnostic strategies in cervical carcinoma of an unknown primary (CUP). Eur Arch Oto Rhino Laryngol 2002; 259:325–333.

47. Lonneux M, Lawson G, Ide C, et al. Positron emission tomography with fluorodeoxyglucose for suspected head and neck tumor recurrence in the symptomatic patient. Laryngoscope 2000; 110:1493–1497.

48. Anzai Y, Carroll WR, Quint DJ, et al. Recurrence of head and neck cancer after surgery or irradiation: prospective comparison of 2-deoxy-2-[F-18]fluoro-D-glucose PET and MR imaging diagnoses. Radiology 1996; 200:135–141.

49. Lowe VJ, Dunphy FR, Varvares M, et al. Evaluation of chemotherapy response in patients with advanced head and neck cancer using [F-18]fluorodeoxyglucose positron emission tomography. Head Neck 1997; 19:666–674.

50. Ciernik IF, Dizendorf E, Baumert BG, et al. Radiation treatment planning with an integrated positron emission and computer tomography (PET/CT): a feasibility study. Int J Radiat Oncol Biol Phys 2003; 57:853–863.

51. Grunwald F, Kalicke T, Feine U, et al. Fluorine-18 fluorodeoxyglucose positron emission tomography in thyroid cancer: results of a multicentre study. Eur J Nucl Med 1999; 26:1547–1552.

52. Cohen MS, Arslan N, Dehdashti F, et al. Risk of malignancy in thyroid incidentalomas identified by fluorodeoxyglucose-positron emission tomography. Surgery 2001; 130:941–946.

53. Wagner JD, Schauwecker D, Davidson D, et al. Prospective study of fluorodeoxyglucose-positron emission tomography imaging of lymph node basins in melanoma patients undergoing sentinel node biopsy. J Clin Oncol 1999; 17:1508–1515.

54. Steinert HC, Schulthess GK Von, Reuland P, et al. A meta-analysis of the literature for staging malignant melanoma with whole body FDG PET. J Nucl Med 2001; 42:307P.

55. Von Schulthess GK, Steinert HC, Dummer R, et al. Cost-effectiveness of whole-body PET imaging in non-small cell lung cancer and malignant melanoma. Acad Radiol 1998; 5:300–302.

56. Wong C, Silverman DH, Seltzer M, et al. The impact of 2-deoxy-2-[18F] fluoro-D-glucose whole body positron emission tomography for managing patients with melanoma: the referring physician's perspective. Mol Imaging Biol 2002; 4:185–190.

57. Avril N, Rose CA, Schelling M, et al. Breast imaging with positron emission tomography and fluorine-18 fluorodeoxyglucose: use and limitations. J Clin Oncol 2000; 18:3495–3502.

58. Samson DJ, Flamm CR, Pisano ED, et al. Should FDG PET be used to decide whether a patient with an abnormal mammogram or breast finding at physical examination should undergo biopsy? Acad Radiol 2002; 9:773–783.

59. Wahl RL, Siegel BA, Coleman RE, et al. Prospective multicenter study of axillary nodal staging by positron emission tomography in breast cancer: a report of the staging breast cancer with PET Study Group. J Clin Oncol 2004; 22:277–285.

60. Kamel EM, Wyss MT, Fehr MK, et al. [18F]-Fluorodeoxyglucose positron emission tomography in patients with suspected recurrence of breast cancer. J Cancer Res Clin Oncol 2003; 129:147–153.

61. Cook GJR, Houston S, Rubens R, et al. Detection of bone metastases in breast cancer by 18 FDG PET: differing metabolic activity in osteoblastic and osteolytic lesions. J Clin Oncol 1998; 16:3375–3379.

62. Gallowitsch HJ, Kresnik E, Gasser J, et al. F-18 fluorodeoxyglucose positron-emission tomography in the diagnosis of tumor recurrence and metastases in the follow-up of patients with breast carcinoma: a comparison to conventional imaging. Invest Radiol 2003; 38:250–256.

63. Shreve PD, Grossman HB, Gross MD, et al. Metastatic prostate cancer: initial findings of PET with 2-deoxy-2-[F-18]fluoro-D-glucose. Radiology 1996; 199:751–756.

64. Larcos G, Maisey MN. FDG-PET screening for cerebral metastases in patients with suspected malignancy. Nucl Med Commun 1996; 17:197–198.

65. Lardinois D, Weder W, Hany TF, et al. Staging of non-small-cell lung cancer with integrated positron-emission tomography and computed tomography. N Engl J Med 2003; 348:2500–2507.

66. Bar-Shalom R, Yefremov N, Guralnik L, et al. Clinical performance of PET/CT in evaluation of cancer: additional value for diagnostic imaging and patient management. J Nucl Med 2003; 44:1200–1209.

67. Hany TF, Steinert HC, Goerres GW, et al. PET diagnostic accuracy: improvement with in-line PET-CT system: initial results. Radiology 2002; 225:575–581.

68. Delgado-Bolton RC, Fernandez-Perez C, Gonzalez-Mate A, et al. Meta-analysis of the performance of 18F-FDG PET in primary tumor detection in unknown primary tumors. J Nucl Med 2003; 44:1301–1314.

69. Alberini JL, Belhocine T, Hustinx R, et al. Whole-body positron emission tomography using fluorodeoxyglucose in patients with metastases of unknown primary tumours (CUP syndrome). Nucl Med Commun 2003; 24:1081–1086.

70. Rees JH, Hain SF, Johnson MR, et al. The role of [18F]fluoro-2-deoxyglucose-PET scanning in the diagnosis of paraneoplastic neurological disorders. Brain 2001; 124:2223–2231.

71. Bleeker-Rovers CP, de Kleijn EM, Corstens FH, et al. Clinical value of FDG PET in patients with fever of unknown origin and patients suspected of focal infection or inflammation. Eur J Nucl Med Mol Imaging 2004; 31:29–37.

72. O'Doherty MJ, Barrington SF, Campbell M, et al. PET scanning and the human immunodeficiency virus-positive patient. J Nucl Med 1997; 38:1575–1583.

73. Bol A, Melin JA, Vanoverschelde JL, et al. Direct comparison of ^{13}N ammonia and [15]O water estimates of perfusion with quantification of regional myocardial blood flow by microspheres. Circulation 1993; 87:512–525.

74. Sand NP, Bottcher M, Madsen MM, et al. Evaluation of regional myocardial perfusion in patients with severe left ventricular dysfunction: comparison of ^{13}N-ammonia PET and ^{99m}Tc sestamibi SPECT. J Nucl Cardiol 1998; 5:4–13.

75. Haas F, Augustin N, Holper K, et al. Time course and extent of improvement of dysfunctioning myocardium in patients with coronary artery disease and severely depressed left ventricular function after revascularization: correlation with positron emission tomography. J Am Coll Cardiol 2000; 36:1927–1934.

76. Radtke RA, Hanson MW, Hoffmann JM, et al. Temporal lobe hypometabolism on PET: predictor of seizure control after temporal lobectomy. Neurology 1993; 43:1088–1092.

77. Theodore WH, Sato S, Kufta C, et al. Temporal lobectomy for uncontrolled seizures: the role of positron emission tomography. Ann Neurol 1992; 32:789–794.

78. Brooks DJ, Ibanez V, Sawle GV, et al. Differing patterns of striatal [^{18}F]-Dopa uptake in Parkinson's disease, multiple system atrophy and progressive supranuclear palsy. Ann Neurol 1990; 28:547–555.

Index

Note: labeled radiopharmaceuticals are listed at the beginning of alphabet groups.